RECENT ADOLESCENT HEALTH

"Knowledge is as wings to man's life, and a ladder for his ascent. Its acquisition is incumbent upon everyone. The knowledge of such sciences, however, should be acquired as can profit the people of the earth, and not those which begin with words and end with words..."

Federation of Obstetric and Gynaecological Societies of India

RECENT ADVANCES IN ADOLESCENT HEALTH

Editors

Roza Olyai MS MICOG FICMCH FICOG
National Chairperson, Adolescent Health Committee, FOGSI (2009-2011)
National Trainer, Adolescent Health, FOGSI-IMA-IAP and WHO
WHO Consultant, Expert Panel ASRH, WHO – Geneva (2010)
Convener, Adolescent Friendly Health Centers, India
Olyai Hospital, Hospital Road, Gwalior, Madhya Pradesh, India

Dilip Kumar Dutta MD PhD MAMS FICOG FIMCH MAAGL MAFS Dip in High
High Risk Pregnancy (USA), Dip in Pelviscopic Surgery (Germany)
Vice President, FOGSI (1997-98)
Chairman, Safe Motherhood Committee, FOGSI (1998-2002)
Chairman, Adolescent Committee, ISOFERB (2005-2007)
Director, GICE Hospital
Kalyani, Nadia, West Bengal, India

Foreword

Hamid Rushwan

A FOGSI Publication

JAYPEE BROTHERS MEDICAL PUBLISHERS (P) LTD

New Delhi • St Louis • Panama City • London

Published by

Jaypee Brothers Medical Publishers (P) Ltd

Corporate Office

4838/24, Ansari Road, Daryaganj, **New Delhi** 110 002, India
Phone: +91-11-43574357, Fax: +91-11-43574314

Offices in India

- **Ahmedabad,** e-mail: ahmedabad@jaypeebrothers.com
- **Bengaluru,** e-mail: bangalore@jaypeebrothers.com
- **Chennai,** e-mail: chennai@jaypeebrothers.com
- **Delhi,** e-mail: jaypee@jaypeebrothers.com
- **Hyderabad,** e-mail: hyderabad@jaypeebrothers.com
- **Kochi,** e-mail: kochi@jaypeebrothers.com
- **Kolkata,** e-mail: kolkata@jaypeebrothers.com
- **Lucknow,** e-mail: lucknow@jaypeebrothers.com
- **Mumbai,** e-mail: mumbai@jaypeebrothers.com
- **Nagpur,** e-mail: nagpur@jaypeebrothers.com

Overseas Offices

- **North America Office, USA,** Ph: 001-636-6279734
  e-mail: jaypee@jaypeebrothers.com, anjulav@jaypeebrothers.com
- **Central America Office, Panama City, Panama,** Ph: 001-507-317-0160
  e-mail: cservice@jphmedical.com, Website: www.jphmedical.com
- **Europe Office, UK,** Ph: +44 (0) 2031708910
  e-mail: info@jpmedpub.com

Recent Advances in Adolescent Health

First Edition: **2011**

ISBN 978-93-5025-227-7

Typeset at JPBMP typesetting unit

Printed at Rajkamal Electric Press, Plot No. 2, Phase-IV, Kundli, Haryana.

Dedicated to

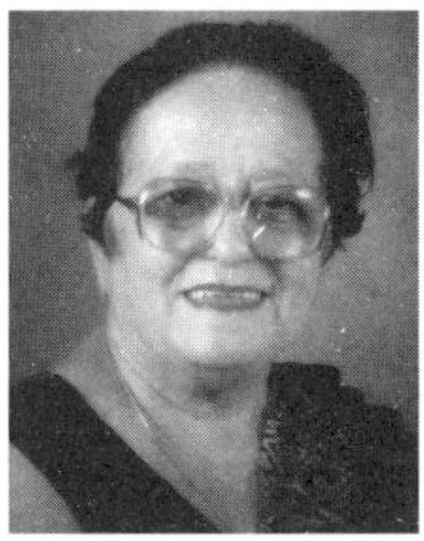

Late Prof Dr (Mrs) Perin Olyai
Professor Emeritus
Ex Head of the Department of Obstetrics and Gynecology
Gajra Raja Medical College, Gwalior, Madhya Pradesh, India
For her genuine love and dedication towards service to humanity

CONTRIBUTORS

Abha Singh
Professor and HOD
Obstetrics and Gynecology
Raipur Medical College
Raipur, Chhattisgarh, India
ajab_2k@yahoo.com

AK Khanna
Chief Operating Officer and Executive Director—Member Board of Directors
Emcure Pharmaceuticals Ltd
Pune, Maharashtra, India
arun@emcure.co.in

Alka Kriplani
MD FRCOG FAMS FICOG FICMCH FIMSA
Professor, Head unit II
Obstetrics and Gynecology
AIIMS
New Delhi, India
kriplanialka@gmail.com

Anita Budania
MS (Obs-Gyn) Fellow in ICOG certificate course
NILES and AAKAR IVF Center
Mumbai, Maharashtra, India

Annie Hawkins
Senior Trainee
Queen Charlotte's, and Chelsea and Westminster Hospitals
London, United Kingdom

Archana Kumari
Assistant Professor
Rajendra Institute of Medical Sciences
Ranchi, Jharkhand, India
dr_karchana@yahoo.co.in

Aruna Kumar MBBS MS
Professor and HOD
Obstetrics and Gynecology
Sultania Zanana Hospital
Gandhi Medical College
Bhopal, Madhya Pradesh, India
profhodszh@yahoo.co.in

Arushi Singh
Programme Officer—Adolescents and Young People
International Planned Parenthood (IPPF)
South Asia Regional Office
New Delhi, India
asingh@ippfsar.org

Atul Kanikar
Consultant
Adolescent care pediatrician
Nasik, Maharashtra, India
akanikar@gmail.com

Basab Mukherjee MD MRCOG
Executive Committee Member
Adolescent Health Committee FOGSI
Kolkata, West Bengal, India
basabm@gmail.com

CP Bansal MD FIAP PGD-AP
Consultant Adolescent Pediatrician
Chairperson Adolescent Health Chapter
Gwalior, Madhya Pradesh, India
cpbansal@gmail.com

Deepa Joshi
Assistant Professor
SAIMS
Indore, Madhya Pradesh, India
drdeepamundra@yahoo.co.in

Deepti Gupta MBBS MS
Assistant Professor
Obstetrics and Gynecology
Sultania Zanana Hospital
Gandhi Medical College
Bhopal, Madhya Pradesh, India
deepteag@rediffmail.com

Dilip Kumar Dutta
MD PhD MAMS FICOG FIMCH MAAGL MAFS
Director
GICE Hospital
Kalyani, Nadia
West Bengal, India
drdilipdutta@yahoo.com

Divya Awasthi MBBS MS
Senior Resident
Obstetrics and Gynecology
AIIMS
New Delhi, India

Gita Guin MS (Obs-Gyn) LLB
Associate Professor
Obstetrics and Gynecology
Govt NSCB Medical College
Jabalpur, Madhya Pradesh, India
gita_guin1966@yahoo.in

Indranil Dutta
Kalyani, Nadia
West Bengal, India
drdilipdutta@yahoo.com

Jayam Kannan
Professor Emeritus
South Zone Coordinator, Adolescent Health Committee, FOGSI
Chennai, Tamil Nadu, India
jayamkannangfc@yahoo.com

Jayeeta Roy
Kalyani, Nadia
West Bengal, India

JS Tuteja MD DCH PGD-AP
Consultant Adolescent Pediatrician
Co-Chairperson
Adolescent Health Chapter
Director Suhani-Dishayen
Teens World Guidance Program
Indore, Madhya Pradesh, India
drtuteja@yahoo.com

Kat Watson
Youth Officer (Access)
International Planned Parenthood Federation (IPPF), 4 Newhams Row
London, United Kingdom
kawatson@ippf.org

Kate Maclaran
Research Fellow
Queen Charlotte's, and Chelsea and Westminster Hospitals
London, United Kingdom

Kavita N Singh
Associate Professor
Obstetrics and Gynecology
NSCB Medical College
Jabalpur, Madhya Pradesh, India
drkavitasingh@rediffmail.com

Kirti Sharma
Postgraduate student
Obstetrics and Gynecology
VMMC and Safdarjung Hospital
New Delhi, India

Krishna Kavita Ramavath MD (Obs-Gyn)
Assistant Professor
KGH Obstetrics and Gynecology
Andhra Medical College
King George Hospital
Visakhapatnam, Andhra Pradesh, India
Mayo clinic
Visiting Clinician
Department of Gynecology
Gynecological surgery
Scottsdale, Arizona
United States of America
drkavita18@gmail.com

Laxmi Maru MS FICOG FICMCH
Professor and HOD
Obstetrics and Gynecology
MGM Medical College
Indore, Madhya Pradesh, India
drlaxmimaru@gmail.com

Lola Ramachandran DNB (Obs-Gyn)
Associate Professor
Obstetrics and Gynecology
Jubilee Mission Medical College
Thrissur, Kerala, India
lola.ramachandran@gmail.com

Madhuri Alwani
Assistant Professor
SAIMS
Indore, Madhya Pradesh, India
drmadhuri_2007@rediffmail.com

Malathi G Prasad MD MRCOG
Director
IS Hospital
Trichy; Tamil Nadu, India
malathi_prasad@hotmail.com

Nick Panay BSc MRCOG MFSRH
Consultant Gynecologist, Subspecialist in Reproductive Medicine and Surgery
Imperial College
Healthcare NHS Trust and Chelsea and Westminster Hospital NHS Foundation Trust
London, United Kingdom
Honorary Senior Clinical Lecturer
Imperial College, London, United Kingdom
Queen Charlotte's, and Chelsea and Westminster Hospitals
London, United Kingdom
nickpanay@msn.com

Prakash Trivedi
Professor and HOD
Obstetrics and Gynecology
Rajawadi Hospital and DY Patil Medical College (Clinical)
Mumbai, Maharashtra, India
Director
NILES and Aakar IVF-ICSI Centre
Dr Trivedi's Total Woman's Health Care Centre, Mumbai, Maharashtra, India
Consultant Endoscopist
ART and Urogynecology
Jaslok and BARC Hospital
FOGSI Sr Vice President 2008
FOGSI Infertility Committee Chairman 2003-2007
Ghatkopar (East)
Mumbai, Maharashtra, India
dr.ptrivedi@gmail.com

Prashanth K Adiga
Associate Professor
Obstetrics and Gynecology
KMC
Manipal, Karnataka, India
dradiga@yahoo.co.in;
adiga.prashanth5@gmail.com

Pratibha Singh
Associate Professor
Obstetrics and Gynecology
SAIMS
Indore, Madhya Pradesh, India
kulpra@hotmail.com

Pratima Mittal
WHO-GOI coordinator program
Adolescent Health
New Delhi, India
drpratima@hotmail.com;
drpratimamittal@gmail.com

Preeti M Galagali MD PGD AP
Director and Consultant Adolescent Physician
Bangalore Adolescent Care and Counselling Centre
Bengaluru, Karnataka, India
himanidev@yahoo.com

Priti Bala Sahay
HOD
Obstetrics and Gynecology
Rajendra Institute of Medical Sciences (RIMS)
Ranchi, Jharkhand, India
pritisahay@rediffmail.com

Rajiv Mohta
Mohta Children Hospital and Adolescent Centre
Nagpur, Maharashtra, India
reach13@yahoo.co.in

Ratna Thakur
HOD
Obstetrics and Gynecology
SAIMS
Indore, Madhya Pradesh, India
ashokumarthakur@gmail.com

Roza Olyai MS MICOG FICMCH FICOG
National Chairperson
Adolescent Health Committee, FOGSI
National Trainer
Adolescent Health, FOGSI-IMA-IAP and WHO
WHO Consultant, Expert Panel ASRH, WHO – Geneva (2010)
Convener, Adolescent Friendly Health Centers, India
Hon. Secretary
Family Planning Association of India, Gwalior
Founder Secretary
Indian Menopause Society, Gwalior
Olyai Hospital, Hospital Road
Gwalior-474009, Madhya Pradesh, India
rozaolyai@gmail.com

Saria Tasnim
FCPS MMEd Diploma in Community Epidemiology
Associate Professor
Obstetrics and Gynecology
Institute of Child and Mother Health
Matuail
Gulshan, Dhaka, Bangladesh
sariatasnim2007@gmail.com

Shashi Khare
Professor and HOD
Obstetrics and Gynecology
NSCB Medical College
Jabalpur, Madhya Pradesh, India
drshashikhare@rediffmail.com

Shilpa Sapre
Assistant Professor
SAIMS
Indore, Madhya Pradesh, India
shpimple@yahoo.com

Shilpa Thaker MD DGO PhD DHHM
Executive member
Adolescent Health Committee, FOGSI
Rajkot, Gujarat, India
dr.shilpathaker@gmail.com

Somen Bhattacharjee MD FICMCH
Assistant Professor
Obstetrics and Gynecology
MGM Medical College
Indore, Madhya Pradesh, India
drsomenmd@yahoo.com

Sunita Mishra MBBS DGO
Sri Aurobindo Institute of Medical
College and Hospital
Indore, Madhya Pradesh, India
dr_sunitamishra_16@yahoo.co.in

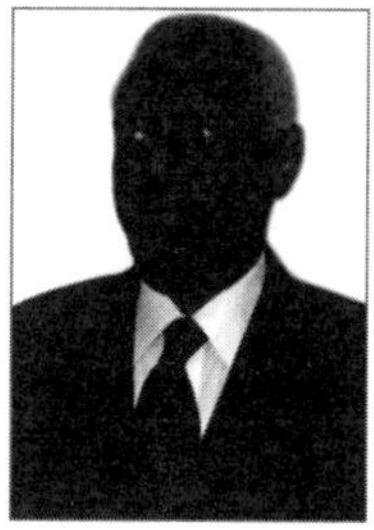

Foreword

I am delighted to introduce the superb work *Recent Advances in Adolescent Health*, a publication from the Adolescent Health Committee of FOGSI.

It provides the very latest update on this critical and highly topical issue, of enormous relevance to gynecologists and obstetricians worldwide.

The International Federation of Gynecology and Obstetrics (FIGO), of which I am the Chief Executive, recognizes that the area of Adolescent Sexual and Reproductive Health (ASRH), especially in low- and middle-resource countries, is a matter of concern for all those working within our profession.

FIGO has long been involved in highlighting the complexities and challenges of ASRH; its specially commissioned studies have been the inspiration behind several recent ground-breaking FIGO ASRH Workshops, funded by the United Nations Population Fund (UNFPA), including one held in Bengaluru, India last April. These popular, highly successful events have been bringing together committed representatives from numerous countries for an opportunity to focus and collaborate on how national professional organisations and national member associations can contribute effectively in the promotion of ASRH.

The eventual findings have provided much food for thought: It is clear that there are notable health and social challenges facing youth of all countries, and it is time to improve our understanding of them, and to focus our energies on the alleviation of these problems. Obstetricians and gynecologists, through their national associations and through FIGO at the international level, have an important role to play in the advancement of ASRH services.

FOGSI's production of this succinct and timely publication ensures that the Society—a longstanding and important FIGO member, is at the very forefront of professional analysis and debate. The launch at the prestigious All India Congress will ensure that the book's contents receive a wide and appreciative audience. I have no doubt that it will be an invaluable point of reference in the future for everyone connected to, and interested, in this fascinating area of health.

Dr Roza Olyai (Chairperson of FOGSI's Adolescent Health Committee) and Dr Dilip Kumar Dutta; in their respective roles as Editor and Co-Editor, have done a commendable work in bringing this valuable project to fruition.

My very best wishes.

Hamid Rushwan MD, FRCOG
Chief Executive
International Federation of Gynecology
and Obstetrics (FIGO)
United Kingdom

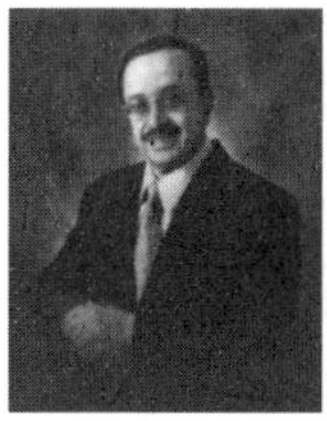

Message from the Desk of President, FOGSI

Adolescence is a period of transformation from childhood to adulthood and is a phase which demands specific attention and intervention. The conventional medicine curriculum has not been able to provide as yet with a specific reference to this particular age group and many a clinician is found wanting for a ready reckoner for understanding the reproductive needs of this age group.

Targeting this age group with awareness and early corrections of matters related to Adolescent Sexual Reproductive Health issues would help us yield a healthy society and empowered youth ready to face the challenges of life further on. I congratulate Dr Roza Olyai for her efforts in bringing out this book which I am sure will help the reader profoundly in clinical practice. I wish this endeavor a great success and may it fulfill the goals for which it was created.

Dr Sanjay Gupte
President FOGSI

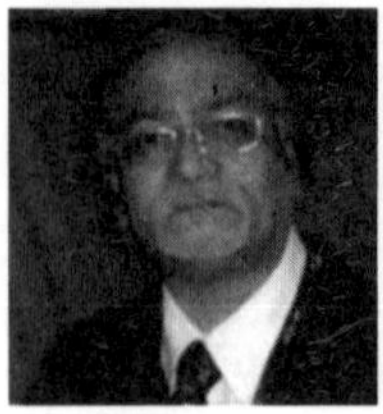

Message from the Desk of Secretary General, FOGSI

It is indeed a matter of pride for FOGSI that the much-awaited book "*Recent Advances in Adolescent Health*" is being published under its banner. If you are looking for complete information on various physiological and pathological aspects of an adolescent, here is one. It is a complete package of knowledge on Adolescent Health put together for the reader. Adolescent health is an important topic especially in a country like ours where not much is discussed or written about it in depth.

I congratulate Dr Roza Olyai, Chairperson of Adolescent Health Committee of FOGSI and editor of this publication as well as Dr Dilip Kumar Dutta, co-editor of this work, for bringing out an interesting and informative book for not only obstetricians and gynecologists but also for all interested in improving the health of younger generation of the world.

Dr PK Shah
Secretary General
FOGSI

PREFACE

It gives us great pleasure to share with you the book, *Recent Advances in Adolescent Health.*

Adolescents experience many challenges in their sexual and reproductive lives, therefore, appropriate and timely specialist advice and care can do much to alleviate problems and misconceptions, and enable young people to move forward with their lives in confidence. Not many doctors are familiar with the delicacy and sensitivity an adolescent girl needs to be treated with as she needs special attention and a quiet, friendly environment.

The Adolescent Health Committee of FOGSI aims to achieve this task by establishing Adolescent Friendly Health Centers. Our mission is to sensitize the youth of our country, through various projects we will be dealing in different aspects of health, i.e. physical, mental, social, spiritual, reproductive and sexual health and well-being, throughout their lives.

We aim to *"help young people form a strong moral identity in their early adolescent years and empower them to contribute to the well-being of their communities..."*

Disseminating knowledge and helping our adolescents to be empowered has been the goal of the Adolescent Health Committee, FOGSI and one such endeavor would hopefully reach to our colleagues through this book. We have selected different topics related to ASRH for the interest of our readers who will invariably face the dilemma of counseling the young adolescents and relieving them of the stress related with their normal pubertal changes. The preventive health section covers the social aspect of health as not many doctors will be well-versed in treating difficult adolescents, peer pressure and introducing life skills to them.

Teenage pregnancy has its own complications and knowledge about contraception is lacking amongst the adolescents which is a major cause of concern globally with complications of unsafe abortion.

Premarital counseling, vaccines and knowledge about STDs are important aspects of reproductive sexual health. Menarche at early age and ovarian tumors are cause of concern not only to the adolescents but to their mothers as well, hence a special section will deal with this area. To update our knowledge and learn about laparoscopic and robotic surgery will be a delight for our readers as these are upcoming recent trends in adolescent gynecology.

For further enhancement of knowledge on adolescent issues, you may kindly visit the website: http://adolescenthealthindia.org/

Roza Olyai
Dilip Kumar Dutta

ACKNOWLEDGMENTS

We are specially honored that Prof Hamid Rushwan, Chief Executive, International Federation of Gynecology and Obstetrics (FIGO), UK has graciously consented to write the foreword.

We are thankful to Dr Sanjay Gupte, President FOGSI and Dr PK Shah for their support and encouragement by sharing their message with our readers.

We would like to thank all our contributors for their generous contribution towards this book. We have selected contributors from different parts of India and from abroad from various specialties and organizations.

We are very grateful to Jaypee Brothers Medical Publishers (P) Ltd for publishing this book and help spread the message. We would also like to thank Mr Narendra Katore for designing the cover page.

Last but not least, we are greatly indebted to our parents who have given us the courage to face challenges of the world by inculcating good attributes in us, to our spouses and children for their tolerance and understanding of the time away from them during our own careers and in editing this book and being the backbone to our progress.

CONTENTS

SECTION 6: SOCIAL ISSUES, LIFE SKILLS AND COUNSELING

SECTION 7: ADOLESCENT FRIENDLY HEALTH SERVICES: BUILDING CAPACITY

Plate 1

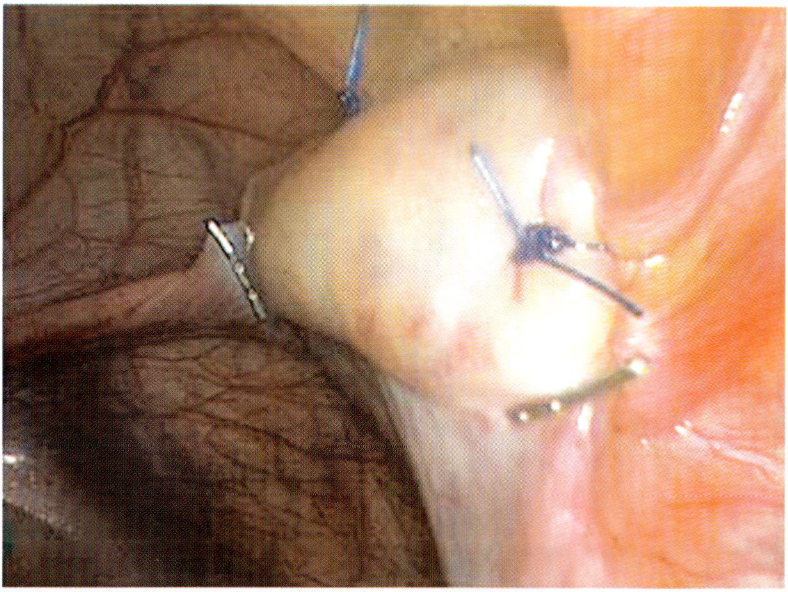

Fig. 14.1: Ovariopexy-ovary is fixed as far as possible from the midline. Clips are placed to allow ovary localization during radiotherapy

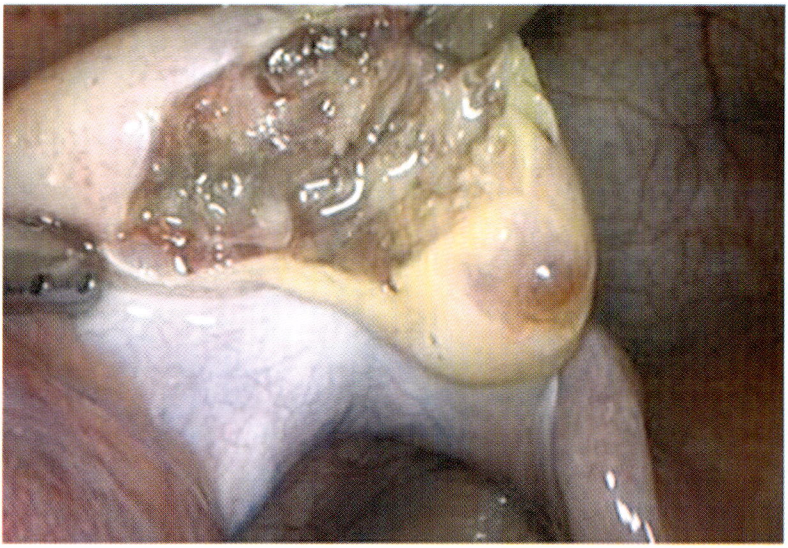

Fig. 14.2: Cortical ovarian biopsy from a 12 year old girl. The posterior part of the left ovarian cortex (2.5 × 1.5 cm) is removed

Plate 2

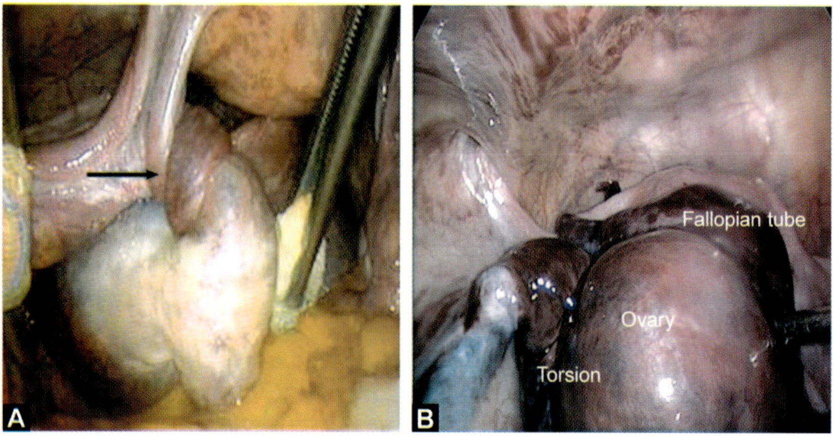

Figs 14.4A and B: (A) Ovarian torsion without gangrene, (B) Ovarian torsion with gangrene

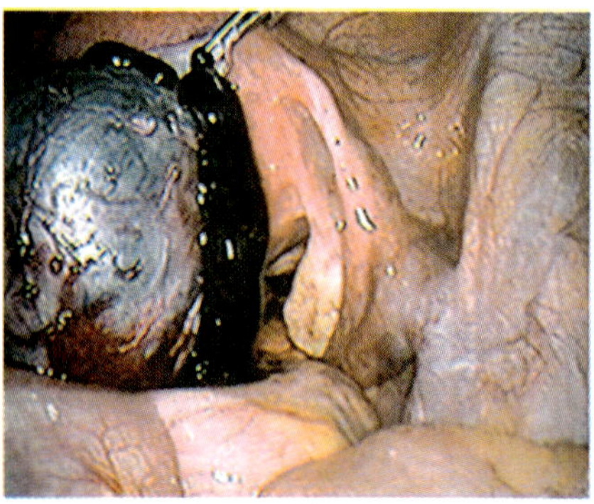

Fig. 18.1: Endoscopic view of ruptured chocolate cyst in the left ovary

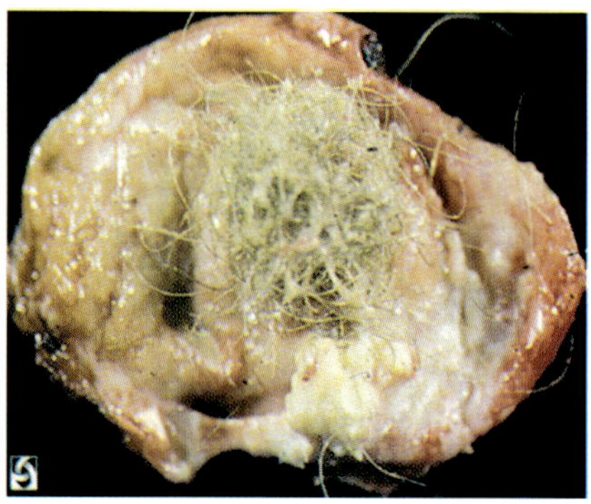

Fig. 18.2: Cut section of dermoid cyst showing pellet of hair

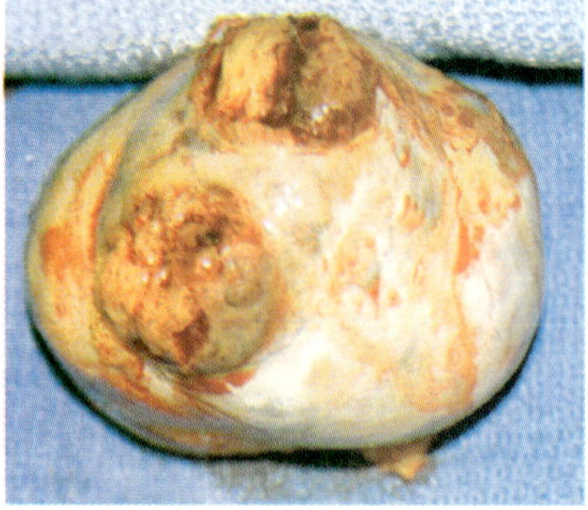

Fig. 19.1: Dysgerminoma (*Courtesy:* img.medscape.com/.jpg)

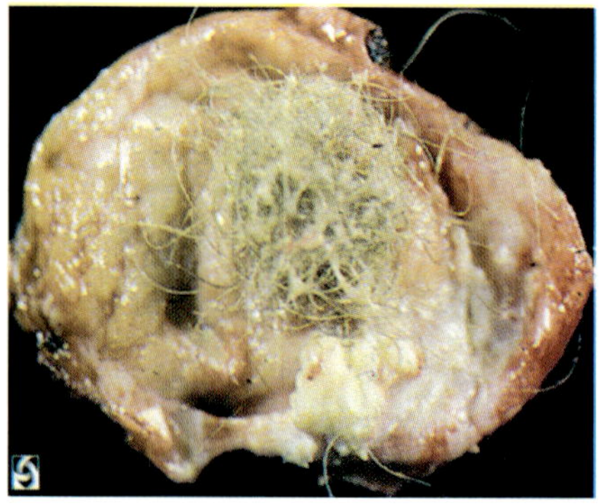

Fig. 19.2: Dermoid cyst (*Courtesy:* theovariancystcure.com)

Plate 3

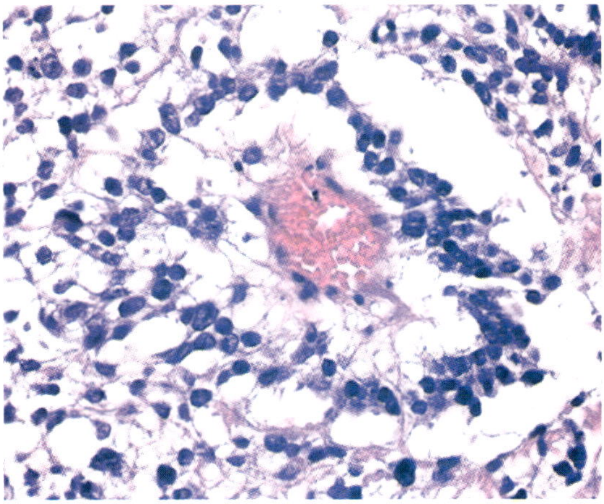

Fig. 19.3: Schiller-Duval body (*Courtesy*: web pathology-visual survey of surgical pathology)

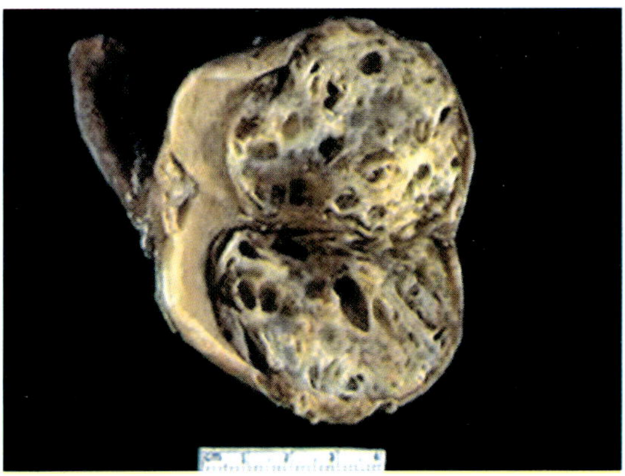

Fig. 19.4: Embryonal carcinoma of the ovary (*Courtesy*: Chad A Hamilton, MD, Walter Reed Army Medical Center emedicine:webmed)

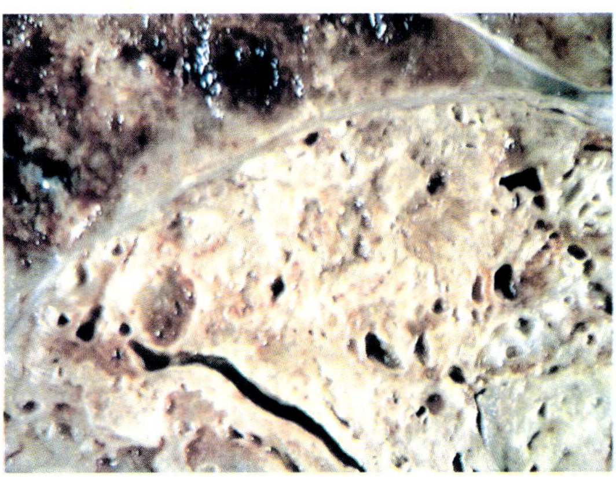

Fig. 19.5: Choriocarcinoma of the ovary (*Courtesy:* Cancercare)

Plate 4

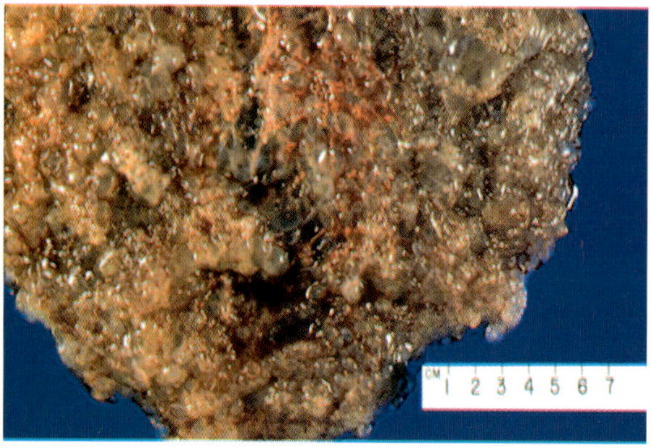

Fig. 19.6: GTD (*Courtesy:* cancer care)

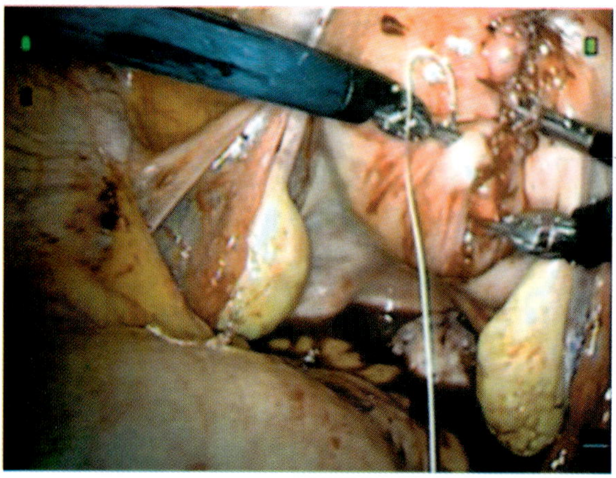

Fig. 19.7: Robotic surgery of RMS (*Courtesy*: Intuitive Surgical Systems, Sunnyvale, CA)

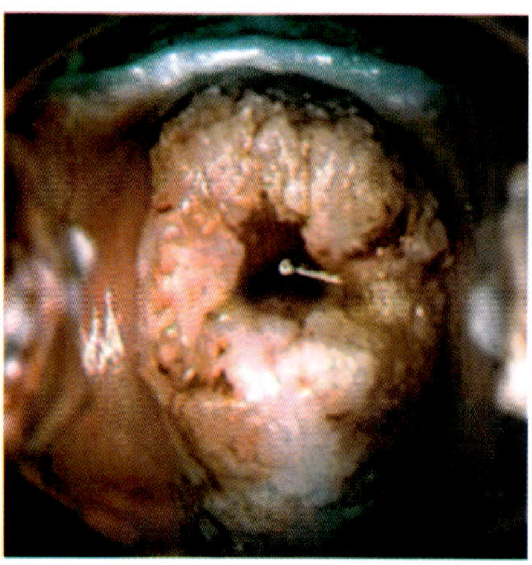

Fig. 19.8: Cervical cancer

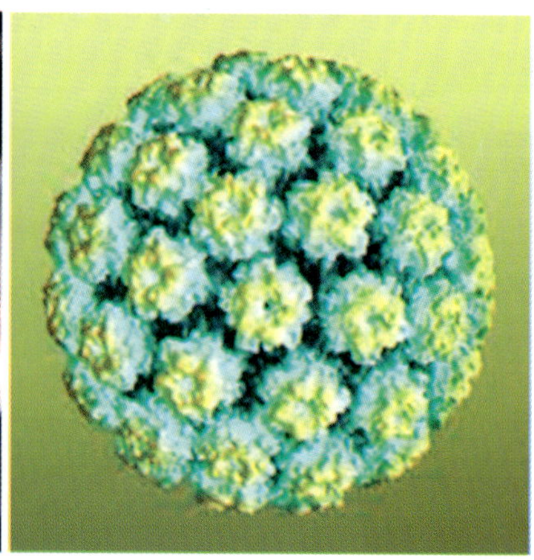

Fig. 19.9: HPV (*Courtesy*: Citizendium, citizens compendium)

Plate 5

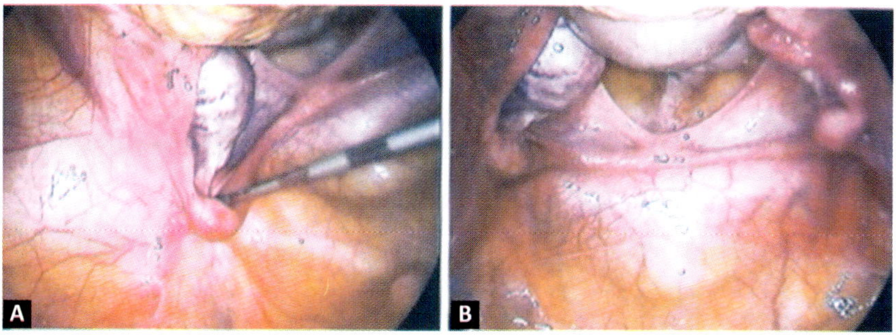

Figs 21.7A and B: Laparoscopic finding of an adolescent girl presenting with primary amenorrhoea and blind vagina showing full length of fallopian tubes and a strip of uterus

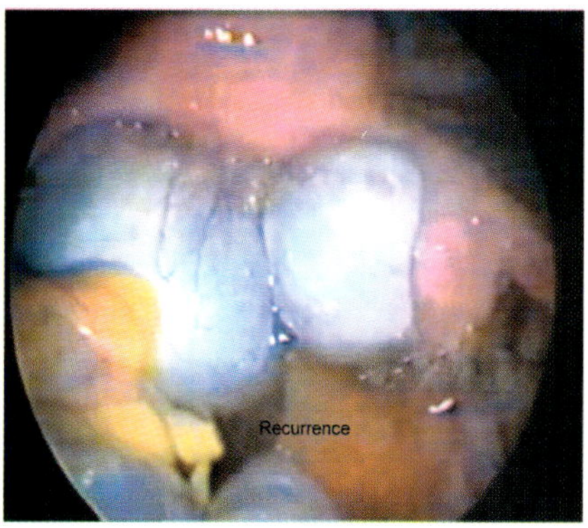

Fig. 23.1: Bilateral recurrent endometrioma

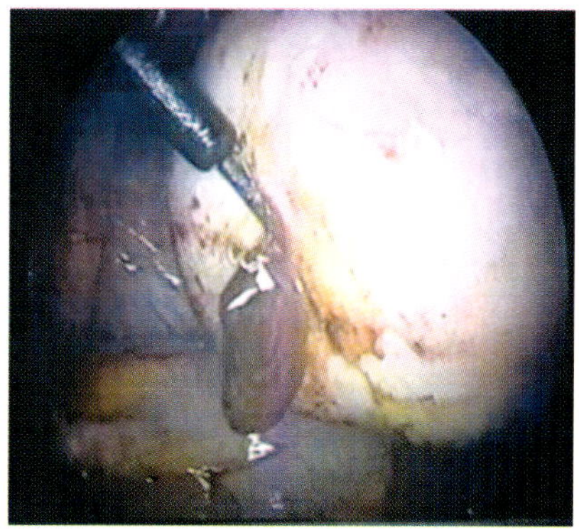

Fig. 23.2: Opening the endometrioma

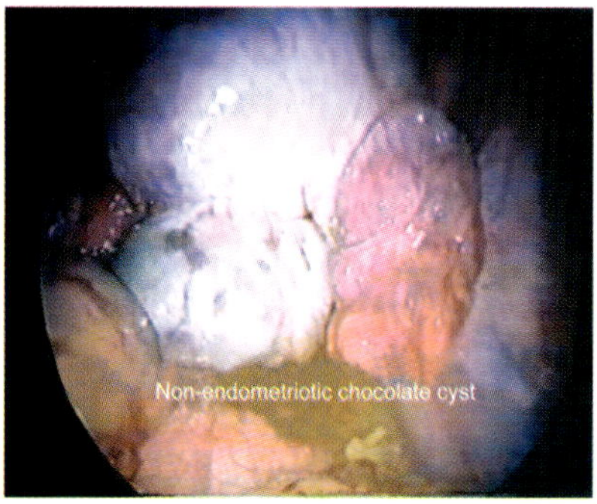

Fig. 23.3: Non-endometriotic chocolate cyst

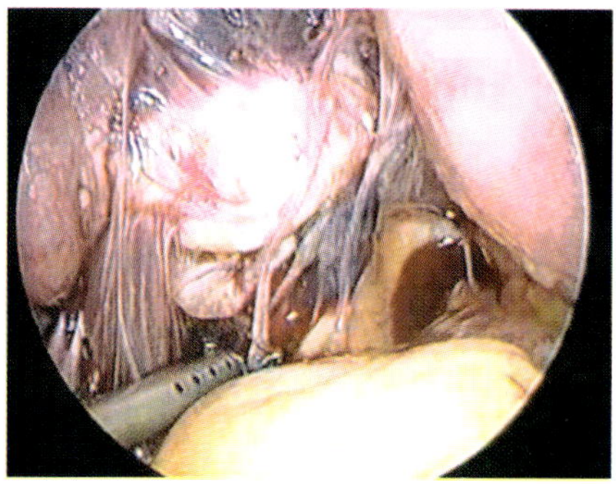

Fig. 23.4: Peritubal and peri-ovarian

Plate 6

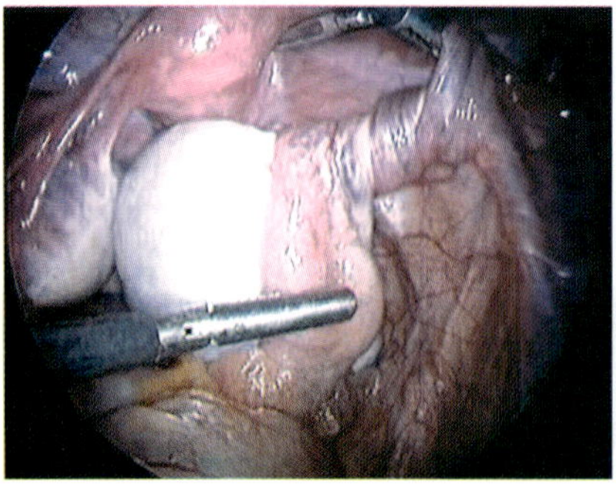

Fig. 23.5: Twisted ovarian cyst

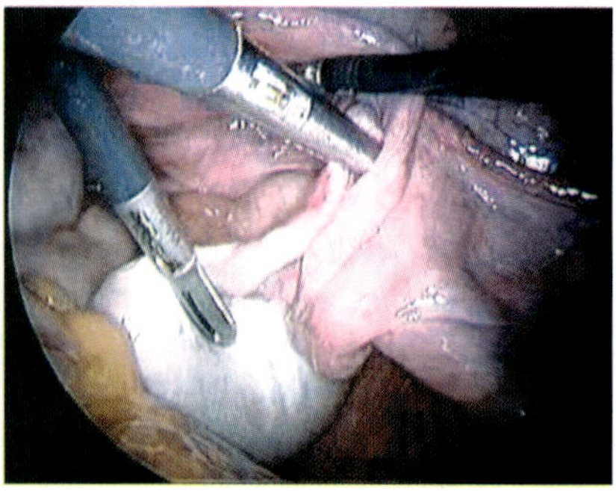

Fig. 23.6: Untwisted ovarian cyst

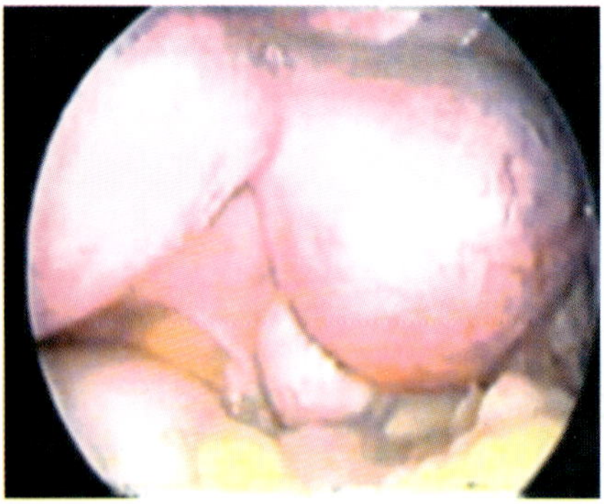

Fig. 23.7: Active rudimentary horn

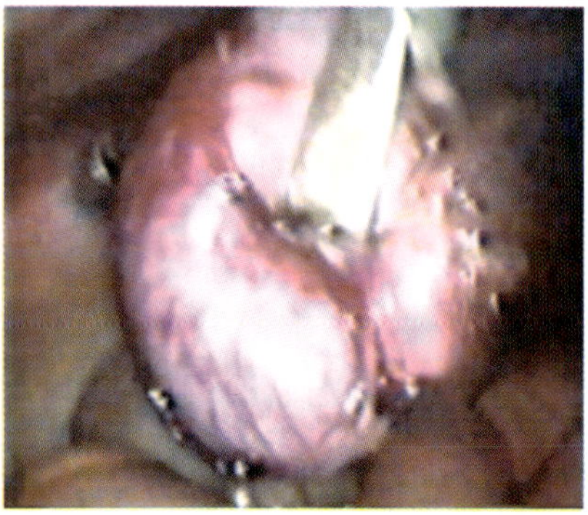

Fig. 23.8: Excision and removal

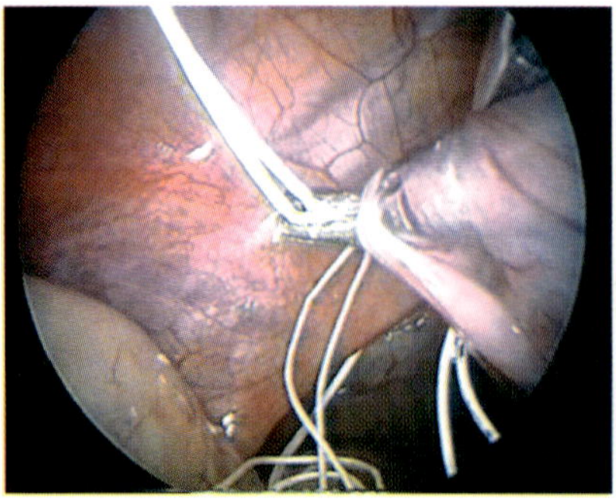

Fig. 23.10: Extraperitoneal traction

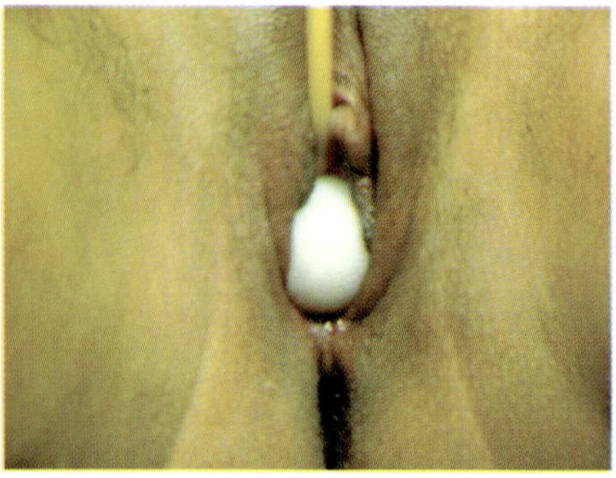

Fig. 23.11: Ball in the vaginal dimple. Suture pulled on the right side. Under traction from above.

Plate 7

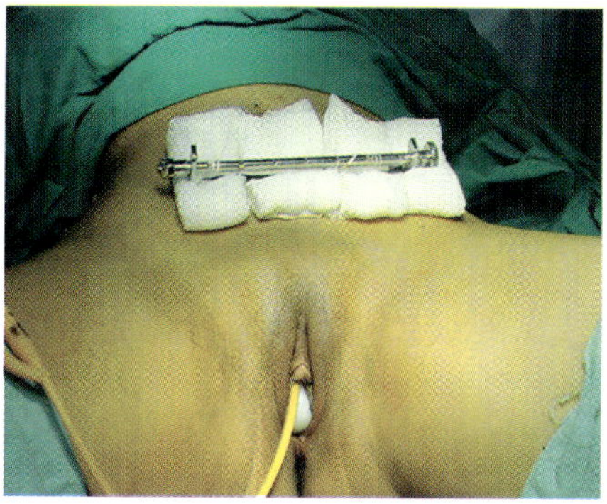

Fig. 23.12: Gradually escalating the traction

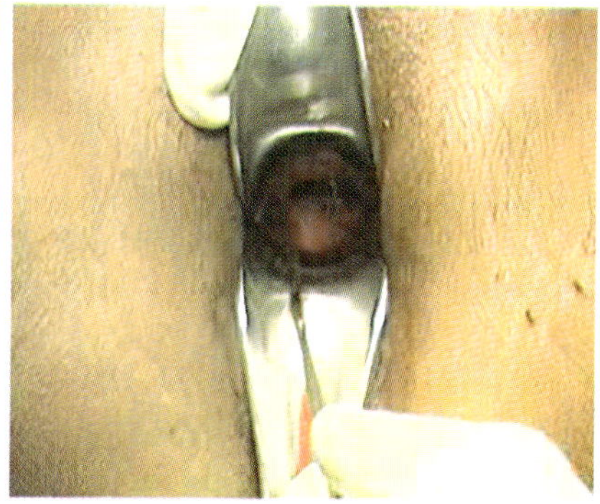

Fig. 23.13: Final result with good depth of vagina

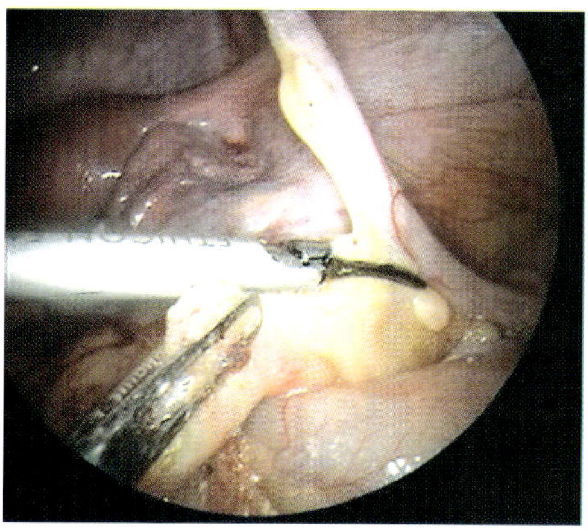

Fig. 23.14: Harmonic ace dissection

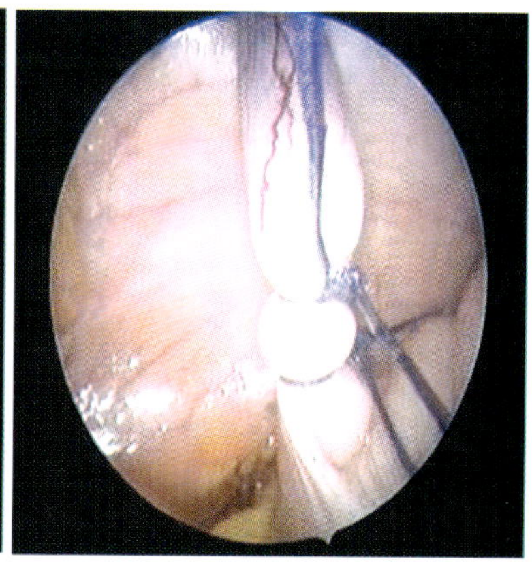

Fig. 23.15: Selfmade endoloops

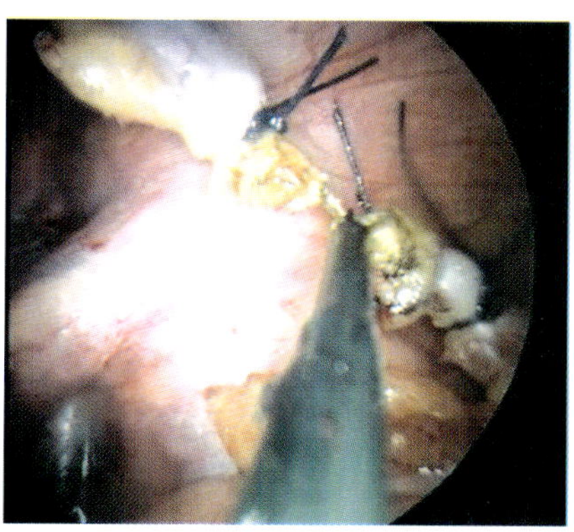

Fig. 23.16: Separation of appendix

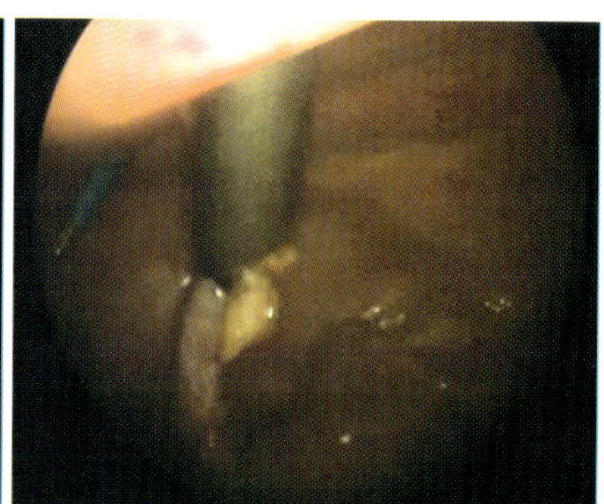

Fig. 23.17: Removal from 10 mm port

Plate 8

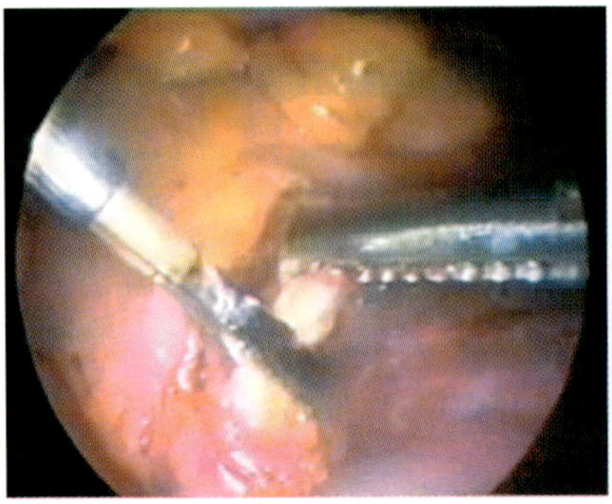

Fig. 23.18: Dissection of the presacral nerve

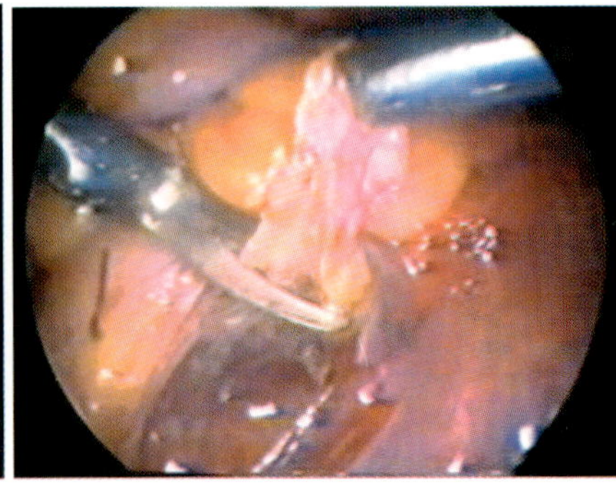

Fig. 23.19: Presacral neurectomy

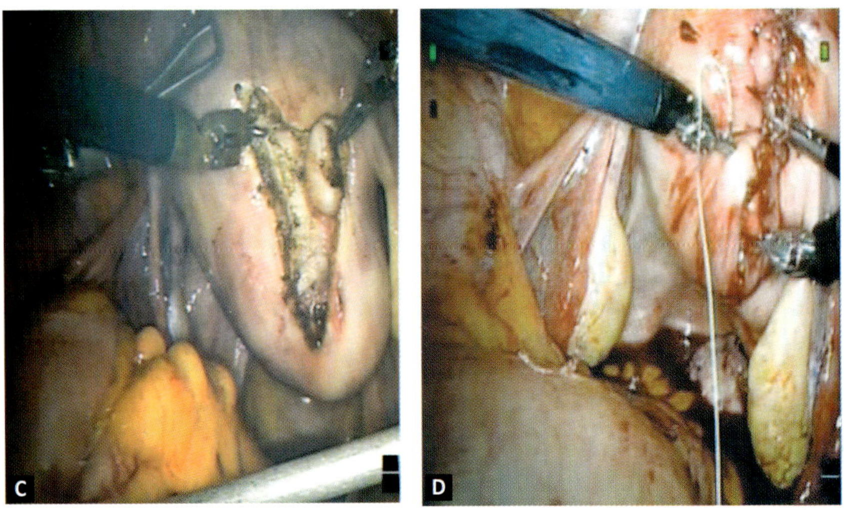

Figs 24.6C and D: Robotic surgery (*Courtesy*: Paul D Indman, OBGYN.NET)

Section 1

PHYSIOLOGICAL AND DEVELOPMENTAL ISSUES

1 Normal Puberty

Laxmi Maru

INTRODUCTION

Puberty is the phase of life during which secondary sexual characteristics develop, menstruation begins and capability of sexual reproduction is attained. It is the phase of transition from a child to a mature adult. The word puberty is derived from the Latin word *pubertas* which means adulthood. The physical changes accompanying pubertal development result directly or indirectly from maturation of the hypothalamus, stimulation of the sex organs and secretion of sex steroids. Alterations in circulating gonadotropin rhythms occur and a positive estrogen feedback loop is established which controls the monthly rhythm. The classic negative gonadal steroid feedback loop is reset. It generally starts earlier in girls than in boys.

TIMING OF PUBERTY

The major determinant of the timing of the onset of puberty is no doubt genetic and a number of other factors like general health, nutritional state, geographic location, exposure to light and psychological state.

The age of puberty is declining for girls, with more girls developing breasts by age 7 than in years past, according to a new study by Dohney published in the journal Pediatrics. This undoubtedly is a reflection of improved nutritional status and healthier living conditions.

Researchers from the University of California at Berkeley noted differences in the girls' ethnic backgrounds, body mass index and family income. Moderately obese girls (20-30% over normal weight) have earlier menarche than normal weight girls. Conversely, anorectics and intense exercisers (low weight or low percentage fat component of weight) have delayed menarche or secondary amenorrhea. Pubertal changes begin earlier in children who live in urban settings, closer to the equator and at lower altitudes than those who live in rural areas, farther from the equator and at higher altitudes. According to official Journal of the American Academy of Pediatrics, 2009, girls from higher income families without a biological father at home are more likely to hit puberty earlier than their peers.

Menarche occurs earliest in obese girls, followed by normal weight girls, then underweight girls and lastly anorectic girls.

The study was published in the American Journal of Pediatrics 1997, violence and antisocial behavior increase during puberty.

THE PHYSIOLOGY OF PUBERTY

By ten weeks of gestation, gonadotropin releasing hormone (GnRH) is present in the hypothalamus and luteinizing hormone (LH) and follicle stimulating hormone (FSH) are present in the pituitary gland. At birth, separation of the newborn from its sources of maternal and placental estrogen and progesterone, releases the newborn FSH and LH from this negative feedback. A prompt rise in gonadotropin and sex steroid concentrations occur at birth, but the levels decline during the first several weeks of life and remain low during the prepubertal years until at least 8 years of age. The hypothalamic-pituitary unit appears to be suppressed by the extremely low levels of gonadal steroids present in childhood (estradiol concentration in these years remains low at 40 pmol/L) (Fig. 1.1). Gonadal suppression of gonadotropin secretion is demonstrated by higher gonadotropin levels in children with gonadal dysgenesis and those who undergo gonadectomy before puberty.

The Prepubertal Period

As puberty approaches, three important changes occur:

Adrenarche

Increased adrenal androgen secretion is important in stimulating adrenarche, the appearance of pubic and axillary hair, in both boys and girls. Pubarche specifically refers to the appearance of pubic hair. A pituitary adrenal androgen stimulating factor formed by cleavage of a high molecular weight precursor, proopiomelanocortin (POMC) has been suggested as the agent stimulating adrenarche is reset.

Onset of 'Gonadarche'

Several hormonal changes associated with pubertal development begin before any of the physical changes are obvious. Early in puberty there is increased sensitivity of LH to GnRH. Sleep related increases in both LH and FSH can be documented early in puberty. In boys, the nocturnal increases in gonadotropin levels are accompanied by simultaneous increases in circulating testosterone levels. In contrast, in girls, the night time increases in circulating

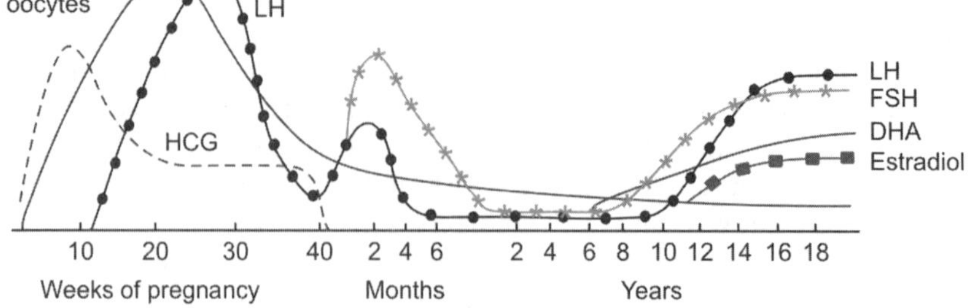

Fig. 1.1: Hormonal fluctuations throughout gestational, neonatal, childhood, pubertal, adolescent and adult life

gonadotropin levels are followed by increased secretion of estradiol next day. This delay in estradiol secretion is believed to be due to the additional synthetic steps required in the aromatization of estrogens from androgens. Basal levels of both FSH and LH increase through puberty (Fig. 1.2).

Puberty

In girls, estradiol secreted predominantly by the ovaries increases steadily during puberty. Estrone, which is secreted in part by the ovaries and in part from extraglandular conversion of estradiol and androstenedione, also increases early in puberty but plateaus by mid-puberty. Thus, the ratio of estrone to estradiol decreases throughout puberty, indicating that ovarian production of estradiol becomes increasingly important and peripheral conversion of androgens to estrone becomes less important during maturation. Episodic peaks of estradiol result and menarche appears. By mid to late puberty, maturation of the positive feedback relationship between estradiol and LH is established, leading to ovulatory cycles.

Breast budding, estrogenization of the vaginal mucosa and lengthening and enlargement of the uterus occur with estrogen exposure. The physiologic vaginal discharge of puberty is the result of the desquamation of epithelial cells and mucus from the estrogenized mucosa. The pubertal process is accompanied by a growth spurt, both growth hormone and sex-steroids appear to contribute to the growth spurt. The levels of growth hormone and IGF-l increase during puberty, largely dictated by the rise of serum estrogen. In boys, the increase in growth hormone is dependent on aromatization of testosterone to estradiol and reflects increasing sex-steroid production at puberty. Nonetheless, there are profound sex differences in growth hormone

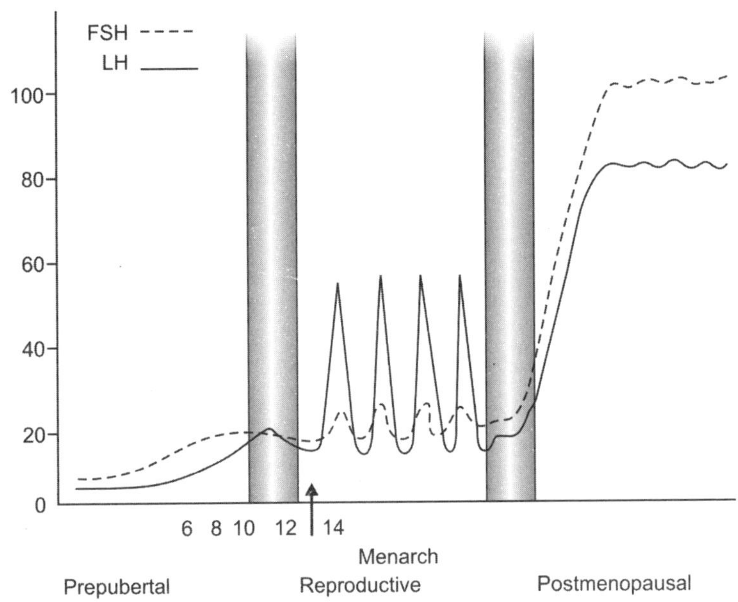

Fig. 1.2: Gonadotropin levels from the age of 6 years to menopause

secretion during puberty. Girls have higher basal levels of growth hormone throughout puberty, reaching maximal levels around the time of menarche and decreasing thereafter. In contrast, basal concentrations of growth hormone remain constant throughout puberty in boys.

Growth hormone stimulates production of insulin like growth factor 1 (IGF-l) in all tissues, with concentrations found in circulation spilling over from the liver. In the final stages of puberty in both boys and girls, growth hormone secretion begins to diminish, returning to prepubertal levels in adult life, despite continued exposure to high levels of gonadal steroids.

Leptin, a hormone secreted by adipose tissue, plays an important role in reproductive physiology. Ankaberg-Lindgren and colleagues found a positive correlation between both estradiol and testosterone and leptin in girls throughout puberty, while no correlation was noted between estradiol and leptin in boys or between testosterone and leptin in pre- or early pubertal boys.

PHYSICAL CHANGES DURING PUBERTY

The typical sequence includes thelarche, adrenarche, growth spurt and menarche.

Thelarche

The first sign of puberty is the development of the breasts. Breast budding usually appears between the ages of 9-11 years, it is indicative of the competency of the hypothalamic-pituitary-ovarian axis. The adolescent breast development is divided into 5 stages (Figs 1.3A to E).

B1—It denotes the prepubertal breast. At this infantile stage, only the papilla is elevated.

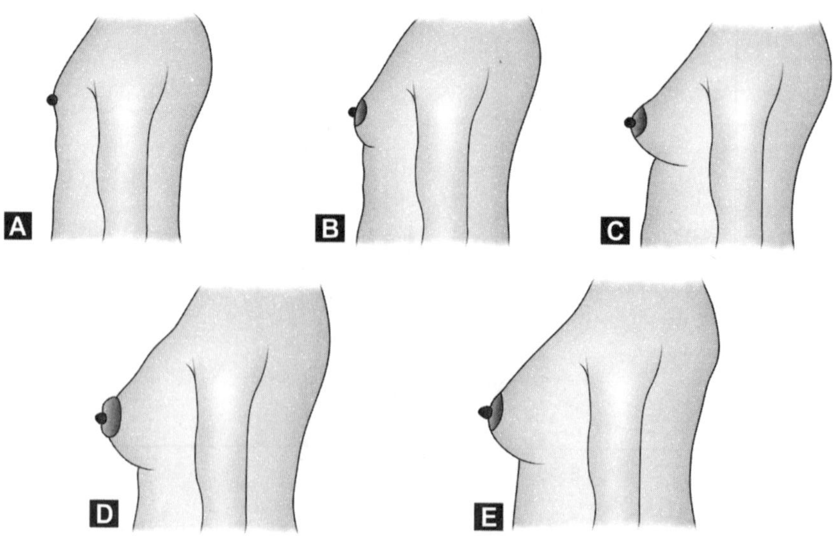

Figs 1.3A to E: Tanner stages of breast development

B2—It denotes thelarche. The breast buds are palpable, the areola enlarges and the breast is elevated like a small mound.

B3—There is further enlargement of the breast and its areola without separation of their contours.

B4—Preferential growth of the areola and nipple leads to formation of a secondary mound over the mound of the breast.

B5—Formation of the mature adult breast. There is recession of the areola into the general contour of the breast because of greater growth of the breast tissue.

Asymmetry of breast development is not uncommon.

There is a recent decline in age at breast development according to the Copenhagen Puberty Study (Pediatrics Vol. 123, No. 5, May 2009).

Adrenarche

Axillary hair development. The sequence of axillary hair development is as follows:

Al—Prepubertal stage. No axillary hair present.

A2—Appearance of sparse axillary hair.

A3—Adult distribution of thick, coarse, dark pigmented hair.

Growth Spurt

At about the age of 12 years, a growth spurt expressed as velocity of growth in height in cm/year occurs. In normal puberty, the growth hormone continues to be secreted at the same earlier constant rate assuring a growth rate of 4 cm/year. Steroids secreted after pubarche superimpose a further acceleration of growth rate of 5 cm/year at the peak of the growth spurt.

Menarche

The first menstrual period generally follows thelarche by about 2 years, when growth development is almost complete and breast development reaches the adult mature stage. An average increment of about 5.0 cm occurs after menarche. The initial menstrual cycles are generally anovulatory for about 12-18 months after menarche.

Skeletal Age

Sexual maturation correlates more with bone age than chronological age. Determination of bone age provides a better marker for prediction of the remaining growth potential.

Pubarche

The adrenals are the main source of androgens which are responsible for the growth of pubic and axillary hair. Pubic hair generally make their appearance about 6 months after thelarche at the B4 stage. Axillary hair generally make their appearance 1-2 years after pubarche.

The stages of pubic hair growth are as follows (Figs 1.4A to E):

P1—Prepubertal stage when there are no coarse pubic hair present, the vellous hair present over the pubic area are similar to the ones seen over the abdominal wall.

P2—Pubarche denotes the appearance of long or slightly curved and pigmented hair sparsely over the labia.

P3—Darker, coarser and curly hair are seen spread over the mons pubis.

P4—The preadult stage when thick dark growth of curly hair are seen covering the area short of the inverted triangle.

P5—Adult inverted triangular distribution of thick, coarse, dark curly hair spreading out to the medial aspects of the thighs is evident.

Stages of Pubarche

Growth hormone secretion is highly pulsatile and during puberty, the amplitude of the pulses increases, especially during sleep. Growth hormone secretion is regulated by growth hormone releasing hormone which has a stimulatory effect and somatropin release inhibiting hormone which has an inhibitory effect. At puberty, growth hormone secretion is highly sensitive to the stimulatory effect of estrogens and growth hormone levels increase before any signs of sexual development appear.

SUMMARY OF PUBERTAL EVENTS

Puberty is a transition from childhood to adulthood. An understanding of the physiology of puberty and menarche is essential for all healthcare providers so that they can give accurate information and help dispel myths. A 'central nervous system program' is responsible for initiating puberty. Development of the hypothalamo-pituitary-gonadal axis in girls during puberty is a two stage process. Firstly, in early puberty, the sensitivity to the inhibitory negative effects of the low levels of circulating sex-steroids

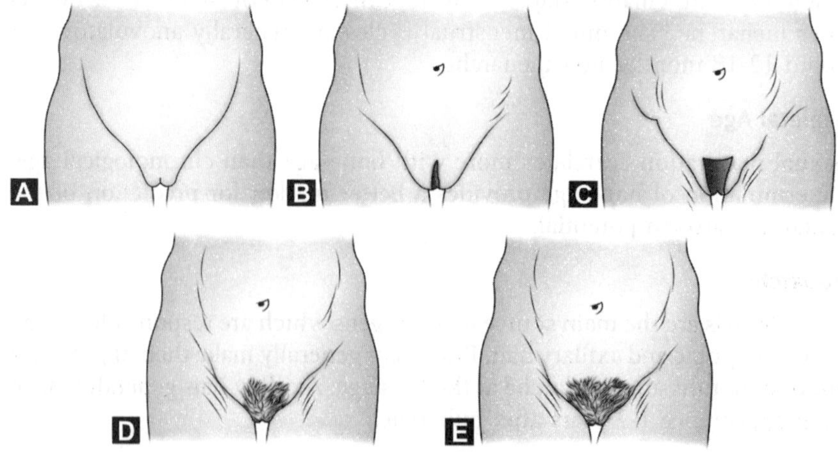

Figs 1.4A to E: Tanner stages of development of female pubic hair

decreases. Secondly, in late puberty, there is maturation of the stimulatory positive feedback response to estrogen leading to mid cycle surge and ovulation.

SUGGESTED READING

1. Altie KM, Ramierez NR, Conte FA, et al. The pubertal growth spurt in eight patients with true precocious puberty and growth hormone deficiency: Evidence for a direct role of sex steroids.J Clin Endocrinol Metab 1990;71:975-80.
2. Boyar RM, Rosenfeld RS, Kapen S, et al, Synchronization of augmented LH hormone secretion with sleep during puberty. New England J Med 1972;54:609-18.
3. Conte FE, Grumbach MM, Kaplan SL. A diphasic pattern of gonadotrophic secretion in patients with syndrome of gonadal dysgenesis. J Clin Endocrinal Metab 1975;40:670-74.
4. Culter GB Jr. The role of estrogen in bone growth and adolescence. J Steroid Biochem Mol Biol1997;61:141-44.
5. DR Pescovitz OH, Barnes, et al. Dissociation of adrenarche and gonarche in precocious puberty and in isolated hypogonadotrophic hypogonadism J Clin Endocrinal Metab 1987;64:1174-78.
6. Ducharme JR, Forest MG, DePeretti E, et al. Plasma adrenal and gonadal sex steroids in human pubertal development J Clin Endocrinol Metab 1976;42:468-76.
7. Frisch RE body fat, menarche and reproductive ability. Semin Reprod Endocrino 1985;3:45-9.
8. Gordan CM, Nelson CM. Amenorrhoea and bone health in adolescent and young women Curr Opin Obstet Gynecol 2003;15:377.
9. Grumbach MM. The neuroendocrinology of puberty. In: Krieger DT, Huges JC, Eds. Neuroendocrinology, Sunderland MA: Siauer Associates 1980;249-58.
10. Judd HL, Parker DC, Siler TM, et al. The nocturnal rise in plasma testosterone in pubertal boys. J Clin Endocrinol 1974;38.
11. Maclure M, Travis LB, Willett W, et al. A prospective study of nutrition intake and age at menarche.
12. Marshall WA, Tanner JM. Variation in patterns of pubertal changes in girls. Arch Dis Child 1969;44:291-303.
13. Marshall WA, Tanner JM. Variation in patterns of pubertal changes in boys. Arch Dis Child 1970;45:13-23.
14. Neinstein LS, Kaufman FR. Normal physical growth and development. Philadelphia: Lippincott Williams and Wilkins, 2002.
15. Parker LN, Liftak AT, Odell WD. A 60,000 molecular weight glycoprotein stimulates androgen secretion. Endocrinology 1983;113:2092-98.
16. Raj B. Mishra R. Normal puberty. In: Krishna U, Salvi V, (Eds)Adolescence. Orient Longman, 2000:10-21.
17. Rose SR, Municchi, Barnes KM, et al. Spontaneous growth hormone secretion increases during puberty in both girls and boys. J Clin Endocrinol 1991;73.
18. Ross JL, Lond LM Sherda, et al. Effect of low dose estradiol on 6 months growth rates and predicted height in patients with Turner syndrome 1986;109:950-54.
19. Sharma K. Age at menarche in northwest Indian females and a review of Indian data. Ann Human Biol1990;17(20):159-62.
20. Tanner JM. Growth in Adolescence. 2nd ed. Oxford, UK; Blackwell Scientific Publication, 1962.
21. Weaver CM. Adolescence: The period of dramatic bone growth Endocrine 2002;17: 43-8.
22. Zacharias L, Wurtman RJ. Blindness: Its relation to age of menarche. 1964;144:1154-55.
23. Zacharias LR, WM Wurtman RJ. A prospective study of sexual development and growth in American girls.The statistics of menarche. Obstetrics Gynaecol Survey1976; 31:325-30.

2

Precocious Puberty

Ratna Thakur, Roza Olyai, Pratibha Singh

INTRODUCTION

Adolescence (Latin: to grow) is the period of life during which the carefree child is in the path of becoming a responsible adult. In other words, it is a period in which a bud blossoms to a fragrant flower. Puberty is the state of becoming functionally capable of procreation. This is usually accepted as occurring at age of 12 years in girls and 14 years in boys.

In precocious puberty, premature activation of hypothalamo-pituitary-gonadal axis occurs, this is defined as the developments of pubertal signs in girls before 8 year[2] and in boys before 9 years taking a mean standard deviation of +/-2 of the normal range.[1]

Incidence

Precocious puberty, in general, is more frequent in girls (20 times more common in girls than in boys), the majority of girls have idiopathic precocious puberty.

CAUSES/ETIOPATHOGENESIS

Traditionally, precocious puberty is divided into:

a. **GnRH-dependent precocious puberty (True or central)**— Also known as true precocious puberty. It includes complete, isosexual, central precocity. Early activation of hypothalamo-pituitary-ovarian axis occurs.
b. **GnRH-Independent precocious puberty (precocious pseudopuberty or peripheral)**—Incomplete, isosexual or heterosexual, peripheral or precocious psuedopuberty.

Sexual maturation in these instances is due to extrapituitary secretion of HCG or sex-steroid secretion independently of hypothalamo-pituitary-ovarian gonadotropins stimulation.

Classification and relative occurrence of precocious puberty:[3]

1. GnRH-dependent (True precocity)	
Idiopathic/constitutional	74%
CNS problem	7.0%
2. GnRH independent	
Ovarian cyst/tumor	11%
McCune-Albright syndrome	5.0%
Adrenal feminizing	1.0%
Ectopic gonadotropin production	0.5%

It can also be classified as:

1. **Isosexual**—Where the features are due to excess production of estrogen.
2. **Heterosexual**—Where features are due to excess production of androgen (from ovarian and adrenal neoplasm).

Causes of precocious puberty

1. GnRH-dependent—80% (complete, central, isosexual or true)
   - constitutional—most common
   - Juvenile primary hypothyroidism
   - Intracranial lesions (trauma, tumor or infection)

   Incomplete
   - Premature thelarche
   - Premature pubarche
   - Premature menarche.
2. GnRH-independent
   Peripheral on precocious psuedopuberty)
   (Excess estrogen/androgen)
   Ovarian:
   - Granulosa cell tumor
   - Theca cell tumor
   - Leydig cell tumor
   - Chorionic epithalamia
   - Androblastoma
   - McCune-Albright syndrome
   - Adrenal-hyperplasia, tumor
   - Liver-Hepatoblastoma
   - Iatrogenic-estrogen or androgen intake

The evaluation of precocious puberty dictates certain priorities:

1. Rule out life-threatening disease: Includes neoplasms of CNS, ovary and adrenal.
2. Define velocity of the progress: Is it progressing or stabilized?—Helps in formulating management decisions.
3. Isolated, nonendocrine cause of vaginal bleeding due to trauma, foreign body, vaginitis, genital neoplasm must be excluded.
4. Physical diagnosis
5. Special findings
6. Laboratory diagnosis.

It involves following diagnostic steps:

I. **Physical Diagnosis**
   1. Record of growth—Tanner stages, height and weight percentiles.
   2. External genitalia changes.
   3. Abdominal, pelvic, neurologic examinations.
   4. Signs of androgenization.
   5. Special findings: McCune-Albright syndrome, hypothyroidism.

II. **Laboratory Diagnosis (Table 2.1):**
   1. Basal gonadotropin levels is the first step in the evaluation of a child with sexual precocity.
   2. Bone age (always to be assessed)—X-ray of hand and wrist.
   3. Thyroid function tests (TSH and free T4)[4]
   4. Steroids (srDHEAS, testosterone, estradiol, progesterone, 17-hydroxyprogesterone)
   5. Head MRI to exclude intracranial lesion. MRI, USG of abdomen and pelvis to exclude ovarian pathology.
   6. Inhibin levels.
   7. GnRH testing.

Table 2.1: Laboratory diagnosis

	Gonadal Size	*Basal FSH/LH*	*Estradiol or Testosterone*	*DHEAS*	*GnRH Response*
Idiopathic	↑	↑	↑	↑	Pubertal
Cerebral	↑	↑	↑	↑	Pubertal
Gonadal	Unilateral ↑	↓	↑	↑	Flat
Albright	↑	↓	↑	↑	Flat
Adrenal	Small ↑	↓	↑	↑	Flat

McCune-Albright syndrome

- Inherited GS alpha deficiency
- Polyostotic fibrous dysplasia of bone
- Irregular café au lait spots on skin
- Hyperfunctioning endrionopathies
- Sexual Precocities[5]—autonomous early production of estrogen by ovary
- Adult Height—normal, Fertility—unimpaired
- Hormonal: Decreased LH/FSH, poor response to GnRH stimulation
- **Treatment**—Testolactone. Competitive inhibitor of aromatose which converts androgen to estrogen.

An approach to the child presenting with premature or atypical puberty:
Initial assessment
1. Clinical history and physical examination
2. Pubertal milestones and growth chart
3. Radiograph of left wrist for bone age.

Unremarkable	Normal variation
1. Clinical evaluation remarkable Early but otherwise (n) puberty (normal) milestone sequence	Clinical evaluation—unremarkable
2. Bone age is less than chronological age	Bone age is consistent with chronological age

Contd...

Contd...

3. Diagnosis: True, idiopathic precocious puberty	Diagnosis: Benign premature adrenalarche, benign premature thelarche, benign premature menarche
4. *Action:* 1. Observation/re-evaluation 2. Consider additional assessment (LH, FSH, estradiol , TSH, HCG levels) to confirm diagnosis of idiopathic precocious puberty or MRI to exclude any pathologic cause *Treatment* 1. Psychologic support 2. Consider suppression of FSH and LH with GnRH analog in selected patient	*Action:* 1. Observation/re-evaluation 2. Consider additional assessment to confirm the diagnosis. *Treatment* Reassurance for patient and parents

TREATMENT

Objectives

- Reassurance, counseling, sex education of both adolescent and parents to prevent pregnancy.
- Arrest maturation of bone until normal pubertal age.
- Attenuate and diminish established precocious characteristics.
- Diagnose and treat intracranial disease.
- Avoid abuse, contraception if necessary.
- GnRH agonist given for 2 to 4 weeks.
- Monitor therapy at regular intervals (1 to 3 months) with serial gonadal ultrasonography, serum sex steroid determination.

Goal

Reduction of pituitary gonadal activity to prepubertal levels (LH < 7.5 IU/L, FSH < 4 IU/L, Estradiol < 9 µg/ml)

The drugs used are:

1. GnRH agonist therapy
2. Medroxy progesterone acetate
3. Cyproterone acetate
4. Danazol

GnRH agonist therapy is the drug of choice in cases GnRH dependent precocious puberty.[6]

These can be administered subcutaneously, nasaly daily or in long-acting depot forms:

1. Buserlin: Subcutaneously 20 to 40 µg/kg/day; intranasal: 1200 to1500 microgram/day
2. Naferin acetate: Subcutaneously 4 µg/day; intranasal 800 to 1600 microgram/day in 3 to 4 doses
3. Medroxyprogesterone acetate: 50 to 200 mg/m^2
4. Cyproterone acetate :100 to 150 mg/m^2 oral in three divided doses

Side Effects

1. Estrogen flare
2. Vasomotor symptoms
3. Psychological symptoms
4. Bone loss: 3 to 5% following 6 months course. It is reversible.

Add-Back Therapy for:

- Effect of GnRH therapeutic effect on original disease process
- Effect on hyperestrogenic syndrome
- Effect on bone
- Effect on lipid profile.
  Dose of GnRH agonist can be monitored by measuring estradiol levels, objective being to maintain estradiol less than 10 pg/ml (in prepubertal range).
- Treatment is maintained until the epiphyses are fused or until appropriate pubertal and chronological ages are matched.
- GnRH agonist treatment is not effective for non-central forms of precocious puberty as McCune-Albright syndrome, GnRH-independent sexual precocity, congenital adrenal hyperplasia.

In above cases, primary treatment is directed towards suppression of gonadal steriodogenesis.

If specific etiology, precocious puberty is identified, it is aimed at curing the underlying disorder:

Hypothalamic, pituitary, cerebral or pineal tumors—Neurosurgical excision.

Of very small size—radiotherapy

Ovarian, adrenal tumors—surgical excision.

Primary hypothyroidism—thyroid replacement prevents further progression of sexual precocity.[5]

Adrenal hyperplasia—treatment with appropriate doses of glucocorticoids and mineralocorticoids (if salt wasting is present) also prevents further progression of pubertal development.

There is no general consensus on the indications for treatment in precocious puberty. However, it is accepted that not all patients with true precocious puberty require treatment. The long term complication of true idiopathic precocious puberty commonly is a compromised adult height.

Part of the decision of whom to treat involves estimating final height. Other criteria include behavioral, psychosocial as possible reasons to treat. Height prediction in precocious puberty is difficult and relies on height prediction algorithms, the most widely used being the bayley method, this estimates adult height based on current height, chronological age and bone age.

Premature pubarche and premature thelarche are too common, benign, normal variant conditions that can resemble precocious puberty but are nonprogressive or very slowly progressive.

Premature thelarche refers to the isolated appearance of breast development, usually in girls younger than 3 years.

Premature pubarche refers to appearance of pubic hair without other signs of puberty in girls or boys younger than 7-8 years. A thorough history, physical examination, and growth curve review can help distinguish these normal variants from true sexual precocious puberty.

Prognosis

Early onset of puberty can cause several problems. The early growth spurt initially can cause tall stature, but rapid bone maturation can cause linear growth to cease too early and can result in short adult stature. The early appearance of breasts or menses in girls can cause emotional distress for some children. The prognosis for precocious puberty depends on the underlying cause. Children with precocious puberty have intellectual, behavioral, psychosexual maturation in keeping with their chronological age, not their physical or pubertal age.

Counseling has to be given about this to parents and children. Children should be counseled that their secondary sexual characteristics are normal a bit early. In rapidly progressing central precocious puberty in girls, gonadotrophin releasing hormone agonists (GnRH agonists) appear to increase final height by about 5 cm in girls treated before the age of eight, but there is no height benefit in those treated after eight years.

SUMMARY

Precocious puberty may be isosexual or heterosexual. It may be GnRH dependent or independent. Growth in precocious puberty is a subject of concern to families and clinicians alike.

In rapidly progressing central precocious puberty in girls, gonadotropin releasing hormone agonists (GnRH agonists) appear to increase final height by about 5 cm in girls treated before the age of eight, but there is no height benefit in those treated after eight years. The decision to treat central precocious puberty should take into account rate of progression of pubertal changes as well as biochemical markers and may need to address other factors (e.g. psychosocial and behavioral issues) as well as height outcome. Investigations must be carried out to rule out any pathology in the CNS, ovary and adrenal. In cases where no cause could be detected, 6-monthly evaluation should be made to detect any life-threatening pathology at the earliest.

REFERENCES

1. Justin S Bromn, Gaery L Warne. Growth in precocious puberty.
2. L Kurt Midjert Moore Sill D Jalobron. Are pubertal changes in girls before age 8 height.
3. Grite Teilmann, Casstenb Pedessen, Tina Kold Jenser, et al. Prevalence and evidence of precocious pubertal development in Denmark: An epidemiologic study based on national registries.

4. GK Indumati/Ganpathy Bantwal, Madhuri Patil. Primary hypothyroidism mutn precocious puberty and bilateral cystic ovaries.
5. Grumbach MM, Kaplan SL. Recent advances in the diagnosis and management of sexual precocity. Acta Paediatr Jpn 1988;30 [Suppl]:155-75.
6. Michael Kappy, Thomas Stuart, Alvin Perelman, Robert Clemons, et al. Children's Health Center of St. Joseph's Hospital (MK, TS), and Phoenix Children's Hospital (AP, RC), Phoenix, Arizona 85013. Suppression of Gonadotropin Secretion by a Long-Acting Gonadotropin-Releasing Hormone Analog (Leuprolide Acetate, Lupron Depot) in Children with Precocious Puberty.

3 Delayed Puberty

DK Dutta, Indranil Dutta, Jayeeta Roy

INTRODUCTION

The ability to diagnose and manage disorder of female pubescence requires a thorough understanding of the physical and hormonal evince that mark the evaluation of the child into a sexually mature adult capable of reproduction. Any abnormalities in this process of development endocrinology to premature, attenuated or delay puberty.

Delayed puberty is a rare condition in girls, and a genetic problem or must be a hypothalamic-pituitary disorder. Delayed puberty represents the end of the normal spectrum of pubertal timing and therefore diagnosis is made by excluding under line condition. Genetic studies will eventually identify the principal and modifying genes that causes constitutional delay of puberty seen in an autosomal-dominant pattern within family.

Definition

Delayed puberty in girls may be defined as the absence of physical manifestations of puberty by the age of 13 years, it is also defined as no menstruation by the age of 16 years in the presence of normal sexual development.

CAUSES OF DELAYED PUBERTY (FIG. 3.1)

Constitutional delay

Constitutional delay—in other words the girl is normal but inherently late in entering puberty—is the commonest cause of delayed puberty. Although these individuals are usually of short stature, and have usually been shorter than their peers for years, their height is generally appropriate for their bone age. All stages of development are delayed. They may be considered to be physiologically immature, with a functional deficiency of gonadotropin-releasing hormone for their chronological age, but not for their stage of physiological development. There is frequently a history of delayed menarche in their mothers.

In these patients, bone age shows a better correlation with the onset and progression of puberty than does chronological age. On attaining a bone age of 11-13 years they can be expected to enter puberty.

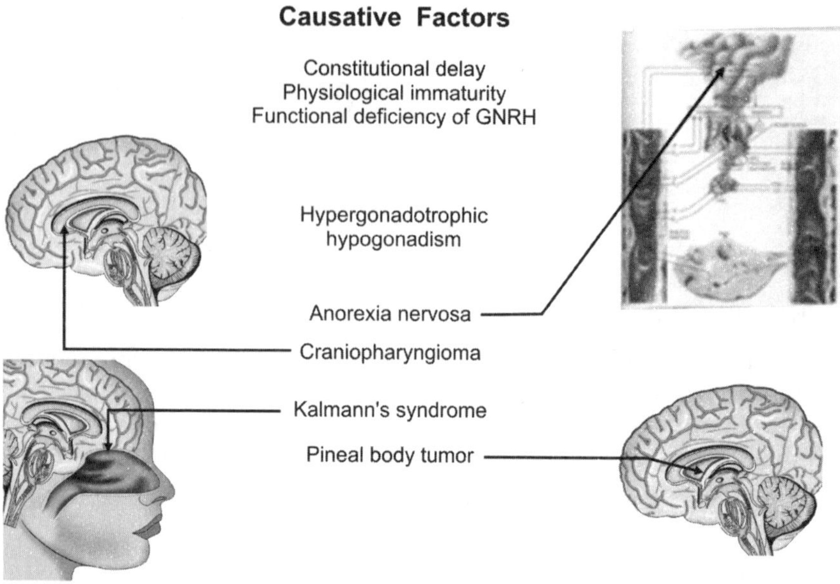

Fig. 3.1: Causative factors of delayed puberty

Hypogonadotropic-Hypogonadism

This arises from a defect of gonadotropin-releasing hormone (GnRH) secretion, and consequently of follicle-stimulating hormone (FSH) and luteinizing hormone (LH). It may be associated with:

- Conditions affecting body weight, such as chronic systemic disease, malnutrition or anorexia nervosa.
- Central nervous system tumors, which may lead to interference with GnRH synthesis or secretion, or with its stimulation of the pituitary gonadotrops. The most common of these rare conditions is craniopharyngioma.
- Isolated gonadotropin deficiency is very rare. Such patients are generally of appropriate height for chronological age, in contrast to patients with central nervous system tumors, who usually have associated growth hormone deficiency, and to those with constitutional delay, who are short for chronological age. The commonest form is Kallmann's syndrome, in which anosmia arising from agenesis or hypoplasia of the olfactory bulbs is associated with GnRH deficiency.

Primary Gonadal Failure (Hypergonadotropic-Hypogonadism)

Although gonadal dysgenesis may occur in isolation, it is most commonly associated with chromosomal anomalies, particularly Turner syndrome. Gonadal failure may also occur following chemotherapy or radiotherapy, as the result of germ cell damage.

Other Causes

These include hyperprolactinemia and hypothyroidism. Table 31.1 gives the incidence of causative factors and Table 3.2 shows differential diagnosis.

DIAGNOSIS OF DELAYED PUBERTY (FIG. 3.2)

The scheme of investigation follows logically from the differential diagnosis discussed above:

1. Plasma FSH, LH, estradiol, prolactin and thyroid function tests
2. Karyotype
3. X-ray for bone age
4. Cranial CT or MRI scan

Table 3.1: Causative factors – incidence[2]

Relative Frequency of Delayed Pubertal Abnormalities		
Hypergonadotropic-Hypogonadism		**43.0%**
Ovarian failure, abnormal karyotype		26 .0%
Ovarian failure, normal karyotype		17.0%
46, XX	15.0%	
46, XY	2.0%	
Hypogonadotropic-Hypogonadism		**31.0%**
Reversible		18.0%
Physiologic delay	10.0%	
Weight loss/anorexia	3.0%	
Primary hypothyroidism	1.0%	
Congenital adrenal hyperplasia	1.0%	
Cushing's syndrome	0.5%	
Prolactinomas	1.5%	
Irreversible		13.0%
GnRH deficiency	7.0%	
Hypopituitarism	2.0%	
Congenital CNS defects	0.5%	
Other pituitary adenomas	0.5%	
Craniopharyngioma	1.0%	
Malignant pituitary tumor	0.5%	
Eugonadism		**26.0%**
Mullerian agenesis		14.0%
Vaginal septum		3.0%
Imperforate hymen		0.5%
Androgen insensitivity syndrome		1.0%
Inappropriate positive feedback		7.0%

Reference: Leon Speroff, Marca Fritz. Clinical Gynaecologic Endocrinology and Infertility. 7th ed. 2005: 384-7)

Table 3.2: Differential diagnosis

	Stature	*Gonadotropins*	*Gonadal Steroids*	*Karyotype*
Constitutional	Short	Pre-pubertal	Low	Normal
Hypogonadotropic hypogonadism	Normal	Low	Low	Normal
Primary Gonadal failure				
Turner syndrome and variants	Short	High	Low	XO and variants
Gonadal dysgenesis	Normal	High	Low	XX or XY

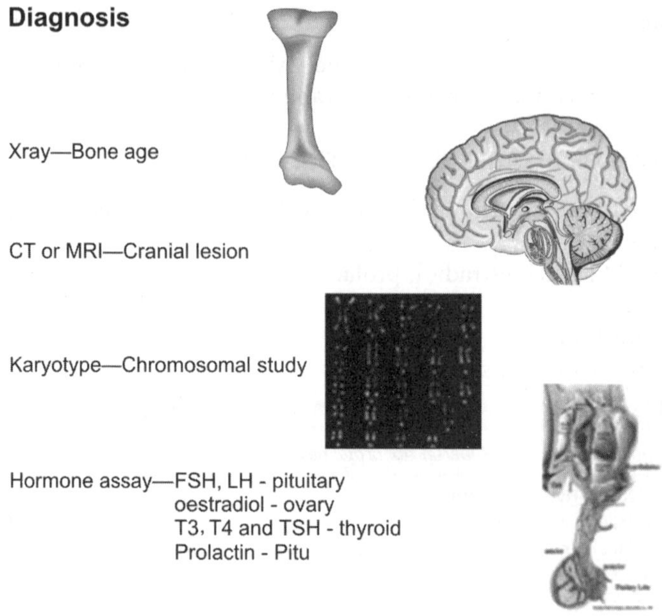

Fig. 3.2: Diagnosis of delayed puberty

MANAGEMENT (FLOW CHART 3.1)

Constitutional delay

Often, reassurance and continued observation are sufficient. It is important to reassure the parents as well as the girl herself. Where psychological problems arise as a result of comparison with her peers, treatment may be indicated. This may take the form of 3 months therapy with low-dose estradiol 2μg daily. If necessary, this can be repeated.

Hypogonadotropic Hypogonadism

In those with low weight, restoration of weight usually results in spontaneous onset of puberty. Those with central nervous system tumors require appropriate neurosurgical treatment.

Where the defect lies at the hypothalamic level, for example with (Kallmann's syndrome, pulsatile administration of GnRH via an infusion pump results in progress through all stages of puberty in the course of 12 months. It is, however, a very demanding form of treatment and in most cases, replacement therapy with estradiol is usually employed for physical maturation. Pulsatile GnRH treatment, however, is necessary if ovulation induction is required.

Primary Gonadal Failure

Girls with pure Turner syndrome or complete ovarian dysgenesis will usually be infertile, although there are reports of successful pregnancies achieved

Flow chart 3.1: Management

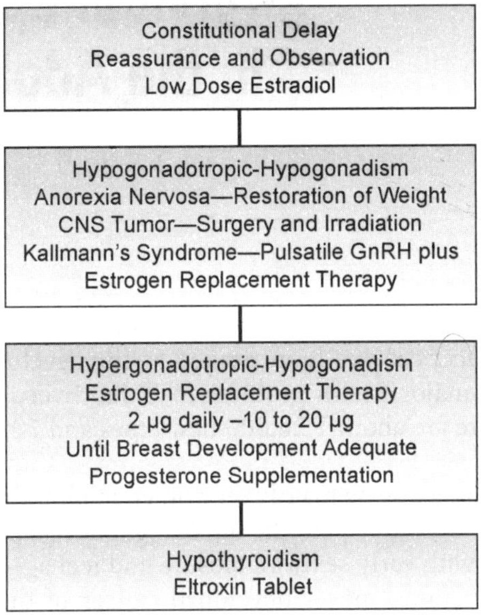

with ovum donation. They will require hormone replacement therapy throughout their lives until the age of 50. The first stage in treatment is to achieve apparently normal progress through puberty, and this is achieved by estradiol replacement therapy. It is commenced at a low dose (2 μg daily) until breast development is adequate. It is important not to begin with higher doses as this may result in poor breast development. Subsequently, higher doses of 10-20 μg daily may be introduced and a progestogen added to avoid unopposed estrogen stimulation of the endometrium. Commonly, ongoing estrogen replacement is with the combined oral contraceptive pill, although hormone replacement therapy can also be used.

CONCLUSION

- Understanding the physical and hormonal events of puberty.
- Detection of any abnormalities during puberty that lead to delayed puberty.
- Estrogen replacement therapy is a treatment of choice for hypergonadotropic hypogonadism.
- Pulsatile GnRH plus estrogen replacement therapy is a treatment of choice for hypogonadotropic-hypogonadism.

REFERENCES

1. Brian Magowan, Philip Jemes Drfe. Clinical Obstetrics and Gynecology 2nd Edition, 2010;43-5.
2. Leon Speroff, Marca Fritz. Clinical Gynaecologic Endocrinology and Infertility. 7th ed. 2005:384-87.

4 Cervical Epithelium in the Adolescents

Kavita N Singh, Shashi Khare

INTRODUCTION

Cervical cancer is the second common cancer in women worldwide. Nearly 86% burden of cancer cervix is contributed by the developing world, and it continues to be a major health problem in India. Every year in India it is estimated that there are about 1,26,000 new cases and 70,500 deaths due to cancer cervix.

Presently, we are focusing mainly on women of reproductive age for early diagnosis of cancer cervix by periodic screening, but real problem starts early in adolescent age, with early sexual exposure and teenage pregnancy.

Virgins (Christian nuns) never developed cancer of the cervix, this was noticed a century ago by Raigoni Stern, this probably provoked Rotkin (1967) into doing his classic epidemiologic study on age at first coitus and its relation to cancer cervix. Early age of sexual initiation and early age at first child birth are known and accepted epidemiological factors. Hence, it is very important to understand the pathophysiology of the cervical epithelium in the adolescent. Every effort must be made to protect it against known and unknown carcinogens. This is part of preventive oncology—a new discipline concerned with gynecology cancer prevention.

Till date, the study of the cervix in adolescence is limited by the fact that studies in normal (non-sexually active) adolescents are difficult since, a speculum examination is not routinely done in gynecological practice. Hence, most of the studies of normalcy are in those adolescent girls who required a speculum examination for medicolegal reasons or are done as postmortem examinations. Unmarried adolescents may not be frank and forthcoming on sexual activity for social reasons. Due to teenage marriages in rural and tribal population, in our medical institution we come across nearly 7-9% adolescents as teenage pregnancy, 12-14% as cases of sexually transmitted disease.

THE TRANSFORMATION ZONE (TZ)

This region of cervix where the columnar epithelium has been replaced by the new metaplastic squamous epithelium is known as the transformation zone. It corresponds to the area of cervix bound by the original SCJ at distal end and proximally by the furthest extent that squamous metaplasia has occurred as defined by the new SCJ.

Few studies are done by Coppelson-Ried (1975) and Singer (1975) were done in state prisons. Singer has divided the adolescent girl population into three groups: virginal group, sexually active but nulliparous group and sexually active and parous group. The transformation zone (TZ) in these three groups were then compared with the transformation zone in adult parous women. Presence of physiological TZ seems to be the most common in all groups and, atypical TZ was more common in sexually active groups (10-44%) giving credence to the hypothesis of early coitus induced carcinogenesis, but was also seen in 12.5% of virgins.

The total area of TZ is also important, Singer (1976) has compared the total area of the TZ in virginal vs. sexually active adolescents and found that area in TZ of the virgin cervix is significantly larger than that of sexually active girls. There are very few other equivalent studies and on the basis of above study and the similar subjective impression by the other investigators, Singer (1976) feels that SCJ probably retracts to within the endocervix as an effect to coitus.

The metaplastic process begins infact from the time of menarche. When the menstrual flow passes through the hymen for the first time, the Doderlein's bacilli enter the vagina and cause it to become acidic. Later on other bacilli invade the vagina.

Pixley (1967-71) conducted a study of 64 (36 pre-menstrual and 28 post menarchal) virginal girls. He classified cervices into two types: Type 1-SCJ at the external os, Type 2 SCJ on the ectocervix with variable amounts of original squamous, columnar and metaplastic squamous epithelium on the ectocervix.

Type 2 predominates 3:1 or more in both groups. The postmenarchal girls tend to have a type 2 cervix to a greater extent than premenarchal girls. Pixley believed that the newly developing vaginal fluid with its acidic pH provides a stimulus for the formation of metaplastic squamous epithelium.

Metaplasia is physiological but should be kept under observation,because exposure to mutagenic agent results in atypical metaplastic process. Once transformed to squamous metaplasia, it is an irreversible process.

In regard to atypical TZ in adolescent virgin and non-virgin girls there seem to be some peculiarities. Atypical TZ was seen in 12.5% of virgins but on histology most of them turned out to be benign.

The colposcopic appearance has been attributed to infiltration and edema in the cervical stroma. In non-virgins, the incidence of an atypical TZ compares equally with the incidence of atypical TZ in adult women. In this group two, precise correlation between colposcopic and histologic findings was found to be difficult. In Singer's series, only 10% of 63 cervical biopsy with an atypical TZ had dysplasia on histology.

Massad and Anoina in 1996 reported on 62 adolescent girls who were under the age of 16 and from low-income group, all had abnormal cytology and were referred for colposcopy. 21% on biopsy revealed atypia and koilocytosis and 21% had moderate dysplasia (CIN2). There was no case of CIN3 or invasive cancer. Unfortunately 66% of girls failed to comply with surveillance.

ASSOCIATION OF HPV WITH CANCER CERVIX

Natural history of transformation is discussed by Reid et al in 1984. The young adolescent had SCJ on ectocervix. The columnar epithelium is thus, exposed to the acid of vaginal epithelium, due to the trauma of coitus, this columnar epithelium undergoes normal metaplasia and then mature squamous epithelium is developed. The SCJ then returns to its normal site at the external os. If however, at this tender juncture, in addition to coitus, the epithelium suffers a persistent HPV infection, the growth goes off at a tangent and may lead to various grades of dysplasia and carcinoma in coming next 2-10 years.

Since the initial reports by Harald Zur Hausen in 1970's suggesting association of HPV with cancer cervix, there have been number of molecular, epidemiological and clinical observational studies implicating HPV as an etiological agent in etiopathogenesis of cancer cervix.

HPV infection can be diagnosed by cytology. The smear shows large cells with a vacuolated cytoplasm and a large bland nucleus. These cells are called koilocytes. There are also clusters of small cells with an orangiophilic cytoplasm and dark, small nuclei called dyskaryocytes. The presence of one or both types of these cells suggest an HPV infection. HPV infection can also be detected by DNA-PCR or Hybrid capture 2 techniques. Further confirmation with colposcopy and histology are mandatory to evaluate its impact, and helps in management plan. HPV vaccines are available as primary prevention against carcinogenic strains HPV-16, 18, 6, 11 but at present availability of vaccine free of cost to rural, slum and high risk group is major concern for developing countries like India.

SIGNIFICANCE OF AGE AT MARRIAGE

Age at sexual initiation plays an important role in carcinogenesis. Rotkin has stated that sexual initiation before the age of 17 years was the most significant factor in all the studies reviewed by him. Saraiya and Lulla (1983) analyzed the age at marriage, in this study, 60% of cancer patients were married before the age of 17 years and only 26% after that age. Similarly Singh K and Khare S (2009) also reported mean age of first coitus at 16.4 years in 355, both negative and positive cases screened by colposcopy for cancer cervix. In India, child marriages are still common although the official age of marriage has risen to 18.

NUTRITIONAL REQUIREMENTS OF THE EPITHELIUM

To maintain the integrity of the epithelium, certain minerals and vitamins are required. Folic acid, vitamin A and its precursors beta carotene, vitamin C and E in adequate amounts will lead to healthy cell growth and division. Anemia adversely affects the body immune system. However, those who are deficient need supplementation with vitamin A, C, E and folic acid. The deficiencies of these also lead to carcinogenesis as young adolescents are found to be in a poor nutritional state, which may be due to poverty, lack of health education or poor eating habits. Due attention needs to be paid to correction of anemia.

CONCLUSION

The understanding of the pathophysiology of the cervical epithelium of the adolescent is necessary to counteract and prevent the process of carcinogenesis. If the incidence of invasive cervical cancer has to come down we must begin with the care of adolescent girl.

Nutrition should be adequate, intake of vitamin A, C and E should be part of health education for all young girls.

Adequate facilities for sexual and menstrual hygiene need to be emphasized. Sexual activity and marriage should be delayed till the age of 18 years. Strict adherence to this law will have an impact on the occurrence of cervical cancer. Child birth should be delayed till the age of 20 years as mature squamous metaplasia would occur by then.

Early detection and prompt treatment of lower genital tract infection will go a long way in maintaining a healthy epithelium. Cervical cancers rarely occur in young girls, hence, routine screening of adolescent girls is not necessary. However, girls who are exposed to multiple partners, who have sexually transmitted diseases and who are used to smoking or tobacco chewing constitute a high-risk group, these girls need to be checked periodically for precursors of cervical cancer.

If we really want to prevent cervical cancer, we must learn to value the girl child and young girls should stick to "late sex, safe sex and vaccination".

SUGGESTED READING

1. ACOG committee on practice bulletins. ACOG practice bulletins: clinical management guidelines for obstetrics gynecologist. Number 45, 2003. Cervical cytology screening (replaces committee opinion 152, March 1995), Obstet Gynecol 2003;102(2):417-27.
2. John W Sellors, R Sankarnarayanan. Colposcopy and treatment of CIN: A beginner's manual. IARC Lyon 2003;1-12.
3. Malcom Fonesca, Saraiya U. Cervical epithelium in the adolescents, its significance in carcinogenesis. The Journal Of Obst and Gyn. of India, 1999;49(5):111-13.
4. Narvekar S, Rao K. Virus and cervical cancer, Recent advances in obstetrics and gynecology-8,2008:106-16.
5. Sankaranarayan RC Mahe. Cervical cancer control in the developing world. Ind J of Gynecologic Oncology 2004;4(2):5-13.
6. Singh Kavita N, Chakma T, Khare S. Colposcopic assessment of the cervix using simplified RCI scoring method, Current Science, 2009;96(3):386-91.
7. Singh Kavita N. Improving prognosis in gynecologic malignancies. Recent trends in obstetrics and gynecology by Pankaj Desai, 2007;117-51.
8. Xavier Bosch F, Salvia de Sanjose. Human papiloma virus and cervical cancer, Burden and assessment of causality, Journal of the National Cancer Institute Monograph no. 31,2003;3-13.

Section 2

MENSTRUAL AND ENDOCRINAL ISSUES

5 Management of Premenstrual Syndrome

Nick Panay, Kate Maclaran, Annie Hawkins

INTRODUCTION

Premenstrual syndrome (PMS) can be defined as a condition which causes distressing physical, behavioral and psychological symptoms, in the absence of organic or underlying psychiatric disease, which regularly recurs during the luteal phase of each menstrual cycle and which disappears or significantly regresses by the end of menstruation.[1] Almost 95 percent of women will experience mild physiological symptoms prior to menstruation, however around five to eight percent experience severe symptoms such that they cause considerable disruption to their lives.[2] Severe PMS is also termed Premenstrual Dysphoric Disorder (PMDD) by the American Psychiatric Association in the DSM-IV classification and has strict diagnostic criteria.[3] The etiology of PMS remains poorly understood. The absence of PMS before puberty, during pregnancy and after the menopause highlights the role of cyclical ovarian activity in its pathogenesis. Women with PMS appear to produce the same levels of gonadal hormones as women without PMS and therefore, it has been suggested that PMS may be due to a differential sensitivity to circulating hormone metabolites rather than abnormal hormone levels.[4] The neurotransmitters serotonin and gaba-aminobutyric acid (GABA) have also been implicated as potential pathways through which abnormal responses to hormone levels may occur.[5,6]

ASSESSMENT AND DIAGNOSIS

Accurate diagnosis of PMS is essential. A careful history should be sought, specifically for a cyclical nature of the symptoms. Premenstrual symptoms may commence up to two weeks prior to menstruation and resolve by the end of menstruation. To make the diagnosis, there should be a symptom-free interval prior to ovulation, however this may often be complicated by physical or psychiatric comorbidities. Ideally, symptoms should be assessed prospectively using symptoms diaries over at least two consecutive months. *Example of symptom diaries can be found at http://www.rcog.org.uk/files/rcog-corp/uploaded-files/GT48ManagementPremensturalSyndrome.pdf.*

PMS can cause a wide range of psychological, behavioral and physical symptoms (Table 5.1). In severe PMS, some form of functional impairment, such as an inability to interact socially or professionally, will be evident.

Table 5.1: Symptoms associated with PMS

Psychological	*Behavioral*	*Physical*
Mood swings	Withdrawal	Bloating
Tearfulness	Lack of control	Pelvic pain
Irritability	Reduced concentration/	Breast tenderness
Depression	Cognitive ability	Headaches
Anxiety	Poor sleep	Food cravings
		Lethargy
		Weight gain

Any underlying conditions as suggested by the history should be excluded and managed appropriately. Common conditions which may cause diagnostic confusion include depression, generalized anxiety disorder, stress, polycystic ovarian syndrome, hypothyroidism, and alcohol or drug abuse.

MANAGEMENT

Once the diagnosis has been confirmed, several management options are available, many of which can be used in the primary care setting. Treatments used are often unlicensed, however, their use is justified when they are of proven efficacy and safety. The National Association for Premenstrual Syndrome (NAPS) has recently published treatment guidelines for PMS which provide a useful clinical tool *(available at: www.pms.org.uk)*.

A potential treatment strategy for PMS is shown in Fig. 5.1.

All women should be given dietary and lifestyle advice on measures which may help reduce symptoms. The prevalence of PMS is increased in

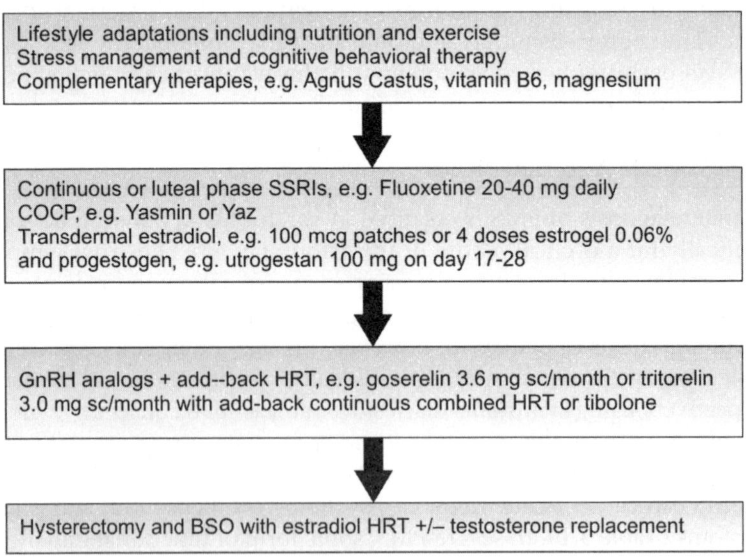

Fig. 5.1: Management strategy for PMS

obese women and those who take less exercise. Weight loss and exercise have been shown to reduce PMS symptoms[7] and therefore, should be recommended. Stress reduction and low glycemic index diets are also likely to be beneficial although no studies have examined these measures directly. Cognitive behavioral therapy has been shown to improve PMS symptoms and should be considered in all women.[8] For further support, women can be referred to the NAPS website: *www.pms.org.uk*.

Some women may choose to use complementary therapies to manage their symptoms. There is some limited evidence to support the use of calcium and vitamin D, magnesium, Agnus Castus or St. Johns wort, however, data for most complementary therapies remains inadequate and the quality control of preparations cannot always be guaranteed. A large placebo effect is generally observed and women should be advised that there is the potential for side-effects and drug interaction.

Serotonin has been implicated in the pathogenesis of PMS[5] and is thought to be associated with symptoms such as irritability and low mood. Selective serotonin reuptake inhibitors (SSRIs) have been used for many years in the management of PMS. A recent meta-analysis has shown SSRIs (fluoxetine, paroxetine, sertraline, citalopram) are effective in reducing premenstrual symptoms in moderate or severe PMS.[9] They have been shown to reduce physical, functional and behavioral premenstrual symptoms and improve quality of life.[9] SSRIs can be given either continuously or in the luteal phase only (i.e. days 15-28); both regimens appear to be of similar efficacy. The advantages of luteal phase treatment include avoidance of dependency and that the regimen is often more acceptable to women concerned about the stigma of using treatments usually associated with psychiatric conditions. Some data exists to the support of the use of the SNRI venlafaxine,[10] however, further large scale studies are needed.

HORMONAL TREATMENT

As LT has already been taking citalopram, the next step may be to try hormonal treatment. This aims to suppress ovulation and stabilize hormonal fluctuations throughout the menstrual cycle.

COCP

There is increasing evidence that new generation COCPs are effective at reducing PMS symptoms. The progesterone component of the COCP has been held responsible for the failure of older COCPs to improve PMS as a common side-effect of progestogens is PMS-like symptoms. The new progestogen drospironone, contained in the preparation Yasmin, has anti-mineralocorticoid and anti-androgenic properties, which may help avoid progestogenic side-effects such as bloating and irritability. The benefit of Yasmin over placebo has been demonstrated for PMS symptoms in a small randomized trial[11] however convincing, large scale data is lacking.

A further advance has been the development of Yaz, which also contains drospironone, but in a 24/4 regimen, in contrast to the traditional 21/7 regimens. The shorter hormone free interval is associated with more profound follicular suppression and more stable hormone levels. Two prospective randomized placebo controlled trials[12,13] have demonstrated the efficacy of Yaz in PMS and it is now licensed in USA for treatment of PMDD.

Estrogen and Progestogen Therapy

Percutaneous hormone replacement therapy in the form of estradiol implants or the transdermal patch has been shown to suppress ovarian activity and improve PMS symptoms.[14,15] Suppression of ovulation usually requires the use of higher doses of estradiol than is used in post-menopausal HRT, for example, 100 mcg estradiol patch.

In non-hysterectomised women, estradiol should be given in combination with a progestogen. Cyclical progestogenic opposition (10-12 days per cycle) is required to protect against endometrial hyperplasia. Unfortunately however, progestogens commonly result in worsening of PMS symptoms and therefore careful consideration should be given to this element of HRT. Fewer side effects are seen with bioidentical progestogens (e.g. Utrogestan), the LNG-IUS or vaginal preparations such as cyclogest pessaries or crinone vaginal gel.

There is no evidence to support the use of synthetic or natural progestogens alone in the management of PMS.[16]

GnRH Analogs

Some women will not respond to the above measures and at this stage referral to specialist services should be made. Inadequate response to treatment may be due to incomplete cycle suppression. GnRH analogs may be considered the next line treatment and can be used to completely suppress the ovarian activity and are of proven efficacy in the treatment of severe PMS.[17] If GnRH analogs are used for longer than six months they must be used in combination with 'add-back' estrogen and progestogen HRT to avoid symptoms of estrogen deficiency and its detrimental effects on bone density. Although the addition of add-back HRT has not been shown to reduce the efficacy of GnRH[17] in a small proportion of women, it may lead to recurrence of their cyclical symptoms, in which case continuous tibolone is an alternative option. For long term GnRH use, yearly assessment of bone density should be undertaken.

Surgical Options

For women with severe PMS, hysterectomy and bilateral oophorectomy will obviously provide permanent cycle suppression. For those with severe PMS who have completed their families, it can be a life changing procedure. It is not without its risks and should only be considered in women who have demonstrated a response to GnRH analogs. Surgical management of PMS is only done in around one percent of patients in the authors unit. Following the procedure, HRT should be given in women below the age of 50 to avoid the effects of estrogen deficiency. Estradiol can be administered via implant, orally or transdermally. Consideration should also be given to testosterone replacement, especially if suffering from symptoms of lethargy and low libido.

CONCLUSION

Severe PMS can cause significant impairment to daily functioning and is often poorly identified and managed. Although the underlying etiology is not well understood a number of treatments with demonstrated efficacy exist. Lifestyle and complementary therapies have an important role, often in combination with psychological or hormonal treatments. Despite advances in treatment options, a small percentage of women will still benefit greatly from surgery management.

PATIENT SUPPORT AND INFORMATION

www.pms.org.uk
www.rcog.org.uk/managing-premenstrual-syndrome-pms-information-you

REFERENCES

1. Magos AL, Studd JWW. The premenstrual syndrome. In: Studd J, editor. Progress in Obstetrics and Gynaecology, Volume 4. London: Churchill Livingstone 1984; 334-50.
2. Panay N. Management of premenstrual syndrome. Journal of Family Planning and Reproductive Health Care 2009;35:187-94.
3. American Psychiatric Association, diagnostic and statistical manual of mental disorders-DSM-IV. 4th ed. American Psychiatric Association, Washington DC 1994.
4. Rubinow DR, Hoban MC, Grover GN, Galloway DS, Roy-Byrne P, Andersen R and Merriam GR. Changes in plasma hormones across the menstrual cycle in patients with menstrually related mood disorder and in control subjects. Americal Journal of Obstetrics and Gynecology 1988;158:5-11.
5. Inoue Y, Terao T, Iwata N, Okamoto K, Kojima H, Okamoto T, et al. Fluctuating serotonergic function in premenstrual dysphoric disorder and premenstrual syndrome: Findings from neuroendocrine challenge tests. Psychopharmacology 2007; 190:213-9.
6. Rapkin AJ, Morgan M, Goldman L, et al. Progesterone metabolite allopregnanolone in women with premenstrual syndrome. Obstetrics and Gynecology 1997;90: 709-14.
7. Prior JC, Vigna Y, Sciarretta D, Alojado N, Schulzer M. Conditioning exercise decreases premenstrual symptoms: A prospective, controlled 6-month trial. Fertililty and Sterility 1987;47:402-08.
8. Hunter MS, Ussher JM, Browne SJ, Cariss M, Jelley R, Katz M. A randomized comparison of psychological (cognitive behaviour therapy), medical (fluoxetine) and combined treatment for women with premenstrual dysphoric disorder. Journal of Psychosomatic Obstetrics and Gynaecology 2002;23:193-99.
9. Brown J, O'Brien PM, Marjoribanks J, Wyatt K. Selective serotonin reuptake inhibitors for premenstrual syndrome. Cochrane Database of Systematic Reviews 2009; 15;(2):CD001396.

10. Cohen LS, Soares CN, Lyster AB, Cassano P, Brandes M, Leblanc G. Efficacy and tolerability of premenstrual use of venlafaxine (flexible dose) in the treatment of premenstrual dysphoric disorder. Journal of Clinical Psychopharmacology 2004; 24:540-3.
11. Freeman EW, Kroll R, Rapkin A, Pearlstein T, Brown C, Parsey K, et al. PMS/PMDD Research Group. Evaluation of an unique oral contraceptive in the treatment of premenstrual dysphoric disorder. Journal of Women's Health and Gender Based Medicine 2001;10:561-9.
12. Pearlstein TB, Bachmann GA, Zacur HA, Yonkers KA. Treatment of premenstrual dysphoric disorder with a new drospirenone-containing oral contraceptive formulation. Contraception 2005;72:414-21.
13. Yonkers KA, Brown C, Pearlstein TB, Foegh M, Sampson-Landers C, Rapkin A. Efficacy of a new low-dose oral contraceptive with drospirenone in premenstrual dysphoric disorder. Obstetrics and Gynaecology 2005;106:492-501.
14. Magos AL, Brincat M, Studd JWW. Treatment of the pre- menstrual syndrome by subcutaneous estradiol implants and cyclical oral norethisterone: Placebo controlled study. British Medical Journal 1986;292:1629-33.
15. Watson NR, Studd JW, Savvas M, Garnett T, Baber RJ. Treatment of severe premenstrual syndrome with estradiol patches and cyclical oral norethisterone. Lancet. 1989;ii:730-2.
16. Ford O, Lethaby A, Roberts H, Mol BW. Progesterone for premenstrual syndrome. Cochrane Database of Systematic Reviews 2009;15(2):CD003415.
17. Wyatt K, Dimmock P, Ismail K, Jones P, O'Brien P. The effectiveness of GnRHa with and without 'add-back' therapy in treating premenstrual syndrome: a meta analysis. British Journal of Obstetrica and Gynaecology 2004;111(6):585-93.

6

Dysmenorrhea in Adolescence

Madhuri Alwani, Ratna Thakur

INTRODUCTION

Dysmenorrhea is a gynecological medical condition characterized by severe uterine pain during menstruation. While most adolescents experience minor pain during menstruation, dysmenorrhea is diagnosed when pain is so severe as to limit normal activities, or requires medication. Dysmenorrhea in adolescents can feature different kinds of pain, including sharp, throbbing, dull, nauseating, burning and shooting pain. Dysmenorrhea may precede menstruation by several days or may accompany it, and it usually subsides as menstruation tapers off. Secondary dysmenorrhea is diagnosed when symptoms are attributable to an underlying disease, disorder, or structural abnormality either within or outside the uterus.

CLASSIFICATION

According to Severity (Recent Method)

Dysmenorrhea can be mild, moderate or severe.

1. Mild—Occurs only on the first day of menstrual bleeding and has few associated symptoms if any. It does not interfere with the daily routine.
2. Moderate—May last for first two or three days, often accompanied by some mild malaise, headache, diarrhea, etc.
3. Severe—There is intense, crampy pain that lasts for 2-7 days and affects the daily routine. Frequent gastrointestinal symptoms are associated. Psychological problems like sexual abuse, rape, and school phobia, personal or family problems may also contribute to decreased threshold to pain.

According to Underlying Cause

Dysmenorrhea can be primary or secondary:

1. Primary dysmenorrhea occurs in young females with no pelvic pathology.
   - It often begins with the onset of ovulatory cycles 6 months to 2 years after the menarche.
   - The pain begins with the onset of the period and may last for 24-72 hours.
   - There is some evidence to suggest that it may occur more frequently, or be more severe in adolescents, whose period starts at an early age.

2. Secondary dysmenorrhea:
   - The pain typically precedes the start of the period by several days and may last throughout the period.
   - Secondary dysmenorrhea may occur as a result of:
     - Fibroids
     - Adenomyosis
     - Endometriosis
     - Pelvic inflammatory disease
     - Adhesions
     - Developmental abnormalities

Secondary dysmenorrhea is a very rare entity in young girls but it may occur sometimes with organic pathology.

CLINICAL MANIFESTATIONS

1. It refers to a syndrome or symptom complex that may encompass nausea, vomiting, headache, nervousness, fatigue, diarrhea, syncope, lower abdominal cramping, bloating and breast tenderness, mood changes and dizziness.
2. The main symptom of dysmenorrhea is pain concentrated in the lower abdomen, in the umbilical region or the suprapubic region of the abdomen. It is also commonly felt in the right or the left abdomen. It may radiate to the thighs and lower back.
3. There may be dizziness, disorientation, hypersensitivity to sound, light, smell and touch, fainting and fatigue.
4. These symptoms appear just before (24-48 hours) or at the onset of menstruation and are maximal during the first 48 hours afterwards.

EPIDEMIOLOGY

- Dysmenorrhea is very common although the precise incidence is not known as it frequently goes unreported.
- Approximately 50% of women will at some stage complain of moderately painful periods.
- Primary dysmenorrhea is the most commonly given reason for absence from school amongst adolescent girls and approximately 15% will complain of severe dysmenorrhea.
- Early menarche, smoking and lengthy periods are all risk factors associated with dysmenorrhea.
- Females who are depressed and/or have poor social support networks are also more likely to experience pain.

PATHOPHYSIOLOGY

Recent theory is that molecular compound called prostaglandins are released during menstruation due to the destruction of the endometrial cells, and the resultant release of their contents and other inflammatory mediators in the uterus cause the uterus to contract. These substances are thought to be a major factor in primary dysmenorrhea. When the uterine muscles contract, they constrict the blood supply to the tissue of the endometrium, which in turn breaks down and dies. These uterine contractions continue as they squeeze the old, dead endometrial tissue through the cervix and out of the body through the vagina. These contractions, and the resulting temporary oxygen deprivation to nearby tissues, are responsible for the pain or "cramps" experienced during menstruation.

Other postulated theories are:

- Role of vasopressin: There is increased vasopressin release during menstruation in women with primary dysmenorrhea. This explains the persistence of pain in cases even treated with antiprostaglandin drugs. The mechanism of action are yet to be explored.
- Endothelins and leukotrienes are vasoconstrictors and stimulate myometrial contractions.
- Platelet activating factor (PAF) is also associated with the etiology of dysmenorrhea as its concentration is high.

MANAGEMENT

A sympathetic approach to the patient including consideration of psychological and behavioral elements will help in a positive outcome.

General Measures

1. Counseling and Reassurance: Patients may be concerned about the possibility of underlying pathology and, when appropriate, reassurance and an explanation of the mechanism of menstrual pain may be helpful.
2. Lifestyle changes: There has been found a clear association between smoking and dysmenorrhea, patients should therefore be informed of this relationship and assisted in any attempts to stop smoking.
3. There also appears to be a link between obesity and dysmenorrhea, although this link is inconsistent, and there is some evidence to suggest that dysmenorrhea is independent of BMI but still it is suggested to loose weight.
4. Previous studies had suggested that there may be a link between alcohol consumption, exercise levels and dysmenorrhea; however, the evidence for this is inconsistent.

Best are Self-help Techniques

The following measures are helpful in relieving the symptoms of dysmenorrhea:

- Intake of tea or mint
- Warmth to the abdomen
- A warm bath
- Abdominal and/or back massage
- Lying in the supine position.

Complementary and alternative medicines—several dietary supplements and herbal remedies have been shown to be effective. These include:

- Calcium and magnesium
- Thiamine
- Ginger
- Fish oil supplements
- Transcutaneous electrical nerve stimulation (TENS)
- Acupuncture
- Toki-shakuyaku-san (TSS)—a Japanese herbal remedy
- Physiotherapy
- Hypnosis
- Acupressure.

Pharmacological

- NSAIDs—Non-steroidal anti-inflammatory drugs (NSAIDs) are the most commonly used drugs for the treatment of dysmenorrhea due to their inhibition of prostaglandin synthesis. This is a class effect and all NSAIDs appear equally effective. Ibuprofen is most often used due to its low incidence of side-effects. Adolescents and young adults with symptoms that do not respond to treatment with NSAIDs for 3 menstrual periods should be offered low dose combined oral contraceptive pills for 3 menstrual cycles.
- Oral contraceptive pills (OCPs) are also used. It is thought that the mechanism of action is reduced prostaglandin release during menstruation. Despite the common use of OCPs in the treatment of dysmenorrhea (and guidance from the Faculty of Family Planning stating it can be used for this purpose from the menarche), recent Cochrane reviews have been inconclusive, due to a lack of evidence from randomized control trials. OCP can also be used to increase cycle length and therefore reduce the frequency of the symptoms.

  Adolescents and young adults who do not respond to this treatment should be evaluated for secondary causes of dysmenorrhea. This is likely in approximately 10% of patients.
- Depo-Provera—In married teenagers, Depo-medroxyprogesterone acetate (Depo-Provera) is also sometimes used as many women achieve amenorrhea within a year of starting treatment.

Surgical Treatment

Surgery is Done in Rare Refractory Cases

Surgery for primary dysmenorrhea is considered:

- When the pain is so severe as to be incapacitating
- When medical treatment has failed
- When a significant psychological or pathological basis is excluded
- It is rarely indicted, and hardly ever before the age of 18 years

Various Surgical Methods

1. ***Dilatation of the cervix:*** The object of this operation is to stretch the fibromuscular tissue at the level of the internal os to such an extent, as to render it hypotonic.
2. ***Injection of the pelvic plexus:*** Injection of the Lee-Frankenhauser plexus with anesthetic agents can be combined with dilatation of the cervix, or carried out alone. The results are equivocal so the treatment has few advocates. It might have a place as a therapeutic test before resorting to sympathectomy.
3. ***Pre-sacral neurectomy:*** The postulated objectives of this operation are to eliminate motor impulses which may be responsible for uterine spasm; to increase the vascularity of the uterus; and to interrupt the sensory pathways from the uterus.The last is probably the main effect.
4. *LUNA:* Currently laparoscopic ultrasound nerve ablation is done in patients along with laparoscopic surgery for the endometriosis, but long-term results are still awaited.

Results

When dealing with a subjective symptom which is prone to spontaneous cure, it is difficult to assess results. Nevertheless, good medical management is effective in 80-95 percent. Otherwise the many forms of treatment recommended, which range from physiotherapy, pharmacology and hypnosis to sympathectomy, give relief in 60 percent of cases, and so do the placebos.

NEWER TRENDS IN DYSMENORRHEA

- Several nondrug therapies for dysmenorrhea have been studied, including behavioral therapy, acupuncture, acupressure, chiropractic care and the use of a TENS unit.
- Behavioral therapies assume that the physiological process underlying dysmenorrhea is influenced by environmental and psychological factors, and that dysmenorrhea can be effectively treated by physical and cognitive procedures that focus on coping strategies for the symptoms rather than on changes to the underlying processes.
- Acupuncture and acupressure are used to treat dysmenorrhea.
- Claims have been made for chiropractic care, under the theory that treating subluxations in the spine may decrease symptoms.
- Treatment with a transcutaneous electrical nerve stimulation (TENS) unit, often used for chronic pain, was indicated as effective in several studies.

CONCLUSION

Dysmenorrhea is a common symptoms complex amongst young adolescent girls, primary dysmenorrhea being the commonest. Secondary dysmenorrhea is very rare. Main etio-pathogenesis implicated is prostaglandin release that leads to uterine cramps due to oxygen deprivation from the uterine musculature. Mainstay of the treatment in majority of the cases is counseling, reassurance and general measures. Some severe cases need drug management. Finally very refractory cases may require surgical interference.

This speaks clearly of the need for pediatricians, gynecologists and generalists to better inform the patients of the help that is available.

SUGGESTED READING

1. ACOG committee opinion: The initial reproductive health visit 2010.
2. Campbell MA, Mchrath PJ. Use of medications by adolescents for the management of menstrual discomfort. Arch Paediatrician1997;151:905.
3. Carol S Havens, Nancy D Sullivan. Manual of outpatient gynaecology 4th edition.
4. Clinical casae in gynaecology Shrish N Daftary.
5. Herweck SP. DUB, OBG Clinic North America 1992;19:129.
6. Iap textbook of paediatrics. page no. 943. 3rd edition.
7. Jeffcoate's principles of gynaecology, 7th edition, 2008;621.
8. Johnson J. Level of knowledge among adolescent girls regarding effective treatment for dysmenorrhoea. J Adolese Health Car 1988;9:398.
9. Klein JR, Litt. IF. Epidemiology of adolescent dysmenorrhea. Paediatrics 1981; 68:661.
10. Rexford, S Ahima. Body fat, leptin hypothalamic amenorrhea. N Engl J med 2004; 351:959-62.
11. Smith RP. Primary dysmenorrhea and the adolescent patients 1988;1:23-30.
12. VG Padubidai, Shrish and Daftary. Shaws textbook of Gynecology, 13th edition.

7 Abnormal Uterine Bleeding in Adolescents

Somen Bhattacharjee

INTRODUCTION

The normal menstrual cycle results from a complex feedback system involving the hypothalamus, pituitary, ovary, and uterus. Menstrual disorders and abnormal uterine bleeding (AUB) are among the most frequent gynecologic complaints of the adolescent.[1,2]

AUB refers to bleeding that is excessive or occurs outside normal cyclic menstruation.[3] Abnormal uterine bleeding is a common clinical problem in adolescence and may also be a potentially difficult condition to treat.

The most common cause of AUB in adolescents during the initial 19 months of menstruation is anovulatory cycle, which is related to immaturity of the hypothalamic-pituitary-ovarian axis.[3,4]

Other common causes include pregnancy, infection, the use of hormonal contraceptives, stress (psychogenic or exercise induced), bleeding disorders, and endocrine disorders (e.g. hypothyroidism, polycystic ovary syndrome).

The treatment for these disorders ranges from observation to pharmacologic and/or surgical therapy. Potential sequel of AUB includes anemia[5] and endometrial cancer.[6,7] With appropriate management of the underlying problem, these sequels may be prevented. Thus, it is crucial to establish the correct diagnosis before any therapy is administered.[8] Frequently, the bleeding problems observed in adolescence require evaluation and intervention.

Menstrual irregularities are a common gynecologic problem; especially in adolescents. AUB is any form of bleeding that is irregular in amount, duration, or frequency. It can be characterized by excessive uterine bleeding that occurs regularly (menorrhagia), by heavy bleeding at irregular times (metrorrhagia), or a combination of both (menometrorrhagia). It can also be intermittent bleeding or sparse cyclical bleeding (oligomenorrhea).

Dysfunctional uterine bleeding (DUB) is a subset of AUB and is defined as excessive, prolonged, or unpatterned bleeding from the endometrium without an organic cause and is frequently used synonymously with anovulatory bleeding.

In adolescents, up to 95% of AUB is DUB. However, because DUB is a diagnosis of exclusion, other potential causes of abnormal bleeding must be ruled out. Here we discuss the physiology, evaluation, diagnostic testing, and treatment of anovulatory bleeding in the adolescents.

The normal menstrual cycle usually consists of a mean interval of 28 days (± 6 days) with a mean duration of 4 days (±2 to 3 days). Normal blood loss is approximately 30 ml per cycle, with an upper limit of 60 to 80 ml. Thirty percent of women who present with a complaint of AUB have clinically significant menorrhagia.[9]

PHYSIOLOGY

The normal menstrual cycle is divided into proliferative, ovulatory, and secretory phases. Normal ovulatory cycles involve regular cyclic production of estradiol, initiating ovarian follicular growth and endometrial proliferation. After ovulation, stability of the endometrium is maintained by progesterone.

In adolescents, a state of "unopposed" continuous estrogen secretion occurs without ovulation. This stimulates excessive dilation of the spiral arterial supply in the endometrium and abnormal endometrial growth without adequate structural support. The consequence is spontaneous breakage and sloughing of the endometrium with unpredictable bleeding. Eventually, continued elevated estrogen levels have a negative feedback effect on the hypothalamic-pituitary-ovarian axis, causing a decrease in FSH, LH, and estrogen.[10,11] This results in a vasoconstriction and collapse of the thickened hyperplastic endometrial lining with heavy and often prolonged bleeding,

Anovulatory cycles may last up to 5 years in adolescents.

Besides physiologic causes, anovulation can also have organic pathologic causes. These include hyperandrogenic states (e.g. polycystic ovary syndrome [PCOS]), hypothalamic dysfunction (e.g. anorexia nervosa and excessive exercise), endocrinopathies, and premature ovarian failure. Occasionally, the bleeding is caused by an anatomic cause (e.g. polyps or fibroids), although this is very rare in adolescents. Therefore, the differential diagnosis of DUB in adolescents prioritizes differently than does the differential diagnosis in adult women (Flow chart 7.1).[12]

COAGULATION DISORDER

Teens with irregular heavy menses should be evaluated for coagulopathies, since 20% to 30% have a major bleeding diathesis.[13]

Blood loss in the normal menstrual cycle is self-limited due to the action of platelets and fibrin. Individuals with thrombocytopenia or coagulation deficiency may have excessive menstrual bleeding. Several studies of the incidence of coagulopathy in teenagers admitted or evaluated for menorrhagia found Coagulopathies in 12 to 33% in all admissions for menorrhagia.[14-16] The most common coagulation disorders include thrombocytopenia, due to idiopathic thrombocytopenic purpura (ITP), von Willebrand's disease, which affects up to 1% of the population, and platelet function defects.[17] Of the adolescents presenting with severe menorrhagia or hemoglobin less than 10 g/dL, 25% were found to have a coagulation disorder. In those presenting with menorrhagia at the first menses, 50% were found to have a coagulation disorder.[16]

Flow chart 7.1: Differential diagnosis of AUB in adolescents

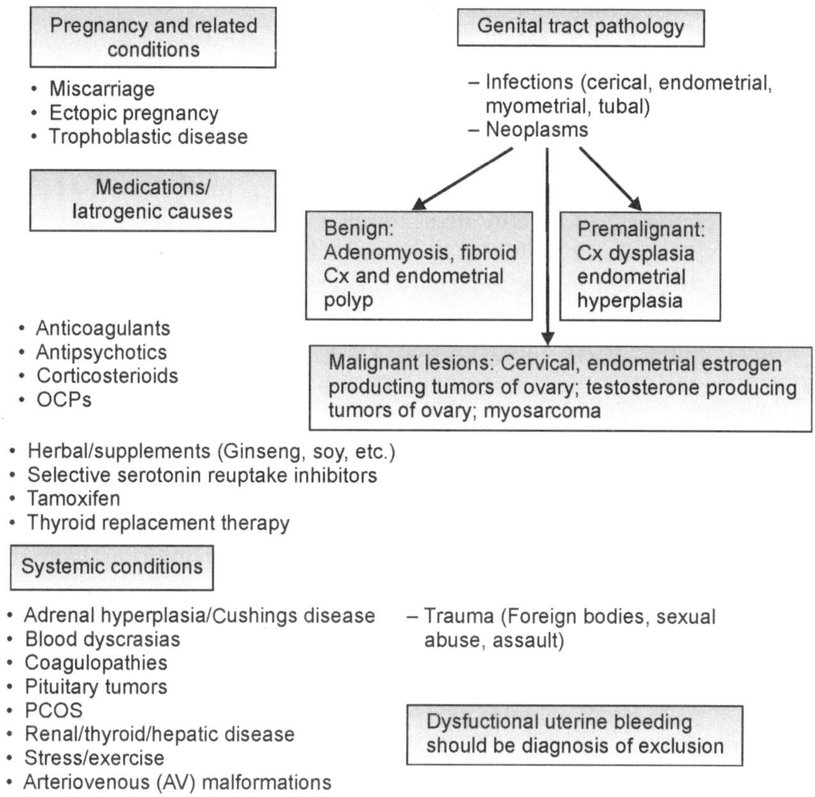

PREGNANCY COMPLICATIONS

The possibility of pregnancy should be considered in any adolescent with abnormal bleeding, and a pregnancy test is mandatory even if the client denies sexual intercourse. Any bleeding in early pregnancy should lead to suspicion of miscarriage or ectopic pregnancy.[18]

Reproductive Tract Pathology

Any trauma, infection, or neoplasm can cause AUB. Infections, such as *Chlamydia*[19] or pelvic inflammatory disease (PID), may present with abnormal bleeding. Vaginal trauma or a foreign body may cause bleeding that might be assumed by the adolescent to be uterine in origin. Women with a foreign body in the vagina generally present with a bloody, odorous discharge. Cervical polyps, cervical carcinoma, and cervical inflammation can cause bleeding. Cervical cancer is fairly rare in adolescents but may be encountered in those who had sexual experiences at a very early age (including those with a history of sexual abuse). Ovarian estrogen-producing tumors need to be excluded in the adolescent with very heavy persistent bleeding. Finally, although rare, uterine pathology, such as polyps and fibroids, may lead to abnormal bleeding.

Endocrinopathies

The most common endocrine disorder to cause abnormal bleeding is thyroid disease.[20] In general, hypothyroidism presents with menorrhagia, and hyperthyroidism presents with hypomenorrhea. Hyperprolactinemia caused by a prolactinoma[21] or certain medications, such as neuroleptics, can also cause anovulation and AUB. PCOS is underdiagnosed in adolescents and should be suspected in obese teens with hirsutism, acne, and continued irregular cycles.[22] There is some recent evidence that PCOS is more common in women with epilepsy.[23] Other diseases to consider are congenital adrenal hyperplasia, Cushing syndrome, hepatic dysfunction, and adrenal insufficiency.

OTHERS CAUSES OF AUB IN ADOLESCENTS

Other causes of AUB (most commonly amenorrhea) in adolescents are eating disorders, stress, excessive exercise, and weight loss. In addition, common medications, which increase the cytochrome P450 enzymatic processes in the liver, may induce the more rapid metabolism of steroid hormones, thereby decreasing their bioavailability and result in AUB that is secondary to a relative insufficiency of estrogen or progesterone (e.g. anti-seizure medications).[24]

EVALUATION

The initial goal in the approach to evaluation of an adolescent with abnormal bleeding is to determine hemodynamic stability, locate the origin of bleeding, identify any organic causes and classify whether the bleeding is ovulatory or anovulatory.

An accurate and complete menstrual history is critical. The history should include age at menarche, frequency, amount, and duration of menses, pain with menses, and last menstrual period. A menstrual calendar can accurately and prospectively keep track of the cycles, especially because adolescents often have difficulty remembering exactly the dates of their cycles. Menstrual flow needs to be assessed in detail, including number of pads, the passage of clots and the soaking of clothes and bedding. Some have advocated a pictorial chart, but more recent research has found that to be unreliable.[25]

In addition, family history should be obtained to rule out any familial diseases including bleeding disorders.

Special attention should also be paid to a careful sexual history because pregnancy and sexually transmitted infections (STIs) can also present with abnormal bleeding.

Medications should also be carefully recorded.

A thorough review of systems should be obtained, with particular emphasis on symptoms of bleeding abnormalities, endocrine disorders, and eating disorders, exercise and sport participation. Because many questions address sensitive areas that may require confidentiality between the adolescent and her health care provider, the young woman can be interviewed without her parents in the room.

A thorough physical examination should include height and weight and evaluation of overall health.

Any signs of hyperandrogenism, such as acne or hirsutism, should be noted. The thyroid gland should be assessed for enlargement and the neck for acanthosis nigricans (a marker for insulin resistance, sometimes found in PCOS).

The breasts should be examined, not only for pubertal staging but also for nipple discharge (galactorrhea) to screen for hyperprolactinemia.

The abdomen should be assessed for masses and hirsutism.

The decision to perform a pelvic examination primarily depends on the sexual history. If the client denies sexual activity, it may not be possible or necessary to perform a pelvic examination. She should have an evaluation of the external genitalia, looking for signs of clitoromegaly or hirsutism. If indicated, a rectoabdominal examination can be done. This is usually well tolerated and can be very helpful in girls with severe dysmenorrhea, to rule out an obstruction in the genital tract, endometriosis in the cul-de-sac, or a pelvic mass. All sexually active girls should have an internal examination with a narrow speculum, screening for sexually transmitted diseases, a Papanicolaou smear (if not done in the last 12 months), and a bimanual examination to assess for masses.

If there is any evidence of coagulopathy, an endocrine abnormality, such as severe hirsutism, acanthosis nigricans, an enlarged thyroid, galactorrhea, or physical evidence of thyroid abnormalities, the patient should be referred to a physician for further evaluation.

A pelvic ultrasound can be obtained if there is a high level of suspicion for an anatomic abnormality or if it impossible to perform a pelvic examination.

Initial laboratory studies should include a complete blood count (CBC) with platelets and a thyroid-stimulating hormone (TSH) or prolactin, if indicated. A pregnancy test should also be obtained, even if the patient denies sexual activity. A coagulation profile, including prothombin time, partial thromboplastin time, and a bleeding time, is recommended if the patient is having acute hemorrhage or has hemoglobin of less than 10 g/dL. Experts recommend a von Willebrand panel, including von Willebrand factor antigen and Ristocetin cofactor activity, if a bleeding disorder is highly suspected. A referral at that time is indicated.

TREATMENT OF AUB

The goals of therapy for AUB in adolescent women are threefold.

The first goal is to assess how serious the abnormal bleeding is, while ruling out any anatomic or pathologic causes.

The second goal is to find out what her expectations and needs are. It is important to realize that often adolescent women may have a different goal for an office visit than she articulates to her parents or office staff; for example, she may have a need for birth control more than she needs regulation of her cycles.

The third goal is to educate about normal irregular bleeding in adolescents. If she is not anemic or does not have symptoms that warrant a referral for medical evaluation and she does not need birth control, then reassurance and education may be all the treatment required. Prospective charting of menses will help to document cycle frequency.

Although anovulation is very common in teens, excessive bleeding leading to anemia is not uncommon in developing countries like India. The goals of therapy for menorrhagia, once pathology has been ruled out, are to:

- Stop the bleeding
- Restore synchrony to the endometrium
- Replenish iron stores.

Most often, this can be achieved with estrogen and/or progesterone therapy. The treatment proper depends upon the hemodynamic stability and the extent of bleeding.

Hemoglobin is Normal or > 10 g/dL

If the bleeding is irregular, but not heavy enough to cause disturbance of the normal activities, reassurance and education should be offered. Prostaglandin inhibitors (ibuprofen or mefenamic acid), which alter the balance between thromboxane and prostacyclin, may relieve cramping and reduce flow volume by 20 to 50%.[26] Oral contraceptives will establish regular menses and regulate blood loss. Adolescents with DUB should be offered this treatment option, which should be explored with the adolescent in a private conversation. Some parents are uncomfortable with adolescents being on "the pill," and it is important to provide thorough information about side effects and non-contraceptive benefits. Anticipatory education about side effects and consistent self-administration are important, because the discontinuation rate in adolescents is high.[27]

A pelvic examination and Papanicolaou smear are not absolutely necessary to prescribe birth control pills. Expert consensus developed in the last decade supports initiating hormonal therapy in adolescents as safe when based on a careful review of medical history and blood pressure measurement alone. Performing a Papanicolaou smear and pelvic examination is important to screen for STIs and cervical cancer in women prior to prescribing oral contraceptives for birth control, but these examinations do not provide information necessary to identify women who should avoid hormonal contraceptives.[28]

However, it is important to emphasize that oral contraceptives do not protect against STIs.

Hemoglobin < 10, But No Active Bleeding

If the patient is clearly anemic, oral contraceptives are the treatment of choice, and a 30- or 35-mcg preparation is usually adequate. Because restoration of synchrony is a goal of therapy, a monophasic preparation is preferred. Oral contraceptives and prostaglandin inhibitors both reduce menstrual flow in patients with a normal uterus. Supplemental iron should be encouraged. Re-evaluation in 3 to 6 months is recommended. The length of treatment should be dependent on the severity of the anemia but will generally be 1 to 2 years (or as needed for contraception).

Progestins alone are also an effective treatment for anovulatory bleeding. Medroxyprogesterone acetate may be prescribed in a dose of 5 to 10 mg per day or micronized progesterone 100 to 200 mg per day for 10 to 14 days, starting on day 16 of the cycle, to induce stromal stability, which is then followed by a withdrawal flow. Disadvantages of this treatment are that the patient is not protected from pregnancy if she is sexually active and irregular bleeding can occur if the patient ovulates. In addition, cyclic progestins, unlike oral contraceptive pills, will not reduce acne or stop the progression of hirsutism, if these are concomitant problems. The side effects of the progestins can include moodiness, depression, and weight gain.

Recently, the role of drospirenone is been evaluated for overweight girls with hyperandrogenism.

Hemoglobin < 10, With Active Bleeding

If the patient had prolonged bleeding and is still bleeding at the time of her visit, but is hemodynamically stable, outpatient therapy with short-term follow-up is adequate. Prolonged asynchronous breakage and shedding results in a thinned endometrium (measurable by ultrasound) and will require higher doses of estrogen to rebuild tissue and replace progesterone receptor sites. Progestin therapy alone will generally not stop the bleeding in this case. Physician consultation is advisable. A cascade of oral contraceptives is started as soon as possible, if the client has no contraindications to the use of estrogen. This should be a 30- or 35-mcg ethinyl estradiol monophasic pill, to be given at high doses with a slow decline. An easy formula is one pill q.i.d. for 4 days, then one pill t.i.d. for 4 days, then one pill b.i.d. for 4 days, then one pill o.d. Nausea may need to be taken care of. With this cascade, the client should have significant slowing of the bleeding in 48 to 72 hours and should be instructed to call if this is not the case or if the dosage is not tolerated. Once the cascade regimen is completed, the severity of the bleeding and the degree of anemia will dictate how long oral contraceptive use is recommended at regular dosing intervals. Conjugated estrogens IV (Premarin) 25 mg IV every 4 to 6 hours is also an option until bleeding ceases or for 24 hours; then OCP is started.[31] Recent studies indicate that prolonged episodes of continuous oral contraceptives are efficacious in the treatment of menorrhagia.[29] If the patient has a contraindication to estrogen, an acute physician referral should be obtained. Depot medroxyprogesterone is an alternative, if long-term amenorrhea is desired. Antifibrinolytic agent such as tranexamic acid (1 gram four times daily) reduces the amount of blood loss by 50%. Its use is usually well tolerated by the patients. Side-effects of tranexamic acid include nausea, and vascular headache. Due to the possible risk of thrombosis, it should be used during the time of heavy bleeding and for a few days per cycle only.

Acute Hemorrhage

Refer immediately to physician for admission and treatment. Often intravenous estrogen is used. Surgery is rarely indicated.[12] DDAVP (desmopressin acetate) nasal spray is been used in managing menorrhagia in adolescents with documented type I vWD with reasonable effectiveness.[32]

PROGNOSIS

The majority of adolescents with AUB will spontaneously convert to normal menstrual cycles within 1 to 2 years, and this information and reassurance should be relayed to her. A 25-year prospective evaluation of adolescents with dysfunctional uterine bleeding showed that of those who continued to have abnormal bleeding after 2 years, persistent problems were noted in 50% after 4 years and in 30% after 10 years.[30]

PATIENT EDUCATION

- After initial treatment and resolution of an episode of AUB, patients need to be educated that, most often, chronic therapy is mandatory to prevent further episodes.
- Reassure patients that most bleeding would stop with the appropriate hormonal therapy. Explain the physiologic reason for the anovulatory bleeding pattern. This is particularly true for the adolescent patient who establishes a predictable ovulatory type of menstrual pattern over time.
- Perhaps the best measure of successful treatment is a good menstrual calendar. Encourage patients to keep a calendar to record daily bleeding patterns. This will serve to document severity of blood loss and impact on daily activities.

CONCLUSION

Abnormal uterine bleeding is a common clinical problem in adolescence but also a potentially difficult condition to treat. Furthermore, most diagnostic criteria and treatment algorithms were optimized for adults and not validated for adolescent population. It is important for clinicians to have an understanding of bleeding patterns of adolescents, the ability to distinguish normal menstruation from abnormal one, and the skill to evaluate the young female patient appropriately. Routine evaluation should include a careful history, physical examination as indicated and permitted, and laboratory studies including a pregnancy test and a complete blood cell count. Quantifying the level of anemia and degree of bleeding along with managing expectations will provide basis for a more successful treatment plan that can almost always avoid surgical methods.[33]

REFERENCES

1. Caufriez A. Menstrual disorders in adolescents: Pathophysiology and treatment. Horm Res 1991;36:156.
2. Deligeoroglou E, Tsimaris P, Deliveliotou A, et al. Menstrual disorders during adolescence. Pediatr Endocrinol Rev 2006;3(Suppl 1):150.
3. APGO educational series on women's health issues. Clinical management of abnormal uterine bleeding. Association of Professors of Gynecology and Obstetrics May 2002.
4. Lemarchand-Beraud T, Zufferey MM, Reymond M, Rey I. Maturation of the hypothalamo-pituitary-ovarian axis in adolescent girls. J Clin Endocrinol Metab 1982; 54:241.
5. Hallberg L, Hogdahl AM, Nelsson L, et al. Menstrual blood loss—a population study. Acta Obstet Gynecol Scand 1966;45:320.
6. Coulam CB, Annegers JF, Kranz JS. Chronic anovulation syndrome and associated neoplasia. Obstet Gynecol 1983;61:403.
7. Southam AL, Richart RM. The prognosis for adolescents with menstrual abnormalities. Am J Obstet Gynecol 1966;94:637.
8. Bayer SR, DeCherney AH. Clinical manifestations and treatment of dysfunctional uterine bleeding. JAMA 1993;269:1823.
9. Prentice A. Healthcare implications of dysfunctional uterine bleeding. Best Pract Res Clin Obstet Gynecol 1999;13:181-8.
10. McLachlan RI, Cohen NL, Dahl KD, Bremner WJ, Soules MR. Serum inhibin levels during the periovulatory interval in normal women: Relationships with sex steroid and gonadotrophin levels. Clin Endocrinol 1990;32:39-48.
11. Marshall JC, Case GD, Valk TW, Corley KP, Sauder SE, Kelch RP. Selective inhibition of follicle-stimulating hormone secretion by estradiol. Mechanism for modulation of gonadotropin responses to low dose pulses of gonadotrophin-releasing hormone. J Clin Invest 1983;71:248-57.
12. ACNM Clinical Bulletin 6. Abnormal and dysfunctional uterine bleeding. J Midwifery Women's Health 2002;47:207-13.
13. Claessens E, Cowell CA. Acute adolescent menorrhagia. Am J Obstet Gynecol or 1981;139:277-80.
14. Smith YR, Quint EH, Hertzberg RB. Menorrhagia in adolescents requiring hospitalization. J Pediatr Adolesc Gynecol 1998;11:13-5.
15. Duflos-Cohade C, Amandruz M, Thibaud E. Pubertal menorrhagia. J Pediatr Adolesc Gynecol 1996;9:16-20.
16. Claessens EA, Cowell CA. Acute adolescent menorrhagia. Am J Obstet Gynecol 1981;139:277-80.
17. Bevan JA, Maloney KW, Hillary CA, Gill JC, Montgomery RR, Scott JP. Bleeding disorders: A common cause of menorrhagia in adolescents. J Pediatr 2001;138: 856-61.
18. McKennett M, Fullerton JT. Vaginal bleeding in pregnancy. Am Fam Physician 1995; 51:639-46.
19. Krettek JE, Arkin SI, Chaisilwattana P, Monif GR. Chlamydia trachomatis in patients who used oral contraceptives and had intermenstrual spotting. Obstet Gynecol 1993; 81:728-31.
20. Koutras DA. Disturbances of menstruation in thyroid disease. Ann NY Acad Sci 1997;816:280-84.

21. Nishio S, Morioka T, Suzuki S, Takeshita I, Fukui Mo, Iwaki T. Pituitary tumours in adolescence: Clinical behavior and neuroimaging features of seven cases. J Clin Neurosci 2001;8:231-34.
22. Gordon CM. Menstrual disorders in adolescents. Excess androgens and the polycystic ovary syndrome. Adolesc Gynecol Part I 1999;46:519-44.
23. Bilo L, Meo R, Valentino R, Di Carlo S, Striano S, Nappi C. Characterization of reproductive endocrine disorders in women with epilepsy. J Clin Endocrinol Metab 2000;86:2950-56.
24. Isojarvi JL, Laatkainen TJ, Pakarinen AJ. Menstrual disorders in women with epilepsy, receiving carbamazepine. Epilepsia 1995;36:676-81.
25. Reid PC, Coker A, Coltart R. Assessment of menstrual blood loss using a pictoral chart: A validation study. Br J Obstet Gynaecol 2000;107:320-22.
26. Bonnar J, Sheppard BL. Treatment of menorrhagia during menstruation: randomized control trial of ethamsylate, mefenemic acid and tanexamic acid. BMJ 1996;313: 579-82.
27. Burke AE, Blumenthal PD. Successful use of oral contraceptives. Semin Reprod Med 2001;19:313-21.
28. Stewart FH, Harper OC, Ellertson CE, Grimes DA, Sawaya GF, Trussell J. Clinical breast and pelvic examination requirements for hormonal contraception: Current practice vs evidence. J Am Med Assoc 2001;285:2232-39.
29. Sulak PJ, Cressman BE, Waldrop E, Holleman S, Kuehl TJ. Extending the duration of active oral contraceptives to manage hormone withdrawal symptoms. Obstet Gynecol 1997;90:257-63.
30. Southam AL, Richart RM. The prognosis for adolescents with menstrual abnormalities. Am J Obstet Gyencol 1966;94:637-45.
31. Am Fam Physician. Copyright 2004 American Academy of Family Physicians 2004;69:1915-26,1931-32.
32. Amesse Lawrence S, Pfaff-Amesse, Teresa, et al. "Oral Contraceptives and DDAVP Nasal Spray: Patterns of Use in Managing vWD-Associated Menorrhagia: A Single-Institution Study." Journal of Pediatric Hematology/Oncology: July 2005 –Vol-27-Issue 7;357-63.
33. Park HT, Kim YT. Abnormal uterine bleeding in adolescence; J Korean Med Assoc. 2009;52(8):779-86.

8 Amenorrhea and Oligomenorrhea in Adolescence

Shilpa Sapre, Deepa Joshi, Sunita Mishra

AMENORRHEA

Introduction

Pubertal development is associated with physical, psychological and emotional changes in the life of an adolescent, hence it needs special attention. The attainment of menarche is influenced by genetic, environmental, nutritional, psychological and various other factors. Delay or failure to attain menarche is of great concern to the parents and the gynecologist as well.

Amenorrhea means absence of menstruation. Interaction between hypothalamus-pituitary-ovarian-uterine axis is required for initiation of menstrual function. It is a symptom, not a disease and so has varied causes. Amenorrhea was arbitrarily classified as: **Primary Amenorrhea** (Absence of menses by 14 years of age in the absence of secondary sexual characters or by 16 years of age in the presence of normal secondary sexual characters) and **Secondary Amenorrhea** (Absence of menstruation for more than 3 cycle intervals or consecutive 6 months in a previously menstruating women[3]) or **False or cryptomenorrhea and True amenorrhea** which could be physiological (constitutional, pregnancy, lactation, etc.) or pathological.

ETIOLOGY

Primary amenorrhea is usually the result of a genetic or anatomic abnormality. The most common etiologies are:

- Chromosomal abnormalities causing gonadal dysgenesis
- Abnormalities of hypothalamic-pituitary axis:
  a. Hypogonadotrophic hypogonadism: Constitutional delay
     functional (stress, exercise, anorexia, etc.)
     Kallmann's syndrome
     CNS tumor
  b. Hypergonadotropic-hypogonadism: Gonadal dysgenesis
     Primary ovarian failure
     Environmental toxins.
- Anatomic abnormalities: Imperforate hymen
  Transverse vaginal septum
  Mayer-Rokitansky-Kuster-Hauser syndrome
  Absent vagina.

- Steroid receptor abnormalities and deficiencies in enzymes of steroidogenesis:
  - 5α–reductase deficiency
  - 17, 20 desmolase deficiency.
- Medical disorders: Chronic illness
  - Juvenile diabetes
  - Tuberculosis
  - Thyroid dysfunction

Secondary amenorrhea is more common than primary amenorrhea. The commoner causes in adolescents can be divided into:

- Hypothalamic dysfunction: Stress
Weight gain/ loss
Tumors.
- Pituitary diseases: Adenoma
Cushing's disease.
- Ovarian disease: PCOS
Premature ovarian failure.
- Uterine disease: Tubercular endometritis.
- Medical diseases: Thyroid dysfunction
Chronic illness.
- Others: Pregnancy.

Menstruation depends upon the proper functioning of hypothalamic-pituitary-ovarian-uterine axis.[4,5] Abnormality at any level can be the etiology for amenorrhea. A logical approach to the woman with either primary or secondary amenorrhea is to consider disorders based upon the level of control.

Etiopathogenesis of Primary Amenorrhea

Hypothalamic and Pituitary Disease

- **Functional hypothalamic amenorrhea**—Functional hypothalamic amenorrhea is characterized by:
  - Abnormal hypothalamic GnRH secretion leading to decreased gonadotropin pulsations
  - Low or normal serum LH concentrations, normal FSH levels
  - Low serum concentrations of estradiol
  - Anovulation, and low serum concentrations of estradiol
  - Associations occur in patients with eating disorders such as anorexia nervosa, exercise, and stress.
- **Congenital GnRH deficiency**—It results in hypogonadotropic hypogonadism which may be:
  - Idiopathic
  - Kallmann's syndrome (amenorrhea with anosmia, isolated GnRH deficiency)
  - Low serum gonadotropin concentrations due to the absence of hypothalamic GnRH.

- **Constitutional delay**—Characterized by:
  - Delayed adrenarche and gonadarche
  - Completely normal pubertal development, but at a later age
  - Familial
- **Hyperprolactinemia** —A rare cause
  - Prolactin-secreting pituitary adenomas and cranial tumors cause pituitary stalk compression
  - Stress, sleep, exercise, intercourse, and meals can raise serum prolactin concentrations transiently. However, serial determinations are important
  - In prolactinomas usually the levels are more than 100 ng/dL
- **Others**—Many infiltrative diseases and tumors of the hypothalamus and pituitary can result in diminished GnRH release or gonadotrope destruction and amenorrhea; these include craniopharyngioma, germinoma, and Langerhans cell histiocytosis.

Ovarian Causes

The most common cause of primary amenorrhea is gonadal dysgenesis caused by chromosomal abnormalities that result in premature depletion of all ovarian oocytes and follicles.

- **Gonadal dysgenesis**—Patients have elevated FSH levels due to the absence of ovarian oocytes and follicles leading to a reduction in negative feedback on FSH from estradiol and inhibins A and B. The largest number of patients with primary amenorrhea and ovarian failure have Turner's syndrome (45 X) followed by:
  - 46, XX gonadal dysgenesis and rarely,
  - 46, XY gonadal dysgenesis.[10]
- **Turner syndrome**—Women with Turner's syndrome are usually missing all of one X chromosome (45, X gonadal dysgenesis). The ovaries are replaced with fibrous tissue and do not produce much estrogen, the external female genitalia, uterus, and fallopian tubes develop normally until puberty when estrogen-induced maturation fails to occur. Characteristic physical findings include webbing of the neck, widely spaced nipples, and short stature, cardiac defects, poorly developed secondary sexual characters, cubitus valgus. Mosaicism also occurs in patients with Turner's syndrome. Serum gonadotropins are high, serum estradiol is low, resulting in hypergonadotropic hypogonadism.

Congenital Anatomic Lesions of the Uterus and Vagina

Account for 20 percent of cases of primary amenorrhea. Pelvic or lower abdominal pain which is usually cyclical is the main complaint.

- **Imperforate hymen**—Presents with cyclic pelvic pain and a perirectal mass from sequestration of blood in the vagina (hematocolpos). These can also present with an abdominal lump, pressure symptoms and malaise. It is actually false or hidden amenorrhea.

- **Transverse vaginal septum**—One or more transverse vaginal septae can occur at any level between the hymenal ring and the cervix.
- **Vaginal agenesis/Müllerian agenesis or Mayer-Rokitansky-Küster-Hauser (MRKH) syndrome**—Congenital absence of the vagina with variable uterine development resulting from agenesis or hypoplasia of the müllerian duct system. Urinary tract abnormalities can occur in association.

Receptor Abnormalities and Enzyme Deficiencies

- **Complete androgen insensitivity syndrome**: Chromosomally 46, XY subjects appear as normal women. These patients are resistant to testosterone due to a defect in the androgen receptor and so the external genitalia are typically female in appearance, but testes may be palpable in the labia or inguinal area. At puberty, breast development occurs, but the areolae are pale and pubic and axillary hair are sparse.

  The testes should be surgically excised after puberty because of the increased risk of developing testicular cancer.[9]
- **5-α-reductase deficiency**: Chromosomally 46, XY, at birth, neonates may appear female or have ambiguous genitalia. At puberty, virilization due to the normal peripubertal increase in testosterone secretion in males lack dihydrotestosterone (DHT) and as a result, they fail to undergo DHT-dependent enlargement of the male external genitalia and prostate.
- **Others**: 17-α-hydroxylase (CYP17) deficiency, vanishing testes syndrome, absent testis determining factor, etc.
- **Thyroid disease**: Excessive weight gain, dry coarse skin, cold intolerance is suggestive of hypothyroidism. It is associated with raised prolactin levels due to increased sensitivity of prolactin secreting cells to thyrotropin releasing hormone. T3, T4 levels are low and TSH is high.
- **Tuberculosis**: In patients of Indian origin, tuberculosis should be ruled out. TB-PCR of the first day menstrual blood will help in diagnosis.

Investigations

Depending upon the history and examination findings, investigations are short-listed. The important ones are:

- CBC
- Fasting ESR
- Mantoux test
- Hormonal assays, if necessary (serum LH, FSH, T3-4, TSH)
- Karyotyping, when indicated
- Laparoscopy
- Ultrasonogrphy or MRI for mullerian anomalies
- IVP for renal anomalies.

Approach to Patient of Amenorrhea

The single most important step in the evaluation is to determine by physical examination or ultrasonography whether there are any anatomic abnormalities of the vagina, cervix, or uterus.[4]

1. *History taking:* Thorough history taking including age, menstrual history, family history, abnormal weight gain or loss, physical or psychological stress in recent past or present, headache, visual disturbances, past surgical history and medical history, etc. should be elicited.
2. *Physical examination:* Detail examination of patient including stature/ weight/BMI/ Nutrition/anthropometry and growth charts, thyroid/ lymphadenopathy, systemic examination,with special emphasis on secondary sexual characters, breast (Tanners staging, galactorrhea), hair distribution (Pubic/Axillary/Bitemporal baldness) body habitus, inguinal or labial masses should be done. Stigmata of Turner's, tuberculosis, etc. should be looked for.
3. *Pelvic examination:* External genitalia: pubic hair (Tanners staging)/ virilization/ ambiguous genitalia.
   Internal genitalia: Absent or presence of uterus/vaginal septum/ imperforate hymen/blind vagina.
4. Pregnancy should be ruled out.
   Breast/Abdominal examination/ Bimanual examination.
5. Stigmata of tuberculosis should be looked for.

MANAGEMENT AND TREATMENT

Treatment of primary amenorrhea[3] is directed at correcting the underlying pathology, if possible, and to prevent complications of the disease process (e.g. estrogen replacement to prevent osteoporosis).

Presence of Secondary Sexual Characteristics

If an adolescent girl with amenorrhea has breast development and minimal or no pubic hair, the usual diagnosis is androgen insensitivity syndrome. Karyotype analysis is needed to determine proper treatment. If testes are present, they should be removed because of the high risk of malignant transformation after puberty. Definitive treatment aims to create neovagina and regular dilatation for sexual purpose.

If an adolescent girl has normal secondary sexual characteristics, including pubic hair, then ultrasonography or MRI is done to see for the presence of uterus as such patients might be having Müllerian agenesis (the congenital absence of a vagina and abnormal uterine development (usually rudimentary). Mayer-Rokitansky-Küster-Hauser syndrome treatment involves vaginoplasty.

If an adolescent has a normal uterus, outflow tract obstruction should be considered. An imperforate hymen or a transverse vaginal septum can cause congenital outflow tract obstruction leading to cryptomenorrhea or hidden menses that is the girl is menstruating but it is not visible outside. Definitive treatment involves hymenotomy under strict asepsis for imperforate hymen and septal resection for transverse septum.

Absence of Secondary Sexual Characteristics

If an adolescent presents with primary amenorrhea and secondary sexual characters are not developed then a detailed history and examination is warranted.[6] The most common cause of hypogonadotropic-hypogonadism in primary amenorrhea is constitutional delay of growth and puberty. A detailed family history also may help detect this etiology, because it often is familial. Hypogonadotropic hypogonadism associated with constitutional delay of growth and puberty is indistinguishable from that associated with hypothalamic or pituitary failure. Counseling and reassurance is all that is needed for in this situation. Kallmann's syndrome, which is associated with anosmia, also can cause hypogonadotropic-hypogonadism. Menstruation can be induced by estrogen-progestin therapy.

Hypergonadotropic-hypogonadism in patients with primary amenorrhea is caused by gonadal dysgenesis or premature ovarian failure. Turner's syndrome (45, XO karyotype) is the most common form of female gonadal dysgenesis. These patients often have a more normal phenotype with spontaneous onset of puberty and menarche.[8] Estrogen and cyclic progesterone replacement at puberty will result in normal pubertal development: pubic and axillary hair; breast growth; cyclic vaginal bleeding; and growth and maturation of the uterus and external genitalia. Postmenopausal hormone therapy may be preceded by growth hormone therapy to gain maximal height. Pregnancy is possible with oocyte donation, IVF and embryo transfer in such cases of gonadal dysgenesis.

Normogonadotropic Amenorrhea

Most common causes of normogonadotropic amenorrhea are outflow tract obstruction. Women with premature ovarian failure have an increased risk of osteoporosis and heart disease. The condition also can be associated with autoimmune endocrine disorders such as hypothyroidism, Addison's disease, and diabetes mellitus. Patients younger than 35 years should undergo karyotype analysis to rule out the presence of a Y chromosome and the need for removal of gonadal tissue to prevent malignant transformation.

Hypothalamic amenorrhea is associated with abnormalities in gonadotropin-releasing hormone (GnRH) secretion and disruption of the hypothalamic-pituitary-ovarian axis. The condition often is caused by excessive weight loss, exercise, or stress, obesity, negative events in the life specially seen during adolescence. Treatment of hypothalamic amenorrhea depends on the etiology. In women with excessive weight loss screening should be done for eating disorders like anorexia nervosa or bulimia nervosa and treated by multidisciplinary approach involving the adolescent, parents, gynecologist and psychologist as well. Menses usually will return after a healthy body weight is achieved. Young athletes who are into rigorous training present with what is called the female athlete triad that includes an eating disorder, amenorrhea, and osteoporosis. Menses may return after a modest increase in caloric intake or a decrease in athletic training in such patients and should be kept under evaluation as they are at risk of bone loss. In adolescent athletes, the bone loss occurs during peak bone mass development and may not be reversible.Weight-bearing exercise may partially protect against bone loss.

In patients with amenorrhea caused by eating disorders or excessive exercise, the use of oral contraceptive pills might prevent bone loss; however, neither therapy has been shown to significantly increase bone mass. Adequate calcium and vitamin D intake are recommended for these patients.[5]

Secondary Amenorrhea

In adolescents, as mentioned previously, the commoner causes include PCOS, tuberculosis, functional hypothalamic amenorrhea and rarely pregnancy. Thorough history, examination and investigations depending upon the diagnosis is to be done. After normal TSH and serum prolactin levels progesterone challenge test is done for withdrawal bleeding, two possibilities arise:

1. Withdrawal bleeding present—Suggestive of endogenous estrogen and hence anovulation.
2. Withdrawal bleeding absent: Go for estrogen-progesterone challenge test, if bleeding occurs, it is suggestive of low estradiol, estimate serum LH/FSH. If serum FSH is high it suggests gonadal failure but normal or low serum FSH is indicative of pituitary or hypothalamic cause. However in patients with absent withdrawal on estrogen-progestogen drugs, it suggests end organ damage.

Polycystic ovary syndrome (PCOS) is the most common cause of hyperandrogenic chronic anovulation. The diagnostic criterion for PCOS is chronic anovulation and hyperandrogenism with no other identified secondary cause. The primary etiology of PCOS is unknown, however insulin resistance is the basic fault. The diagnosis of PCOS is primarily based on clinical and ultrasound findings. The primary treatment for PCOS is weight control through diet and exercise. Weight loss has been found to be beneficial in restoring, normal menses and decreasing insulin resistance. Oral contraceptive pills or cyclic progestational agents can help maintain a normal endometrium. Insulin sensitizing agents such as metformin can reduce insulin resistance.[7]

Points to Note

1. The evaluation for primary amenorrhea should begin early at 13 years of age in absence and 15 years of age in presence of secondary sexual characters respectively.[1,2]
2. Categorization of amenorrhea into primary, secondary is arbitrary and should not be considered in evaluation.
3. Leptin, Ghrelin, CRH, B-endorphins, allopregnanolone and neuropeptides are found to have a role in functional hypothalamic amenorrhea.[11]
4. ACOG recommends initial reproductive health visit at 13-15 years.[12]
5. Diet, exercise, stress, body composition, use of sedative and hypnotic drugs, intellectual and stressful occupations and other unrecognized nutritional and environmental factors contribute in various proportions to amenorrhea.

6. In Indian scenario, tuberculosis should always be ruled out when patient with amenorrhea comes at any age.
7. Female athelete triad: Eating disorder,osteoporosis and amenorrhea. Athelete with amenorrhea of more than 6 months needs medical and gynec evaluation with stress on caloric intake, calcium intake, decreased training intensity, HRT and close follow-up.
8. Pregnancy should be ruled out in adolescent girl with secondary amenorrhea.

OLIGOMENORRHEA

Oligomenorrhea is infrequent menstruation. More strictly, it is menstrual periods occurring at intervals of greater than 35 days for at least a duration of 6 months in a previously normal cycle. It is a common problem seen in adolescent girls due to anovulation, however, evaluation is needed if clinical history and examination are suggestive of any organic cause.

Causes

PCOS

- Eating Disorders
- Adrenal hyperplasia
- Anxiety disorder
- Thyroid dysfunction
- Pituitary tumor
- Tuberculosis
- Obesity
- Medical disorders
- Others.

Evaluation

History

Should include age of menarche, pattern of bleeding, duration of abnormal cycles, family history, weight loss and gain, headache, visual disturbance, prolonged fever, heat or cold intolerance, etc.

Examination

Vitals, BMI, hair growth, body habitus, skin and hair texture, psychological and physical stress, stigmata of tuberculosis, breast discharge, etc.

Investigations

Depending upon the etiology, the investigation and further treatment is to be outlined as neglecting this problem can have future implications on the health of an adolescent girl. Routine and specific investigations like complete blood count, thyroid function tests, hormonal assays if needed, ultrasonography, etc. can be planned.

MANAGEMENT OF OLIGOMENORRHEA

1. **Hypothalamic**: Patients with physical and psychological stresses having oligomenorrhea, due to defect in the pulsatile secretion of GnRH and hence gonadotropins can be managed by counseling and behavioral therapy. Due to constant rise in the expectations of the parents and the pressure from the society, these problems are frequently seen in the adolescents. Changes in body weight, eating disorders, exercise,intense training in professional career also needs counseling, regarding optimum body weight, lowering of exercise hours and various de-stressing activities.
2. **Pituitary:** From a functional situation, oligomenorrhea of pituitary origin is similar to the hypothalamic form. Patients have low levels of gonadotropins and estradiol. Management of functional causes involves counseling and psychologist opinion. Secondary oligomenorrhea may be a sign of an organic lesion such as a brain tumor. The work-up should include evaluation for pituitary tumors. Management involves surgery.
3. **Hyperprolactinemia**: Hyperprolactinemia is rare in adolescence. An elevated prolactin level more than 100 ng/dL is diagnostic of prolactinomas. Treatment consists of medical using drugs like cabergoline, bromocriptine and definitive surgery for prolactinomas. Hyperandrogenism is a frequent cause of oligomenorrhea in adolescence. The increasing production of androstenedione, testosterone, dehydroepiandrosterone and DHEA-S during the development of the adrenal axis in puberty causes a transient hyperandrogenic state. Persistent hyperandrogenemia is characterized by elevated androgens; in routine assays, testosterone and DHEA-S levels are increased. The most common form is the syndrome of PCOS. Oligomenorrhea with PCOS should be treated to induce regular bleeding with transformation of the endometrium to protect against hyperplasia.

   Treatment involves use of monophasic combined oral contraceptive pills. If features of androgenization such as hirsutism, seborrhea and acne are present then combination of ethinyl estradiol and cyproterone acetate is given because of the antiandrogenic effect of this progestin.
3. **Ovarian origin**: Oligomenorrhea caused due to ovarian factors like radiation exposure, drugs, medical disorders or in autoimmune diseases needs careful attention as it may affect her reproductive potential. These patients have elevated levels of FSH and LH and low amounts of estradiol. Chromosomal analysis should be performed to exclude an abnormal karyotype.

   Polycystic ovary syndrome—The menstrual disturbances in PCOS classically have a peripubertal onset. Two minimal criteria for the diagnosis of PCOS are: menstrual irregularity and evidence of hyperandrogenism, whether clinical (hirsutism, acne, or male pattern balding) or biochemical (high serum androgen concentrations).

   Treatment involves supplementation of estrogen/progestogen combination in a cyclic form to induce regular bleeding and correct the estrogen deficit. A multidisciplinary approach involving gynecologist, dermatologist, cosmetologist, endocrinologist and psychologist is the key in treatment of PCOS adolescents.

4. Others, like tuberculosis, specially in Indian set-up be looked for and treated accordingly, pregnancy due to unprotected intercourse should be ruled out and hence the need for sex education in teenage girls.

CONCLUSION

Menstrual disturbances in an adolescent girl either in form of amenorrhea or oligomenorrhea can be a point of worry both for the patient and the parents as well, hence it should be dealt with utmost care. They should be explained about the normal physiological changes occurring at the time of puberty and the sequence of events. Detailed history taking and examination coupled with investigations can help in arriving at a definitive diagnosis. Constitutional delay can be managed by reassurance and counseling alone, however, conditions like Turner's syndrome or androgen insensitivity needs more careful and extensive work-up as they may affect future reproduction.

Accurate diagnosis, stepwise approach for management of amenorrhea and oligomenorrhea is essential. The menstrual cycle is susceptible to outside influences; thus, missing a single menstrual period is rarely important. In contrast, prolonged amenorrhea might be the earliest sign of a decline in general health or signal an underlying condition, such as a pituitary tumor. Thus thorough evaluation and multidisciplinary approach is needed.

REFERENCES

1. Current evaluation of amenorrhea. Fertil Steril 2006;86:S148.
2. Reindollar RH, Byrd JR, McDonough PG. Delayed sexual development: A study of 252 patients. Am J Obstet Gyneol 1981;140:371.
3. Current diagnosis and treatment, obstetrics and gynecology, 10th edition, chapter 56, 926:929.
4. Jeffcoate's principles of gynecology, 17th edition, chapter 37;579:82.
5. Santoro N, Filicori M, Crowley WF. Hypogonadotropic disorders in men and women: diagnosis and therapy with pulsatile gonadotropin-releasing hormone. Endocr Rev 1986;7:11.
6. Practice Committee of the American Society of Reproductive Medicine. Current evaluation of amenorrhea. Fertil Steril 2004;82:266-72.
7. Revised 2003 consensus on diagnostic criteria and long-term health risks related to polycystic ovary syndrome (PCOS).
8. De Arce MA, Costigan C, Gosden JT, et al. Further evidence consistent with Ygh as an indicator of risk of gonadal blastoma in Y-bearing mosaic Turner syndrome. Clin Genet 1992;41:28.
9. Krasna IH, Lee ML, Smilow R, et al. Risk of malignancy in bilateral streak gonads: the role of the Y chromosome. J Pediatr Surg 1992;27:1376.
10. Lukusa T, Fryns JP, Kleczkowska A, Van den, Berghe H. Role of gonadal dysgenesis in gonadoblastoma induction in 46, XY individuals. The Leuven experience in 46, XY pure gonadal dysgenesis and testicular feminization syndromes. Genet Couns 1991;2:9.
11. Rexford S Ahima. Body fat, leptin, hypothalamic amenorrhea. N Engl J Med 2004; 351-959-62.
12. ACOG committee opinion: the initial reproductive health visit 2010.

9 Polycystic Ovarian Syndrome in Adolescent Girls

DK Dutta, Indranil Dutta

PCOS is a complex and heterogeneous disease. In spite of accumulated literature and remarkable advances in the understanding of polycystic ovary syndrome, the etiology of the PCOS is not clear and the primary mechanism is not known. Evidence suggests that Granulosa cells of PCOS contain high level of EGF receptors indicating that hypersensivity of these cells to EGF/ TAFα, particularly in terms of suppression of aromatase activity and LH receptor formation.

Broadly, treatment depends on the symptoms expressed and whether the therapy is for aesthetic reasons in patient not desiring pregnancy, for infertility or even to prevent long-term complications.

This chapter is not only focused on recent concept of pathophysiology, diagnosis and long-term sequelae of PCOS but also highlights treatment protocol in details.

OVERVIEW

From our present state of knowledge about PCOS it was very difficult to make final consensus regarding definition, pathophysiology, clinical manifestations and treatment modalities. Since last few years, various concepts have emerged which have received agreement.

Consensus now agreed as regards definition that it should be better defined as syndrome rather than disease since actual cause or causes of disease is still not known.[1]

Till date there is no supporting evidence regarding the pathophysiology of PCOS although recently familial cluster of PCOS is reported—suggesting a major component of its etiology. Study was done intensively (Steven Franks) to find the genes involved in androgen production and secretion and action of insulin. The results of both linkage and association studies suggest the involvement of two key genes in the etiology of PCOS, the steroid synthesis gene CYPlla and insulin gene—variable number tandem repeats (VNTR).

Urbanck et al[2] concluded from his study that follistatin gene, found to have the strongest linkage with PCOS from 37 genes, but failed to confirm this finding in large series.

Helen Mason has scientifically setout the possible reasons for the increased follicular number and attenuated apoptosis.

Robert Rosenfield proposes that dysregulation of androgen secretion accounts for this abnormality, probably due to hyperactivity of on enzyme, cytochrome P450c17. A single genetic defect enhancing serine phosphorylation, which would decrease the activity of the insulin receptor could account for both the hyperandrogenism and the insulin resistance of PCOS.

Clinical Manifestation

The concept of wide spectrum of signs (Adam Balen), ranging from single finding of polycystic ovarian morphology (detected by USG), to obesity, menstrual irregularities, infertility, cardiovascular diseases—all are due to metabolic disturbances involving increased level of LH, insulin and androgen and dyslipidemia.

PATHOPHYSIOLOGY

The pathogenic mechanisms of PCO are still not known. It has been suggested that PCOS[3] represents a wide range of disorders rather than a single entity. Hyperandrogenism is however, the most endocrine feature in women with polycystic ovary. The ovary, rather than the adrenal gland is the major source of excessive androgen.

The vicious cycle probably begins as a result of excessive androgen production in the adrenal cortex during puberty and adolescent period. Androgens are then aromatized, particularly in the subcutaneous adipose tissue. This leads to an increase of estrogens, which exert a positive feedback on LH but a negative feedback to FSH concentrations. LH leads to excessive androgen production in theca cells surrounding the follicles. Normally FSH maintains aromatase activity in the granulosa cells. When the concentrations of FSH are low, androgens cannot convert to estrogen. Consequently, excessive amounts of androgen of ovarian origin enter the circulation and the vicious cycle continues.

Basically pathogenesis of PCOS are divided into:

a. Follicle arrest up to 10 mm in diameter
b. Hypersecretion of LH
c. Hypersecretion of androgen
d. Hypersecretion of insulin

a. The large number of follicles up to 10 mm in diameter that have been arrested in their development may be due to a number of factors; hyperfunction of EGF/TGFa, Follistatin, Inhibin-B, all of which would interfere with the action of endogenous.
b. An increased number of LH receptors and increasing the sensitivity of LH may be due to a deficiency of growth differentiating factor 9.
c. The abnormal ovarian steroidogenesis results in excess production of androgens by PCO thecal cells which may originate from several possible sources either alone or in combination:
   1. An intrinsic hyper function of CYP11A encoding for cholesterol side chain cleavage.
   2. Increased stimulation of enzyme P450cl7 and by LH mediated by insulin and IGF-I.

d. A post receptor genetic, unique to PCO, causing abnormality of serine phosphorylation of the insulin receptor[4] may be source of insulin hypersecretion on resistance which may be responsible for increased androgen production, reduced transport of testosterone, menstrual irregularity, anovulation and in long run, factors for increased cardiovascular risk.

GENETIC FACTORS IN THE ETIOLOGY OF PCOS

Two key genes are found to be causative factor for PCOS. The results of both linkage and association studies suggest that the (a) Steroid synthesis gene CYP1la[5] and (b) Insulin VNTR[6] (Variable number tandem repeats) regulatory polymorphism are important factors in the genetic basis of PCOS and may explain, in part, the heterogeneity of the syndrome.

Thus, differences in expression of CYPlla could account for variation in androgen production in women who have PCO. Women carrying class III alleles at the insulin gene VNTR locus may be more likely to be hyperinsulinemic and to suffer from menstrual disturbances.

Environmental factors can alter the clinical and biochemical presentation in those with a genetic predisposition to PCOS.[7] This is illustrated by the effect of obesity on serum insulin lends, insulin sensitivity and menstrual function.

Diagnosis

History

1. *Medical history:* A history of headaches or blurred vision (indicating pituitary tumor), any signs or symptoms of thyroid dysfunction (as a differential diagnosis of amenorrhea), or clinical signs of diabetes (indicating adrenal tumor) need to be elicited. History of acne, hirsutism, deepening of the voice, and increase in muscle mass (without exercise). A rapid onset of these symptoms is rare in a PCOS patient, but if present, they suggest a need for an urgent work-up, as an ovarian tumor or adrenal tumor needs to be ruled out. Also, masculinization is uncommon with PCOS patients and is more suggestive of congenital adrenal hyperplasia.
2. *Family history:* PCOS tends to run in families; it is important to ask about family history. Some believe that if a mother has PCOS and her daughter is showing signs of it, she should be evaluated by her pediatrician or by an endocrinologist.
3. *Social/cultural history:* Ethnic factors must be considered in the evaluation of women who are hirsute. Northern European white women and women of Asia usually have small amount of hair on their face, torso, and extremities. However, Mediterranean white women will frequently have hair on their upper lip, chin, and have dark hair on their arms and legs. Also, certain conditions like pregnancy and

menopause can cause transient hirsutism. An important caveat to remember is the patient may not appear hirsute at the time of the examination as she may be using cosmetic procedures like waxing, shaving, or electrolysis to control it.

4. *Menstrual history:* In addition to obtaining a thorough medical and surgical history, elicit a completed menstrual history, including menarche and family history of PCOS. A history of hirsutism, acne, alopecia, menstrual irregularities, or infertility, especially in the patient's mother, is very important. A diagnosis of PCOS may often be made with a complete history. Particular attention to the onset of menstrual irregularities, as this will usually date back to menarche. Inquire about recent pregnancy status and other reproductive history such as miscarriages.
5. *Drug history:* In addition to asking about the patient's current medications it is important to remember that there are certain medications and classes of medications that can cause transient hirsutism. Examples of these are phenytoin (Dilantin), diazoxide, glucocorticoids, and the phenothiazines.

Clinical Features

1. Evaluate the skin for evidence of hirsutism, acne, alopecia, fat distribution, and pigment changes in the skin, specifically acanthosis nigricans. Hirsutism can be defined as hair in locations in women where it is usually not found. Examples of these locations are upper lip, chin, midline of the body, and in the intermammary region. Hirsutism can be graded using the Ferriman-Gallowey scoring system. This scoring system evaluates 9 key anatomic sites. These sites can be graded from 0 (no terminal hair growth) to 4 (maximal growth).[1] The maximum score is 36. A score of greater than 8 suggests androgen excess.[8-10]

   Even when a PCQS patient has increased levels of androgens, hirsutism may not be present unless there is an increase in peripheral androgen metabolism. This is why some women with PCOS are hirsute and others are not. Temporal balding is usually seen after prolonged exposure to androgens. Frontal balding is associated with a virilizing ovarian or adrenal tumor.
2. Central obesity with a ratio of > 0.85 is associated with cardiovascular disease and is marker for PCOS. A "buffalo hump" on the back or purple striae on the abdomen might suggest Cushing's syndrome.
3. During the pelvic examination, assess for clitoromegaly and pelvic masses. Bilateral pelvic masses would be more consistent with PCOS whereas a unilateral pelvic mass may be more consistent with a neoplasia. Remember, too, that the pelvic exam may not reveal any masses in a patient with

Laboratory Studies Blood Profile

1. **Glucose testing:** Glucose tolerance testing is important. As many as 35

to 45 percent of PCOS patients will have impaired glucose testing and about 7 to 10 percent will have type 2 diabetes mellitus. A fasting glucose to fasting insulin ratio less than 4.5 is predictive of insulin resistance. Values on the 2HR glucose tolerance test are as follows: 2H < 140 mg/dL (normal); 140-199 mg/dL (impaired glucose); and > 200 mg/dL (type 2 diabetes).

Cardiac risk profile: Because PCOS patients have hyper-androgenism, they are at an increased risk of cardiovascular disease. It is imperative that the patients are screened for an abnormal HDL, cholesterol, and triglycerides at 35 years of age. Normal results should be repeated in 3-5 years. If these results are abnormal, these entities can be treated early, thus reducing the risk of cardiovascular disease.

2. **Endocrine screening:** Prolactin and thyroid-stimulating hormone (TSH) levels are tested to rule out pituitary or thyroid disease as an etiology of anovulation. LH and follicle-stimulating hormone (FSH) may be analyzed, and they are usually seen in a ratio of > 2.5 to 3. However, a normal LH/ FSH ratio does not exclude the diagnosis of PCOS. An FSH level will also help rule out premature ovarian failure in a woman with amenorrhea.

   Total testosterone and dehydroepiandrosterone sulfate (DHEAS) are evaluated to rule out an androgen-producing neoplasm. Total testosterone levels of 200 mg/dL are not generally seen in PCOS and suggest a virilizing tumor. DHEAS is a weak androgen that primarily comes from the adrenal glands. A level greater than 800 mcg/dL suggests a virilizing adrenal tumor.

   17-hydroxyprogesterone (17OH-progesterone) is a useful screen for late-onset congenital adrenal hyperplasia (LOGAD). 17OH-progesterone levels less than 2 mg/mL are normal. A level > 5 mg/mL is diagnostic for LOG AD. A value between 2 mg/mL and 5 mg/mL should prompt an investigation with an adrenocorticotropic hormone stimulation test. If there is a suspicion for Cushing's syndrome, may get a 24 hours urine for free cortisol or can do a 1 mg dexamethasone suppression test overnight.

Endometrial Aspiration and Biopsy

Many PCOS patients have unopposed estrogen stimulation for prolonged periods of time and are thus a risk for endometrial hyperplasia or endometrial carcinoma. Any PCOS patient with prolonged oligomenorrhea or amenorrhea or a patient with PCOS who is older than aged 35 years and has irregular bleeding should have endometrial aspiration or biopsy to rule out endometrial carcinoma. An important point to remember is that advancing age is not a factor in deciding to obtain endometrial aspiration in patients with PCOS as it is in non-PCOS patients.

Radiologic Studies

An enlarged uterus or enlarge ovaries palpated on pelvic examination suggests a need for pelvic ultrasound to distinguish uterine fibroids from an adnexal mass. If a patient has elevated DHEAS, adrenal imaging is indicated. An important caveat to remember is that polycystic ovaries can be seen in a number of healthy women who do not have PCOS, and women with PCOS do not always have radiographically demonstrated polycystic ovaries. By ultrasound, 25 percent of "normal" ovulating women would have polycystic-appearing ovaries. Typical USG findings of PCOS ITC (i) No. of cysts = >10 mm, pushed/phenipheny (Necklace pattern), (ii) Abnormal stroma, (iii) Uterine width: ovarian length = < 1. (iv) Increased ovarian roundness index = > 0.7.

Differential Diagnosis

Premature ovarian failure, rapid weight loss, extreme physical exertion, low body mass index (BMI) as in anorexia nervosa, and pregnancy will cause abnormal menstrual cycles. Discontinuation of oral contraceptives may also cause amenorrhea. The letter is called post-pill amenorrhea. A pituitary adenoma, hyperthyroidism, or hypothyroidism will also cause a change in the menstrual cycle. Other important etiologies to consider include congenital adrenal hyperplasia, late-onset adrenal hyperplasia, and Cushing's syndrome. Tumors of the adrenal gland or the ovaries may also present with menstrual irregularities.

SEQUELAE OF PCOS

Long-term sequelae in polycystic ovary is still confused due to lack of evidence, since the cause of disease or syndrome is still not known. However, it is important to know its long-term sequelae because (a) Higher incidence of PCOS in adolescent (20%) and postmenopausal women (37-44%) detected by USG[11] (b) Women having PCOS want to know its significance in future reproductive years.

The Natural History of PCO

The natural history of PCO is not known, PCO or PCOS have been found in young girls and adolescents by USG.[12] During reproductive period it was occasionally found during routine USG at assisted pre-productive clinic, otherwise ovary shows quiescence during lactation, oral contraceptive use, GnRH analog use and hypothalamic gonadism. During postmenopausal period PCO is found in 37 to 44 percent having larger ovaries, higher endometrial thickness. Higher serum concentration of testosterone and triglycerols compared with postmenopausal women with normal ovaries. Postmenopausal women with PCO were found to require lipid modifying drugs more frequently than postmenopausal women with normal ovaries and were more hirsute. The high prevalence of polycystic ovaries found in postmenopausal women, who had history of chest pain and were undergoing coronary angiography by USG.

Complication

a. Short-term sequelae
b. Long-term sequelae

Short-term Sequelae

Obesity, hirsutism, menstrual irregularities (oligomenorrhea, amenorrhea) and infertility were short-term sequelae due to persistent anovulation caused by high level androgen, estrogen, lower level of progesterone, low FSH, High LH, and insulin resistant, etc.

Long-term Sequelae

Diabetes, cardiovascular disease, osteoporosis and cancer may develop in PCO women if not treated early. (Diabetic: Untreated hyperinsulamic women with PCOS may develop diabetes in long run).

Cardiovascular Disease

There have been many reports of metabolic abnormalities in women (both lean and obese) with polycystic ovaries. These include raised serum concentrations of triaglycerol and low-density lipoproteins cholesterol, lowered serum concentrations of high density lipoproteins (HDL) cholesterol[13] and evidence of insulin resistance[14] which are all recognized cardiac risk factors. Obese women with PCOs tending to have higher systolic blood pressure is also reported.

Cancer

Breast Cancer

A study has examined the association between breast cancer and PCO.[7] A count of 34835 cancer free women aged 55-69 years was assembled in 1986 and followed until 1992. A total of 472 (1.35%) women reported a history of PCOS at baseline. During the follow-up period 883 women developed breast cancer, 14 of whom had PCOS, but this study does not entirely answer the question as to whether, any association exists between breast cancer and PCO, because premenopausal women were not included and the prevalence of PCOS was found to be only 1 percent.

Endometrial Cancer

The endometrial cancer that is reported in association with PCO tends to occur in women at the severe end of the PCO spectrum and are generally associated with a favorable prognosis,[15] although the exact risk is probably small. Long episodes of amenorrhea in PCOS may increase the risk of endometrial cancer in untreated cases.

Ovarian Cancer

Ovarian cancer risk was found to be increased 2.5 fold (95% CI, 1.1 to 5.9) among women with PCOS,[16] but this study did not use a histological definition of PCOS. Therefore, more research is needed to confirm its association with PCOS. Dehlgren from Sweden showed that PCO was a definite risk factor for myocardial infarction, and his group estimates that myocardial infarction would be seven times more common in women with PCOS compared with the general population. Mary Bindsall group from Auckland reported that PCO were diagnosed in 42 percent of the women and were associated with hirsutism, previous hysterectory, higher free testosterone, triaglycerol and C-peptid levels and lower HDL cholesterol levels and the number of segments with more than 50 percent stenosis was 1.7 (95% CI, 1.1 to 2.3) compared with 0.82 (CI, 0.54 to 1.1); $P < 0.01$. However, this study did not answer the question as to whether women with PCO died more frequently of cardiovascular disease.

Osteoporosis

Women with PCO with history of amenorrhea or oligomenorrhea, with anovulation, with anorexia nervosa, hypothalamic amenorrhea, exercise induced amenorrhea or hyperprolactinemia anemia, may be at increased risk of osteoporosis. Reassuring evidence shows that women with PCO do not have an increased risk of osteoporosis, may be due to secondary PCO secreting significant quantities of testosterone, estrone and estradiol, all of which prevent against bone loss.

PCO and Mortality

A study was conducted on 842 British women with diagnosis of PCOS, followed until the age of 75 years of age, confirmed that there were fewer deaths than expected in women with PCOS, less than circulatory disease as a cause of death and fewer neosplasms causing death but more cases of diabetes were recorded. These findings conclude that PCOS may be protective against cardiac disease because of excess estrogen in the blood. In conclusion, association with PCOS and its long-term sequelae is still confused since the reported is scanty. Association with breast and ovarian cancer is still doubtful but long episodes of amenorrhea in PCOS may increase risk of endometrial cancer if not treated early. As regards osteoporosis and mortality, no substantial evidence is reported till date.

MANAGEMENT

Till date, PCOS was diagnosed as a syndrome of ovarian hyper-function; influenced by genetic defect causing intrinsic ovarian dysfunction whose degree of symptomatology is largely influenced by extraovarian factors. Causative genes, involved although small in number, have yet to be delineated. Due to above facts, treatment of PCOS remains almost symptomatic.[17]

Basically treatment depends upon various factors:

- Age of girl
- Presence or absence of obesity, hirsutism, acne
- Menstrual irregularity
- Presence or absence of hyperinsulinemia or hyperandrogenism or high LH
- Prevention of long-term sequelae.

Prime importance of treatment:

a. Reduction of weight loss
b. Reduction of insulin level
c. Lowering of LH secretion
d. Lowering of androgen secretion
e. Treatment of hirsutism, acne, if any.

Treatment were divided into:

a. Weight reduction and diet
b. Surgical
   1. Wedge resection of ovary
   2. Laparoscopic ovarian puncture.

Weight Reduction and Diet

Weight reduction[18] often has beneficial effect on menstrual abnormalities and hirsutism.

Short-term (4 weeks) very low-energy diets in women with PCOS resulted in a reduction in (a) Serum free testosterone (b) Insulin and insulin like growth factor I (IGF-I) and increase in SHBG levels. It has been shown that weight loss decreased ovarian P450c17a activity and reduced scrum free testosterone concentration in obese women with PCOS, but in obese ovulatory women.

Weight loss then decreases both hyperinsulinemia and insulin resistance increases SHBG and results in overall reduction of hyperandrogenism.[19] Therefore, low-energy diet and exercise should be encouraged as a form of first-line therapy.

Medical Treatment of Acne and Hirsutism

The individual drugs used in the treatment of hirsutism affect different aspects of androgen metabolism. The idea is:

1. To decrease androgen production
2. Increase metabolic clearance rate of androgens
3. Inhibit androgen receptors
4. Inhibit or block enzymes responsible for peripheral production of testosterone or conversion of testosterone to dehydrotestosterone (DHT)
5. Increase the amount of sex hormone binding globulin (SHBG).

Treatment divided into: (1) Medical management, (2) Other Therapies.

Medical Management: Combined Oral Contraceptive Pill

Estrogen/progesterone oral contraceptive pills is the treatment of choice for mild hirsutism of PCOS. However, 19 nortestosterone derivates (norethindrone, norgestrel, ethynodiol diacetate) in OC is better to avoid as because of androgenic properties. Hence it is better to choose a combination drug estrogen plus cyproterone acetate (CPA) (antiandrogenic effects). Treatment with OC containing 2 mg of CPA had masked beneficial effects on acne, seborrhea and hirsutism. Beneficial effects of low dose combined estrogen-antiandrogen preparation in PCOS:

a. *On hormonal disturbances*
   i. Decrease in LH levels
   ii. Decreased ovarian and adrenal androgen levels
   iii. Increase of SHBG concentration.
b. *On clinical signs:* Decrease in hirsutism, improvement in acne and seborrhea, good control of menstrual cycle.
c. *On ovarian size:* Decrease in ovarian volume, this regimen is found to be better in adolescents with PCOS.

Antiandrogens

Till date no antiandrogen has been shown to be superior in well designed trial on hirsute women. Cyproterone acetate, a steroid derived from 17 hydroxyprogesterone has progestational and antigonadotrophic actions in addition to antiandrogen activity. A 'reverse sequential' regimen is found to be better in CPA (25-100 mg daily is given orally on 5-15 of the cycle and ethinyl estradiol 20-30 mg is given on days 5-26 of the cycle.

CPA (50 mg daily for 10 days) combined with an OC is found to be treatment of choice for women with PCOS because it suppresses LH androstenedione, an drostenedione levels, and increases SHBG. This regimen is a highly effective treatment for severe hirsutism and provided excellent cycle control and contraception. Monotherapy with CPA for l0 days in each cycle or month could be an option for women who do not tolerate estrogens provided adequate contraception is used.

In severe hirsutism, CPA (10 mg) daily can be advocated for 6 month to 1 year, but when satisfactory result is achieved, the dose of CPA may be reduced every 3-6 months, first to 50 mg daily and then to 25 mg daily for the first 10 days of reverse sequential regimen. Alternatively, a regimen with 10 mg CPA during the first 15 days of the OC can be employed in cases of recurrence or less severe hirsutism. When a satisfactory clinical reduction in hirsutism is observed, it is justifiable to continue treatment with a lower dose preparation containing 20 mg of CPA and 35 mg of ethinyl estradiol with no added CPA.

Side-effects of CPA include weight gain, loss of libido, headache and fatigue and mood changes but when ethinyl estradiol is added to CPA, these complaints diminish in frequency. Often hyperinsulinemia and glucose tolerance hepatotoxicity are reported.

Spironolactone

In clinical practice, doses of spironolactone range from 50 to 200 mg daily but most patients require at least 100 mg. This dosage has been associated with significant improvement in 70-75 percent of hirsute women after 6 months.

Serum levels of SHBG, DHEAS and DHEA are unaltered by this regimen but testosterone levels will drop with a few days of treatment. Side-effects are gastrointestinal (20%), menstrual irregularities (27%), increased fasting blood insulin concentrations. It should be avoided in women using drugs such as angiotensin converting enzyme inhibitors or angiotensin II receptor blockers.

Flutamide

Doses of 250 mg—three times daily for 3-6 months.[20] It induces a significant reduction in total free testosterone, 5-dihydro testosterone, DHEA, DHEAS and androstenedione levels and a favorable effect on lipid profile. Side effects include nausea, vomiting, deterioration in liver function tests, cholestetic jaundice and hepatic necrosis.

Finasteride

5 mg daily has clinical effect on hirsutism similar to that of spironolactone and flutamide. The drug is well tolerated and no side effects have been noted in human.

GnRH Agonists

GnRH agonists such as nafarelin, leuprolide or buserelin decrease ovarian steroid production by suppressing LH and FSH secretion. This treatment is highly effective (i) in women with PCOS (ii) ovarian hyperthecosis (iii) severe premenstrual syndrome.

Combination of GnRH agonists with estrogencan prevent bone loss and coronary heart disease (due to decreased level of estrogen). It acts by suppressing androgen and increasing SHBG concentrations.

Ketoconazole

400 mg per day in PCOS as well as with 1000 mg per day in stromal hyperthecosis. Side effects are nausea, vomiting, pruritus and alternations with hepatic functions.

Metformin

Metformin 500 mg three times a day for 6 months is used in the treatment of PCOS. It significantly reduces hyperinsulinemia and hyperandrogenism independent of changes in body weight (obesity). But in thin PCOS if father is diabetic, metformin can be advocated in some selected cases.

Other Therapy

a. *Cosmetic procedures:* All forms of hormonal treatment will benefit from concurrent mechanical hair removal.
b. *Antibiotic and topical therapies:* Tetracycline, erythromycin and tetracycline with conjunction with androgen therapy are the mainstays of therapy of acne.
c. *Psychological interventions:* Psychological treatment in the form of group therapy has important beneficial effects on the management of obese women with PCOS because hirsute women have increased levels of anxiety and depression.

Surgical

i. Wedge resection of ovary
ii. Laparoscopic ovarian puncture.

Wedge Resection of Ovary: Stein and Leventhal described resection of half to three quarters of both of the enlarged ovaries. Out of 1766 patients whose results were published between 1935 and 1983, there was an overall pregnancy rate of 58.8 percent with results ranging from Stein's high of 86.7 percent to a low of 25 percent. Bilateral wedge resection[8] of the ovaries are abandoned long ago because of problems associated with postoperative adhesions.

Laparoscopic Ovarian Puncture: The methods described range from: (i) Multiple ovarian biopsy to remove 0.5-1 mm of tissue, (ii) Electrocautery using a unipolar coagulating current, (iii) Puncture of the ovarian surface with a laser.

With KTP and carbon dioxide lasers: As with electrocautery, the ovarian cortex over follicles is vaporized; the number of punctures is however increased compared with electrocautery. With the Nd: YAG laser, coagulation rather than vaporization is the goal and a wedge of various tissues is coagulated to a depth of 4-10 mm without opening the ovarian cortex.

Laparoscopic Ovarian Puncture Indication

a. Anovulatory
b. LH level is high
c. Women undergoing medical induction or WHO develop solitary cyst formation. This procedure is contraindicated: (a) obesity (b) infertility that cannot be accounted for by an ovulation.

CONCLUSION

PCOS is a complex and heterogeneous disease. Till date there is no supporting evidence regarding the pathophysiology of PCOS, although familial cluster of PCOS is reported—suggesting a major component of its etiology. Treatment depends in the symptoms expressed and to prevent short- and long-term complications.

REFERENCES

1. Roy Homburg. Polycystic ovary syndrome consensus and controversy. PCOS edited by Roy Homburg, 2001;l-9.
2. Urbanek, Legro RS, Driscoll Da, et al. Thirty-seven candidate genes for polycystic ovary syndrome. Strongest evidence for a linkage is with Follistatin. Proc Natl Sci USA 1999;96:8573-78.
3. Franks S. Medical progress article: Polycystic ovary syndrome. N Engl J Med 1995;301-25.
4. Dunaif A. Insulin resistance and ovarian dysfunction. In: Moller D (Ed.): Insulin resistance. John Wiley: New.
5. Gharanin, Wather Worth DM. Battyental association of the steroid synthesis gene CYPlla with polycystic ovary syndrome and hyperandrogenism. Hum Mol Genet 1997;6:397-402.
6. Wather Worth DM, Bennetist, Gharani, et al. Linkage and association of insulin gene VNTR regulatory polymorphism with polycystic ovary syndrome. Lancet 1997;349:986-89.
7. Holte J, Bergh T, Berne C, et al. Restored insulin sensitivity but persistently increased early insulin secretion after weight loss in obese women with polycystic ovary syndrome. J Clin Endocrinol Metab 1995;80:2586-93.
8. MacPannill, MPAS. PA-C; Polycystic ovary syndrome. An overview topic in Advanced Practice Nursing Journal 2(3), 2002.
9. Slowey MJ. Polycystic ovary syndrome. New Perspective on an old problem. South Med J, 2001;94:190-96.
10. Stenchever MA, Droege Muellen W, Henbst AL. Chapter 39. Comprehensive Gynaecology. Third Edition, St. Lonsmo: Mosby; 1997:1087-1112.
11. Farquhar CM, Bindshall MA, Manning P, Mitchell J, France JT. The prevalence of polycystic ovaries on ultrasound scanning in a population of randomly selected women. Aust NZ J Obstet Gynaecol 1994;34(i):67-72.
12. Bridges NA, Hindmansh PC, Cooke A, Brook CGD, Healthy MJR. Standards for ovarian volume in childhood and pulesty. Fentil Steril (1993) 60: 456-60.
13. Wild RA, Alaupovic P, Parken IJ. Lipid and apolipoprotein abnormalities in hirsute women 1. The association with insulin resistance. Am J Obstet Gynecol 1992; 166:1191-97.
14. Banobieni RL. Polycystic ovarian disease. Annu Rev Med 1991;42:199-204.
15. Jafani K, Javaheni G, Ruiz G. Endometrial adenocarcinoma and the Stein-Leventhal syndrome. Obst Gynec 1978;51:97-100.
16. Schildknaut JM, Schwing L PJ, Bastos E, Evanoff A, Hughes C. Epithelial ovarian cancer risk among women with polycystic ovary syndrome. Obst Gynec 1996;88: 554-59.
17. Conway GS, Honour JW, Jacobs HS. Heterogeneity of the polycystic ovary syndrome: Clinical, endocrine and ultrasound features in 556 patients. Clin Endocrinol 1989;40:459-70.
18. Guzick DS, Wing R, Smith D, Berga SL, Winters SJ. Endocrine consequences of weight loss in obese, hyperandrogenic women before and after weight loss. J Clin Endocrinol Metab 1989;68:173-79.
19. Jakubowicz DJ, Nestler JE. 17-alpha-hydroxy-progesterone responses to leuprolide and serum androgens in obese women with and without polycystic ovary syndrome after dietary weight loss. J Clin Endocrinol Metab 1997;82:556-60.
20. Venturoli S, Marescalchi O, Colombo FM, et al. A prospective randomized trial comparing low dose flutamide, finasteride, ketoconazole and cyproterone acetate-estrogen regimens in the treatment of hirsutism. J Clin Endocrinol Metab 1999;84:1304-10.

Section 3

CONTRACEPTION, PREGNANCY AND ABORTION

10 Premarital Counseling and Vaccines

Shilpa Thaker, Roza Olyai

Essence of Marriage

Marriage is regarded as a divine institution; it is not simply a contract between the two parties. Marriage is seen as grace and a benefit from God, a "fortress for well-being," which is both a sacred and eternal bond, and a challenge to be won each day. The true marriage is this, that husband and wife should be united both physically and spiritually, that they may ever improve the spiritual life of each other.

Marriage is a lifelong partnership; the aim should always be to create strong marriages and a stable foundation for the larger structures of society.

PREMARITAL COUNSELING

Premarital counseling is very important and helpful, especially in the developing countries it is seen that many times, young girls and boys plan to marry at an early age not knowing about their health status and consequence of early pregnancy. It is important to strengthen marriage and make it successful. Premarital counseling is a good resource for learning more about each other and this type of therapy is intended to help develop a deeper level of communication. Good communication is important in any relationship but especially in marriage.

The idea behind premarital counseling is that adolescents need to strengthen their relationship before tying the knot so that one can be fully equipped to deal with the challenges and conflicts that every couple inevitably faces at some point in their marriage.

No matter how well they know each other, life after marriage changes with new responsibilities and duties coming in. Thus getting pre-wedding jitters is normal.

Good communication is essential to a successful marriage. During premarital counseling, they learn a little more about each other's communication styles and discuss methods for effective communication. These techniques will greatly improve their chances of having good communication during marriage and their happiness as well.

Premarital Health Screening

Premarital screening consists of a group of tests meant to be done before marriage. The tests will help identify potential health problems amongst prospective life partners. It will also help to detect some of the hereditary diseases, chronic disorders and infections.

Primary Health Screening

This basic health plan includes the minimum array of tests necessary for a conclusive health assessment of an individual. Today's fast-paced, stressful world, however, places a number of more specific health-endangering demands on our bodies.

In fact, in most locations, the standard premarital blood tests check for evidence of syphilis (now or in the past) and rubella (German measles). Screening for other diseases in future newlyweds has in some cases included tuberculosis, gonorrhea, and HIV; of these, only HIV can be detected by blood tests. Only two states have passed legislation requiring HIV testing before marriage, but those laws did not last long at least in part because of very low detection rates.

Why is it important to have the premarital test done?

- This is an opportunity for her to be screened for some tests that she might not have done before.
- Since sickle cell anemia and thalassemia are common hereditary diseases and since these diseases are only inherited from parents to children, the premarital test will determine the risk of her and her future partner having a child with these dangerous blood disorders.
- HIV and Hepatitis B and C viruses are life-threatening diseases. These viral infections can be transmitted by blood, sexual intercourse, and body fluids. Testing for these infections is very important because the viruses may remain dormant for months or even years in carriers without showing any symptoms. Marrying someone who carries these illnesses will put mother and her baby at risk of getting the infection.
- With early diagnosis and proper treatment, carriers of HIV or hepatitis viruses can keep the symptoms under control and reduce the risks of serious complications.

Premarital screening helps to:

- Assess the general health status of both partners
- Detect infectious diseases, e.g. HIV and hepatitis B infection
- Screen hereditary conditions that may effect the future offspring, e.g. thalassemia
- Hemophilia, cystic fibrosis, etc. which are preventable tragedies
- Screening for communicable diseases like TB
- Screening for mental illnesses
- Screening for fertility problems and timely counseling.

The screening tests include:

- Age of the individual whether early or late marriage
- Physical examination including height, weight, BP and secondary sex characters

- Menstrual history and any disturbances related to it
- Vaccination status including hepatitis-B and rubella
- History of addictions to certain recreational drugs, narcotics, marijuana, alcohol, smoking, etc.
- Psychiatric assessment
- Examination for all organ systems for any diseases like TB, diabetes, heart disease, etc.
- Your hereditary status to rule out the genetic disorders.

PREMARITAL VACCINATION

Vaccination programs that focus on infants and children have decreased the occurrence of many childhoods, vaccine-preventable diseases. However, many adolescents, i.e. persons 11-21 years of age continue to be adversely affected by vaccine-preventable diseases (e.g. cancer cervix, varicella, hepatitis B, measles, and rubella), partially because vaccination programs have not focused on improving vaccination coverage among adolescents.

Help Keep Adolescents Healthy and Safe with Immunizations

Changing behavior among adolescents and their parents or guardians will require education and outreach. While younger children have little or no control over healthcare decisions, adolescents often play a key role in decision making. Therefore, it is important that adolescents, as well as their parents or guardians, are educated about the value of vaccines and the seriousness of vaccine-preventable diseases.

Reasons for Targeting Adolescents

There are strong reasons for targeting adolescents for immunization. These may be related to a direct benefit to the adolescents themselves, or they may be part of wider disease control activities. Probably the most compelling reason is to maintain protection acquired by immunization earlier in life.

Adolescents Are Vulnerable to Vaccine-Preventable Diseases

Immunizations can prevent many of the diseases that pose serious threats to adolescents. Vaccines prevent serious morbidity and mortality. Vaccine-preventable diseases can cause serious morbidity and mortality in adolescents and their close contacts.

To Counter a Specific Risk

As for all ages, travel represents a special need for adolescent immunization, indeed may be even more important on the basis that adolescent behavior may place them at increased risk. Adolescents may enter a period of increased risk, for instance from hepatitis B virus, through embarking on a lifestyle that involves drug taking or sexual experimentation with a number of partners.

Immunological Considerations

Immunological considerations also need to be taken into account. In situations where adolescents typically acquire natural immunity to common infections, immunization in this age group is unlikely to be necessary.

Immunization As a Preventive Health Service for Adolescents

Administration of vaccinations should be integrated with other preventive services provided to adolescents. The importance of improving the vaccination levels and of providing other preventive services indicated for adolescents and young adults has been emphasized recently by many national organizations.

Vaccines recommended for adolescents are underused, leaving our nation's teens vulnerable to serious morbidity and even death. Healthcare providers should make every effort to vaccinate adolescents according to our national immunization schedule to benefit adolescents, their close contacts and society at large.

The end of high school/college entry point is a great time to review immunization status and provide necessary vaccines before insurance coverage changes.

Health services can provide adolescents the opportunity for:

a. Ensuring vaccination of those adolescents not previously vaccinated with hepatitis B vaccine, varicella virus vaccine (if indicated), or the second dose of the measles, mumps, and rubella (MMR) vaccine;
b. Administering a tetanus and diphtheria toxoid (Td) booster;
c. Administering other vaccines that may be recommended for certain adolescents; and
d. Providing other recommended preventive services.

Vaccines for Adolescents

Human papillomavirus (HPV)

HPV is a virus that is spread through sexual contact and is the leading cause of cervical cancer in women. It can also cause genital warts and warts in the throat.

HPV is frequently acquired during adolescence. About one in four adolescent girls contracts at least one sexually transmitted infection, the most common being HPV. Although in most cases the body's immune system will keep the virus under control or get rid of it completely, some people develop cell changes that may lead over the course of many years to cervical or other anogenital cancers.

HPV is one of the most common sexually transmitted infections. In the vast majority of cases, however, the infection clears or becomes undetectable within one to two years.

The best time for HPV vaccination is before the first sexual contact, which is why it is recommended for adolescents regardless of whether or not they are sexually active.

HPV is the Primary Cause of Cervical Cancer

Human papillomavirus (HPV), a common sexually transmitted infection, is the primary underlying cause of cervical cancer. Preventing HPV transmission is very difficult. Barrier contraceptive methods are only partially effective because the virus can exist throughout most of the anogenital area (including areas not covered by male condoms) and can remain infectious for years. Although HPV cannot be treated, in the majority of cases, the infection becomes undetectable. In a small percent of women, however, HPV infection persists and leads to precancerous lesions, called dysplasia. Immunocompromised women may be at particularly high risk of persistent infection.

Detectable HPV infection is most common in younger women. Although prevalence varies among region, it generally reaches a peak of about 20 percent among women aged 20 to 24, with a subsequent decline to approximately 8 to 10 percent among women over age 30.

Importance of the HPV Vaccine

Vaccine is highly efficacious in reducing the incidence of cervical, vulvar and vaginal cancers. Vaccine is efficacious during the course of the three doses of vaccination regimen.

Rubella Infections

The majority of rubella infections occur in young adults, who may suffer a slightly longer course of the illness. Most of these adults have not received the rubella vaccine or the Measles, Mumps, Rubella (MMR) vaccination. Others have received the rubella vaccine, but may not have maintained immunity to rubella.

Rubella infection in a pregnant mother is indicated in spontaneous abortion. Congenital rubella contracted from the mother, can cause severe retardation in the unborn child, failure to thrive *in utero*, congenital heart defects, and defects of the eyes. Additionally, the unborn child's liver, spleen and/or bone marrow are affected, may fail to form properly, or fail to function properly.

An infant who has had contracted rubella *in utero*, can often be contagious with the illness for up to a year after birth. Rubella can be shed through excretions from the nose or through urine. An infant with congenital rubella should not be around pregnant women who are not immunized. If the child is in daycare, it is possible for the child to spread the disease to either caretakers who are not immune, or to other children. Parents should notify any potential caregivers about possible contagion, so they can receive the rubella vaccine.

New Vaccines

New vaccines have recently become available and are recommended for all adolescents—meningococcal and pertussis vaccines. Three other vaccines (hepatitis B, varicella, and measles-mumps-rubella) are recommended for adolescents who did not receive them as children. Immunization has the potential to protect not only the health of adolescents but their friends, families, and communities.

Pertussis (Whooping Cough)

- Highly contagious with prolonged cough. If transmitted to infants, may be life-threatening
- New vaccine: Tetanus-diphtheria-acellular pertussis vaccine (Tdap) adds pertussis disease protection while maintaining tetanus and diphtheria protection.
- Adolescents 11–18 years of age should receive a single shot of Tdap. Adolescents who received tetanus-diphtheria booster (Td) should receive Tdap 5 years after they received Td.

Meningococcal Infections

- Extremely serious disease that can rapidly progress to meningitis, pneumonia, and death
- New vaccine: Meningococcal conjugate vaccine (MCV4) provides protection against these infections
- Adolescents should receive a single shot of this vaccine during their 11-12 years old check-up or when they enter high school or college.

Hepatitis B

- Can cause different kinds of liver disease, including cancer
- Adolescents who did not receive the hepatitis B vaccine during childhood should receive the three-shot course of this vaccine.

Varicella (Chickenpox)

- Highly contagious and can be a serious and sometimes life-threatening disease
- Adolescents who have not had chickenpox or the vaccine should receive this vaccine at their 11-12 years old check-up. If anyone is uncertain about having had the disease, a blood test can determine immunity.

Measles, Mumps and Rubella

- Historically among the most serious vaccine-preventable diseases
- Adolescents who did not receive the two-shot course of measles-mumps-rubella vaccine (MMR) during childhood should receive this vaccine at their 11-12 years old check-up.

Additional Vaccines

Some adolescents with specific health risks may need additional vaccines such as hepatitis A, influenza, and pneumococcal.

CONCLUSION

Premarital counseling is very important and helpful especially in adolescents. It is important to strengthen marriage and make it successful. It greatly improves adolescents' chance of having good communication during marriage and their happiness.

Premarital health screening will help them to detect some hereditary diseases like thalassemia, sickle cell anemia, hemophilia, etc. which may affect the future offspring, some sexually transmitted infections like syphilis, rubella, etc. and life-threatening diseases like HIV, AIDS, and hepatitis B, etc. Premarital vaccination protects adolescents from consequences and serious complications of such diseases in their future life.

Adolescents are vulnerable to certain diseases. HPV infection spread through sexual contact and it is the leading cause of cervical cancer. If Rubella infection occurs during pregnancy it may lead to abortion or many congenital malformations and physical or mental retardation in unborn child. Premarital vaccination decreases the occurrence of vaccine preventable diseases like cervical cancer, rubella, hepatitis B, etc. Nowadays vaccines are available against such diseases. Immunization especially of vaccine preventable diseases during adolescent age can prevent serious morbidity and mortality.

SUGGESTED READING

1. Dudgeon JA. Congenital rubella. Pathogenesis and immunology. Am J Dis Child 1969;118(1):35-44.
2. Farber ME, Finkelstein SN. A cost-benefit analysis of a mandatory premarital screening program. N Engl J Med 1979;300:856-59.
3. Gottman J. The marriage clinic: A scientifically based marital therapy (Norton, 1999).
4. Judson FN, Shaw BS, Vernon TM, Jr. Mandatory premarital rubella serologic testing in Colorado. A preliminary report. JAMA 1974;229(9):1200-02.
5. Lieberman E, Faich GA, Simon PR, Mullan RJ. Premarital rubella screening in Rhode Island. JAMA 1981;245(13):1333-35.
6. Orenstein WA, Bart KJ, Hinman AR, Preblud SR, Greaves WL, Doster SW, et al. The opportunity and obligation to eliminate rubella from the United States. JAMA 1984;251(15):1988-94.
7. Povar GJ, Maloney M, Watson WN, McBean AM, Giguere G. Rubella screening and follow-up immunization in Vermont. Am J Public Health 1979;69(3):285-86.
8. Schneider JP, Schneider BH. "Marital satisfaction during recovery from self-identified sexual addiction among bisexual men and their wives". J Sex Marital Ther 1990;16 (4):230-50. PMID 2079706.
9. Schoenbaum SC, Hyde JN Jr, Bartoshesky L, Crampton K. Benefit-cost analysis of rubella vaccination policy. N Engl J Med 1976;294:306-10.
10. Wendy Kline Building a better race: gender, sexuality, and eugenics from the turn of the century.

11 Contraception for Adolescents

Lola Ramachandran

INTRODUCTION

Worldwide women aged 15-19 years give birth to about 17 million of the 131 million children born each year. Women in this age-group have 10% of all abortions (PAI 2001). According to the census 2001, there are 225 million adolescents in India comprising nearly 1/5th (22%) of the population. Out of them 12% belong to the 10-14 age-group and nearly 10% are in the 15-19 age-group (Fig. 11.1).[1]

Contraception for this large number of teenagers presents a lot of problems and is also likely to create a lot of controversies. One may argue that the average Indian teenager, especially those in their early teens are too young to know anything regarding sex and hence it is not proper to give them contraceptive advice. Another argument is that if we give them contraception, then they are more likely to be promiscuous. Studies done in the US have proved that when contraception was made easily accessible to their teenagers, neither sexually transmitted infections nor un-intended pregnancies increased. And the argument that if we teach teenagers regarding safe sex they will become promiscuous is like the proverbial ostrich with its head buried in the sand. There is teenage sexuality in our society and we have to face it.

There is no doubt that, fertility control is essential in the adolescent, even among married women. Since our girls are married off at an early age especially in the northern states like Bihar, Madhya Pradesh, Rajasthan, Uttarakhand, Jharkhand and Orissa, teenage pregnancies are very common in those areas. The advent of an active sex-life will catapult the young girl into the world of the adult woman regarding contraception, pregnancy, abortion and gynecological pathology including STDs and AIDS.

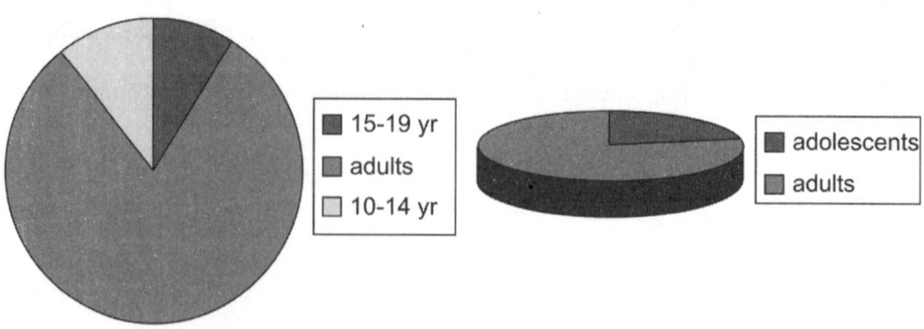

Fig. 11.1: Pie chart indicating the percentage of the age-groups of adolescents in India

A considerable number of the teenagers aged 17-19 years in India are either mothers or pregnant. Another problem is that these young girls tend to delay seeking abortion, thus increasing the risks of the procedure. Teen pregnancy also may have disastrous consequences for the girl, often driving her out of school or college, thus limiting her future options.

There is significant risk associated with sexual activity and child bearing all over the developing world. Teenaged mothers face twice the risk of dying from childbirth as do women in their twenties and their children also are more vulnerable to health risks.

HIV infection disproportionately affects the teenaged, as they often become sexually involved with older infected males. Every year almost half of all new HIV infection and at least 1/3rd of all new sexually transmitted infections occur in younger than 25 years of age (PAI, 2001). Herein lies the special importance of contraception for the adolescents of today.

The ideal contraception for an adolescent girl should be safe, totally reversible, usable from time-to-time just before or just after intercourse, easy to use and well-tolerated. Such a method is not yet available.

Before advising contraception, the teenager should be counseled that:

1. There is no reversible method which is 100% safe although intrauterine devices like ML cu 375,CuT 380 A and LNG 20 (Mirena) and the less used implants and injectable contraceptives have a very low failure rate of 0.5%.
2. There is no method that is highly effective yet, at the same time giving protection against STDs and HIV (AIDS).
3. Contraception is safer than abortion, especially unsafe abortion.
4. If abstinence is not possible, condoms should be used in all sexual encounters to prevent sexually transmitted diseases (STDs).

Broadly put, adolescents are eligible to use any method of contraception. Age alone does not constitute a medical reason for denying any method of contraception to young girls. Though some concerns have been expressed about the use of certain contraceptive methods in adolescents (e.g. the use of progesterone only injectable by those younger than 18 yrs of age), these concerns must be weighed against the advantages of avoiding pregnancy (WHO 2004). However, alternative methods can be advised if they suit the adolescent. Method of choice may be influenced by factors like sporadic patterns of intercourse and the need to conceal such sexual activity and contraception use from the parents or guardians. Proper counseling may address many of the specific problems of this group of people and help them in making informed and voluntary choices.

A girl is more likely to adhere to a choice that she has made of her own free will rather than something which has been forced upon her.

The goal of the clinician who provides care to the adolescent is to prevent un-intended pregnancy and the transmission of sexually transmitted diseases.

Now we will examine each of the commonly used methods of contraception and see how applicable they are in adolescents. For each method, the WHO risk category for use in adolescents will also be mentioned.

These categories are not intended to be used as strict guidelines but as evidence-based recommendations for the development of family planning programmes, based on the reviews of literature.

For all methods of contraception, the WHO assigns categories for use in women under the age of 20 years and then they make a useful adjunct to the evidence presented below. Category 1 is a condition for which there is no restriction for use. Category 2 is a condition where the advantages generally outweigh the risks. Category 3 is a condition where the risks usually outweigh the advantages and category 4 is a condition which represents an unacceptable health risk.

All of the contraceptives reviewed below are given either a category of 1 or 2 for the adolescent population.

BARRIER METHODS OF CONTRACEPTION

The latex condom is the only method of contraception that protects against sexually transmitted infections (STIs) including the human immunodeficiency virus (HIV). Adolescents are at especially high risk for STIs. For this reason, clinicians should advise all adolescents (and all patients) who are at risk for STIs to use a latex condom with every act of intercourse. But condoms are not highly effective methods of contraception under typical use. The typical use failure rate for the first year of use is 15% for the male condoms and is 21% for female condoms. These figures are substantially higher than the perfect-use failure rates of male and female condoms of 2% and 5% respectively. Such a big difference is mainly due to user error, such as failure to use a condom with every act of intercourse. This rate is unacceptably high, especially when there are many more effective means for pregnancy prevention.

Hence, doctors should counsel all adolescents who are at risk for STIs and at risk for unintended pregnancy to use both latex condoms and a more effective method of contraception together.

Other barrier methods of contraception also have high typical use failure rates, 16% for the diaphragm, cervical cap and sponge in nulliparous women. Withdrawal has a 27% typical-use failure rate and spermicides alone can have a 29% typical-use failure rate. The combination of poor protection against pregnancy without the STI protection of condoms makes these methods a poor choice for use by adolescents.

WHO gives barrier methods a category of 1 for all ages but it advises women who are poor risks for pregnancy that barrier methods for pregnancy prevention may not be appropriate for these who cannot use them consistently and correctly because of their relatively higher typical use failure rates.

COMBINED ESTROGEN PROGESTIN METHODS

Most adolescents prefer to use the Oral contraceptive pills (OCPs) more than any other method as their most effective method although the perfect-use failure rate is only 0.3%. The typical-use failure rate is much higher at 8%. Adolescents are notorious for inconsistent use and for discontinuation and therefore for unintended pregnancy. On an average, adolescents miss up to 3 pills per cycle. At least 20-30% of adolescents miss at least 1 pill per month. Factors associated with poor compliance with use of OCP in teens include multiple sex partners, low evaluation of personal health, feelings of hopelessness, ambivalence about becoming pregnant, previous abortion, low socio-economic status, etc.

In addition to inconsistent use, discontinuation of OCPs among adolescents is also common. It has been found to be as high as 50% within the first 3 cycles of use according to a study by Rosenbergh MJ, Burnhill MS and Waugh MS.[2] The most common reason given for OCP discontinuation is the presence of side-effects, including nausea, irregular bleeding, breast tenderness and mood changes. When these side-effects occur, adolescents fear that their health is compromised and also can distrust the doctor who prescribed the OCPs. The solution for this may be thorough and individualized pre-use counseling that focuses on preconceived negative beliefs about the safety of OCPs. Some side-effects may appeal to adolescents. Examples are reduction of dysmenorrhea, regulation of menstrual cycles, lighter menses and decreased acne. The adolescents may be encouraged to use pills regularly for these side-effects.

The monthly vaginal ring that is now available in the Indian market and the progestin patch has longer acting delivery systems and so do not require daily action. Perfect-use failure rate for the vaginal ring is roughly equal to that of OCP, also it has similar health benefits and side-effects as OCPs. The contraceptive ring has better cycle control than OCP and also lesser hormone related side effects probably because of the lower levels of circulating estrogen than OCPs. But the disadvantages of the vaginal ring are increased vaginal discharge and discomfort. Also young girls even if married may not like to put something inside their vagina. They may not mind this so much if they are used to inserting vaginal pessaries or having regular vaginal examinations.

The WHO gives all combined estrogen-progestin contraceptives a category 1 for women up to 40 years. In addition, the WHO guidelines specifically state, "theoretical concerns about the use of combined hormonal contraceptives among young adolescents have not been substantiated".[3]

DMPA

If used perfectly for 1 year, the failure rate of DMPA is 0.3%. The main advantage of this non-oral hormonal method is that its typical use failure rate for 1 year is also extremely low at 3%. This low rate of failure when used in the typical manner is because it is user-friendly. DMPA is easier to use and less prone to user error. In addition, it allows privacy because there is no need of storing (e.g. pills, rings) and it cannot be felt or seen by others like the implant. Cooperation from the sexual partner is also not required. But discontinuation rates are high mainly due to the irregular vaginal bleeding. It can also cause weight gain and many teenage girls won't like this. DMPA also exacerbates depression. Since it is an intramuscular preparation, it cannot be discontinued as soon as one desires. So, adolescents with a history of depression are not good candidates for DMPA. Also adolescent patients who desire an immediate return of fertility after stopping contraception should avoid DMPA since the median return to fertility after injection is 20 months regardless of how long it has been used.

The most controversial topic regarding the use of DMPA by teenagers is its effect on Bone mineral density (BMD). Though it is true that the long term effects of DMPA use on peak bone mass and on the risk of osteoporotic fractures later in life are unknown, the current data do not support denying this highly effective method of contraception to the adolescent population. Also it is important to note that teen pregnancy by itself has an adverse effect on BMD. In a study of 252 women aged 12-34 yrs which examined BMD in and after pregnancy, found the greatest bone loss in teens with an average of 5.5% loss. This was statistically significantly larger than that in adult women with an average of 1.9% loss.[4]

The WHO gives DMPA a category of 2, i.e. the advantages of using the method generally outweigh the theoretical or proven risks of the method for up to 17 years of age and a category 1, no restriction for use, for ages 18-45yrs.[3]

PROGESTERONE ONLY PILL, IMPLANON, NORPLANT

These are the other progestin only hormonal methods available. POPs have a slightly lower effectiveness when compared to combined OCPs in clinical trials. Also it had to be taken at the same time each day. But this problem is no more there with the newly developed desogestrel-only pill. If that is used, a lady can take a pill as much as 12 hours late without reducing its effectiveness.

Implants are not really very popular with adolescents probably because of the requirement of surgery to insert and to remove it. Also it causes irregular vaginal bleeding or amenorrhea and increase in weight, acne, headache, breast tenderness and mood changes as possible side-effects. So, a good counseling about all the effects is a must before prescribing these methods of contraception to the adolescents.

The implants do not have any significant effect on BMD. Though it is said to be a safe, highly effective method for this age-group, more research is needed on the use of implants on adolescents. The WHO gives this method a category of 1 (no restriction) for women of any age.[3]

INTRAUTERINE CONTRACEPTIVE DEVICE (IUD)

Usually IUDs are not considered as a good contraceptive option for adolescent women. This is because of the fear that the IUD may increase the risk of PID and infertility. It is easy to use, highly effective, allows privacy, does not require action at the time of intercourse, does not require partner cooperation and does not require short interval pharmacy or clinic visits. Because of their ease of use, perfect-use and typical-use failure rates are identical. The

CuT 380 A can be used for up to 10 years and contains no hormones. The other highly useful one is Mirena (LNG-IUS) but it is very costly. Though early studies did show a link between IUDS and PID and infertility, the preponderance of evidence now supports the acceptability and safety of IUD. Continued use of modern IUDs does not increase the risk of upper genital tract infection over a woman's baseline risk, however, there is an increased risk of upper genital tract infection in the first 20 days after insertion. This increased rate is probably secondary to insertion techniques or the presence of cervical infection at the time of insertion.[5] So, we should test for cervical infection at the time of insertion or soon before that for all adolescents. In a prospective randomized trial, the LNG IUS protected against upper genital tract infection compared with a Cu IUD.[6] A case control study of 1895 nulliparous women in Mexico provided the strongest evidence against a link between IUD use and subsequent infertility. The study compared cases with tubal infertility with controls having non-tubal infertility and with primigravid controls. Both comparisons showed no associations between tubal infertility and past use of a copper containing IUD.[7]

Another common worry may be that nulliparous women face an increased risk of expulsion and adverse side-effects compared with parous women. A US study that included 3533 women using the CuT 380 A examined this problem in copper IUDs. The study found only a slightly higher expulsion rate of the CuT 380 A in nulliparous women. There were similar rates of removal for bleeding or pain. Further, a study of the LNG IUS that included 129 nulliparous women found the risk of expulsion in this group to be less than 1% per year.[8]

Although the WHO does state that there is concern about expulsion and increased risks of STIs in nulliparous and younger women, respectively, it gives IUDs a category 2 (advantages of using the method generally outweigh the theoretical or proven risks of the method for use) in women younger than 20 years.[3]

EMERGENCY CONTRACEPTION (EC)

No discussion of adolescent contraception will be complete without mentioning EC.

The immediate insertion of a CuT is the most effective means of EC. It reduced the risk of pregnancy by 99%. Combination of estrogen-progestin OCPs in a specific regimen that contains 2 doses of ethinylestradiol 0.1 mg and levonorgestrel 1 mg in each dose, reduced the risk of pregnancy by 75%. We have preparations like I-pill which are specifically for this purpose. It contains 2 levonorgestrel 0.75 mg pills. They are used as 1 tablet as soon, after unprotected intercourse, as possible and the next 12 hours later. There is no change in effectiveness or side-effects when both tablets are taken together as single dose. Taking the pills together makes the dosing easier and may increase compliance as well as correct use. This regimen reduces the risk of pregnancy by 89%. Effectiveness is inversely proportional to the time interval after unprotected intercourse and EC is most effective when used within the first 12 hours though studies have shown effectiveness up to 120 hour afterwards.[9] In addition, use should not be limited to only mid-cycle intercourse, especially in adolescents who often have irregular cycles and so unpredictable ovulation.

I-pill was being promoted as an OTC drug at first but later on this status was withdrawn. Availability of EC should be easy for adolescents who have casual sex or else many unintended pregnancies will occur. Increased access to EC will increase the use of EC among adolescents and the fear that it will increase promiscuity among teenagers is not true. In a study 2117 young women which included 964 adolescents aged 15-19 years found that adolescents were not more likely to increase sexual risk taking behavior such as multiple partners, lack of consistent condom use or unprotected intercourse. There was also no increase in STIs among the population studied.[10] Another point

Flow chart 11.1: Contraceptive care for adolescents

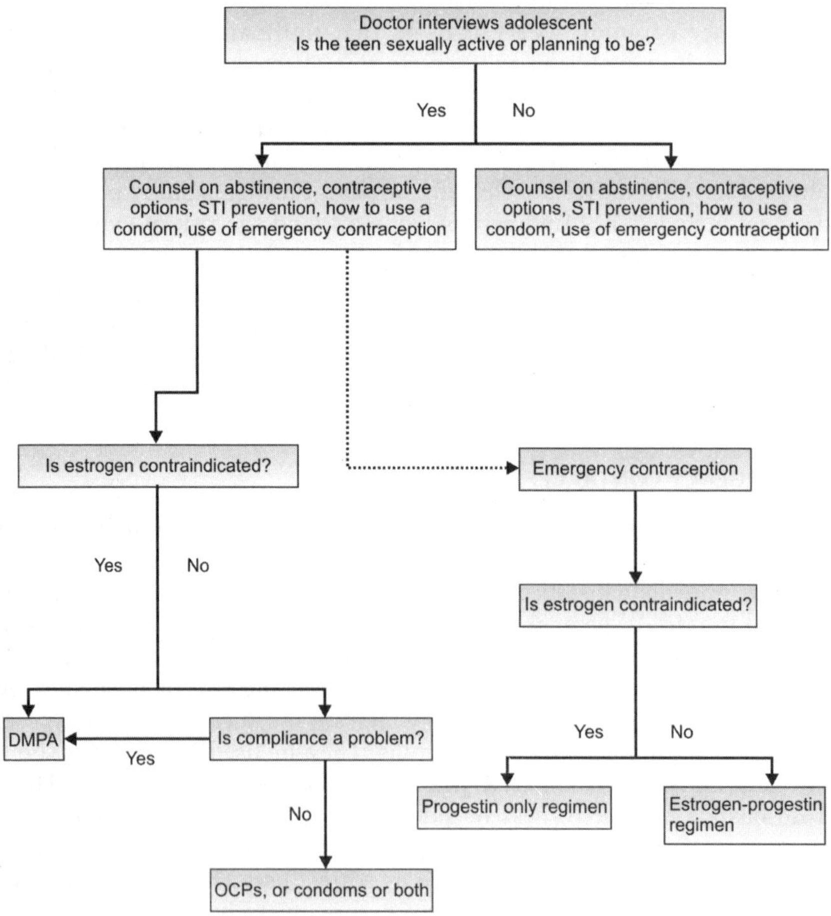

to note is that adolescents are more likely to be using contraceptives of low or medium effectiveness. So they can derive maximum benefit from EC if they are properly able to identify when they are at risk for unintended pregnancy. Thus, counseling adolescents and educating them about when and how to use EC is an essential step in providing it to them. Flow chart 11.1 summarizes the various aspects of contraceptive care for adolescents.

CONCLUSIONS

Adolescent pregnancy rate in India is really high. The factors concerned are many including social as well as economic, geographic and political. We, as concerned citizens of this country, have a responsibility to improve this state of affairs by providing proper counseling and prescribing the appropriate method when we are faced with an adolescent likely to indulge in sexual activity. This will go a long way in decreasing unwanted pregnancies and the resulting maternal mortality and morbidity. Remember that today's adolescents are our citizens of tomorrow.

REFERENCES

1. Census Report, 2001. New Delhi: Government of India, 2001.
2. Rosenbergh MJ, Burnhill MS, Waugh MS, et al. Compliance and oral contraceptives: A review. Contraception 1995;52:137-41.
3. World Health Organization. Medical Eligibility Criteria for Contraceptive Use, 3rd edn. Geneva: World Health Organization; 2004.
4. Sowers MF, Scholl T, Harris L, et al. Bone loss in adolescent and adult pregnant women. Obstet Gynecol 2000;96:189-93.
5. Farley TM, Rosenbergh MJ, Rowe PJ, et al. Intrauterine devices and pelvic inflammatory disease: An international perspective. Lancet. 1992;339:785-88.
6. Andersson K, Odlind V, Rybo G. Levonorgestrel-releasing and Copper- releasing (Nova T) IUDs during 5 years of use: A randomized comparative trial. Contraception 1994;49:56-72.
7. Hubacher D, Lara-Ricalde R, Taylor D, et al. Use of copper intrauterine devices and the risk of tubal infertility among nulligravid women. N Engl J Med.2001;345:561-67.
8. Veldhuis HM, Vos AG, Lagro-Hanssen AL. Complications of the intrauterine device in nulliparous and parous women. Eur J Gen Pract. 2004;10:82-7.
9. Hatcher RA, Trussel J, Stewart F, et al. Contraceptive Technology, 18th edn. New York: Ardent Media; 2004.
10. Harper CC, Cheong M, Rocca CH, et al. The effect of increased access to emergency contraception among young adolescents. Obstet Gynecol 2005;106:483-91.

12 MTP in Adolescents—How to Handle It?

Abha Singh

INTRODUCTION

Adolescents constitute about one-fifth of the world's population (UNFPA, 2003). Only 13% of them live in developed countries, the rest of them belong to the developing countries. The transition from childhood to adulthood takes place during this period. The rate of transition is variable in all individuals.

PREGNANCY IN ADOLESCENTS

WHO has estimated that 16 million adolescents give birth annually. This comprises 11% of all births worldwide. Sub-Saharan Africa has the highest incidence of 50% adolescent deliveries. An added burden to this is the orphaned children suffering AIDS (13 million) who are vulnerable to sexual exploitation. US teen pregnancy and birth rates are the second highest in the world:[1]

Adolescent pregnancy	79.8 per 1000
Adolescent birth	48.7 per 1000
Adolescent abortion	27.5 per 1000

Half of all the adolescent births occur in just 7 countries, namely Bangladesh, Brazil, Congo, Ethiopia, Nigeria, **India** and USA.[2]

Most of the time, the pregnancy is unintended. The intended pregnancy is due to social and cultural norms of the society. Sometimes, unmarried girls see it as the only means of establishing their identity. Unintended pregnancy is likely to end in abortion.

RESPONSIBLE FACTORS

Adolescent pregnancy is a complex and challenging issue. It is one of the important factors for rapid growth in the world population.[3] The following factors are mainly responsible:[4,5]

- Cultural and social
- Lack of education and knowledge
- Lack of information and access to contraceptives
- Sexual abuse
- Early pubertal development
- Younger age at pregnancy
- Poor school performance
- Poverty.

ABUSES OF ADOLESCENT PREGNANCY

The dangers of adolescent pregnancy are much greater than the women who conceive in their second twenties, thirties or forties.[13] Not only the teenage mother is at risk, but their children are also at a greater risk of reduced intellectual and academic achievement, health complications and behavioral problems. The perinatal mortality rate is 50% more in comparison to the pregnant women who deliver in their 3rd decade. In an Indian study, it was found out that 90% of the adolescents were unmarried, 11% came for repeated MTP and 42% sought it in 2nd trimester.[6]

Problems During Pregnancy

1. Poor maternal weight gain
2. Anemia
3. Preterm delivery[7]
4. PIH
5. Placenta previa
6. HIV
7. Sexually transmitted infections
8. Psychosocial problems
9. **Unsafe abortions** (account for 14% of all unsafe abortions).

Problems During Delivery

1. CPD (as the pelvis has not yet fully developed)
2. Obstructed labor
3. Obstetric fistula (65% are due to adolescent pregnancy).

Postpartum Problems

1. Anemia
2. Pre-eclampsia
3. Postpartum depression.

Long-term Consequences

1. Chronic ill health
2. Depression
3. Marital discord
4. Divorce
5. Interrupted career
6. Behavioral problems and **suicide**.

TREATMENT OF ADOLESCENT PREGNANCY

Though there may be many options ranging from giving the infants for adoption after delivery to MTP, this chapter deals with only MTP. The laws of MTP vary greatly from being illegal in Sri Lanka to being permitted in India.

COUNSELING BEFORE MTP

Counseling is the most vital part of MTP. When an adolescent first discovers her pregnancy and comes to the practitioner, one must provide her with all the options varying from MTP to carrying the pregnancy to term. The counselor should always involve the parents and/or guardians. Most often there is lack of parental support because she does not wish to tell her parents.[8] The healthcare provider must help her in planning how to inform them. The counselor should not force any decisions on the adolescent. She should be informed about her legal options and the place where safe and legal abortion is available. One must make sure that she is not forced by her parents/partner into any decision. At the same time, she should be provided with the information about contraception including emergency contraception, HIV and STI prevention.

It is very important to ensure confidentiality and privacy during counseling. No interruption should be there during the session. Repeating her name often throughout the conversation exhibits that one cares for her. A non-judgmental attitude should always be practiced. Answer any question that she might have instead of deferring them for later. Simple words should be spoken as their cognitive skills are still developing. Counselor should provide an emotional support for her during the conversation.[9] Guidelines from Estado on adolescent reproductive health recommend 30 minutes of counseling.[10]

INFORMED CONSENT

As youth-friendly service approach, inform her about the examination and the MTP procedure and obtain a written consent from her parents or guardian. The consent should include the following information:

- The duration of pregnancy
- All the legal options
- Consequences of MTP

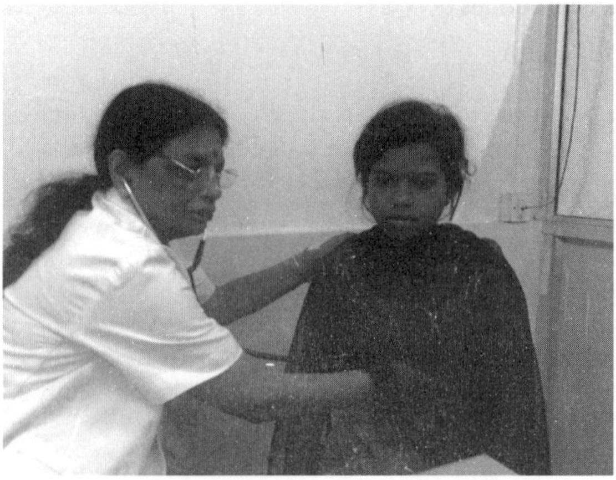

Fig. 12.1: Adolescent counseling

- Complications of the methods involved and permission to treat if required
- Requirement of the necessary investigations
- Anesthesia and its advantages/disadvantages
- Legal requirement of parental/guardian's/judicial consent.

Examination

Always explain her the procedure of examination. She may not be familiar or prepared for the pelvic examination. In case of sexual abuse resulting in a pregnancy, she may not be comfortable with this examination. Sometimes the examination has to be carried out under anesthesia only.

Anemia should always be checked, as it is very common. A follow-up may be required after the MTP if she is anemic.

The uterine size should always be confirmed with USG as she may not cooperate during examination.

Use of a small speculum and asking her to do deep breathing while its insertion, helps to relax her.

At the Time of Procedure

- Understand her pain threshold and give her pain control options
- Explain her the time taken for the procedure
- Use a small size speculum and an ovum forceps/tenaculum (to hold the cervix)
- Keep talking to her and reassure that the procedure is about to finish.

At Discharge

- Explain her in written that she may need to come after a fortnight for a follow-up. In case of pain, continued bleeding and fever or foul smelling discharge, she may come earlier.
- Give her appropriate contraceptive advice.
- Guide her about HIV prevention and treatment and support group if she has suffered sexual assault.

METHODS

1. **Medical abortion.** Not many studies have been conducted especially on adolescents. In a recent study in Cuba 800 mcg misoprostol completed abortion in majority of adolescents.[11] The adverse gastrointestinal side-effects should be counseled beforehand.
2. **Vacuum aspiration.** This has largely replaced D and C at present. It is also recommended by WHO. It can be done under local anesthesia.[12]

CONCLUSION

Children and adolescents are our future. Adolescent pregnancy has become a global health concern. WHO estimates that 2.5 million adolescents have unsafe abortions annually.[12] It is a complex and challenging issue not only for the families but for the gynecologists too. We need to create awareness especially for the negative health consequences and the socio-economic causes. We cannot succeed alone in this endeavor, unless joined by parents, families, politicians and community leaders to discuss the needs and concerns of adolescents and support them. Adolescents with unwanted pregnancies should become one of our important priorities while making the health policies before this problem takes a mammoth form.

REFERENCES

1. Ammie Feijoo, "Adolescent Sexual Health In Europe and US—why the difference? Advocates for youth, 2001 at http://www.advocatesyouth.org/.
2. WHO. MPS notes Vol. No.1 Oct 2008.
3. Senderowitz J, Paxman JM. Adolescence fertility: Worldwide concern. Population bulletin, 1985;40(2):3-51.
4. Haffner DW, (Ed). Facing facts: Sexual health for America's adolescents: The report of the national commission on adolescent sexual health. New York, NY: Sexuality Information and Education Council of the United States; 1995.
5. Brooks-Gunn J, Furstenberg FF Jr. Adolescent sexual behavior. Am Psychol 1989; 44:249-57.
6. Sonia Trikha. Abortion scenario of adolescents in a North Indian city—Evidence from a recent study. Indian Journal of Community Medicine. 2003;26(1).
7. Chhabra S. Perinatal outcome in teenage mothers. J Obstet Gynaecol of India 1991; 41(1):30-32(S).
8. Paul M, Lichtenberg ES, Borgatta L, Grimes DA, Stubblefield PH. A clinician's guide to medical and surgical abortion. New York: Churchill Livingstone 1999.
9. Senderowitz J, Solter C, Hainsworth G. Module 16: Reproductive Health Services for Adolescents. In: Watertown, MA, (Ed). Comprehensive Reproductive Health and Family Planning Training Curriculum. Pathfinder International 2002.
10. Secretaria de Estado de salud Publica y Asistencia Social. Normas nacionales y procedimientos para la atencion integral de adolescents. Dominican Republic 2000.
11. Velazaco A, Varela L, Tanda R, et al. Misoprostol for abortion upto 9 weeks of pregnancy in adolescents. The European Journal Of Contraception and Reproductive Health Care 2000;5:227-33.
12. IPAS. Adolescents, unwanted pregnancy and abortion 1-49.
13. Lum Milton. Hazards of adolescent pregnancy. Malaysia 2010.

13 Teenage Pregnancy

Priti Bala Sahay, Archana Kumari

INTRODUCTION

"The youngest mother whose history is authenticated is Lina Medina, who was delivered by cesarean sectin in Lima, Peru in 1939. Although, her exact age is disputable, she was around 5 years old. Gerardo, who was named for the doctor who performed the cesarean section, was 10 years old before he knew that Lima was his mother. He married at age of 18 years, had two daughters and died in 1979 of an apparent heart attack at age 40."

Teenage pregnancy is universal in all known cultures, past and present. Teenage pregnancy is defined as teenaged or underaged girls (within ages of 13-19 years) becoming pregnant. In UK there is a legal definition whereby a woman is considered to be a teenager pregnant, if she becomes pregnant before her 18th birthday.

As a consequence of decrease in average age of menarche and ovulation, early sexual activity, most obstetric services are witnessing a marked increase in number of extremely young pregnant woman. Teenage pregnancy is associated with adverse perinantal outcome like stillbirth, preterm delivery, LBW babies, IUGR. Maternal complications like toxemia of pregnancy, eclampsia, CPD are also more common in teenagers.

Teenage pregnancy in developed countries is usually outside marriage whereas in developing countries it is usually within marriage and often is a part of social customs.

GLOBAL INCIDENCE

One in four girls in the world becomes a mother before age of 19 years. "Save the Children" found that annually 13 million children are born to females under 20, worldwide, and more than 90% in developing countries. The highest rate of teenage pregnancy in world is in Sub-Saharan Africa where women tend to marry at early age. In the Indian subcontinent, rate is much higher in rural region than urbanized areas.

In the mid 1970s, United States was told to have "epidemic" of teenage pregnancy (Gutmacher, 1976). Ever since then, there has been a general downward trend in teenage pregnancy. But still, US has highest teenage pregnancy and abortion rate among the industrialized nations.

IMPACT OF AGE ON PREGNANCY OUTCOME

Obstetric risks of older teenagers, 16-19 years, are related to socioeconomic factors like poverty, inadequate nutrtion and poor health before pregnancy, rather than maternal age itself. (McAnarney, 1978). In contrast, the teenagers of 15 years or younger have pregnancy complications related to their young age.

It is a common belief that teenage mothers are more likely to experience fetopelvic disproportion as a consequence of incomplete development of bony pelvis. This appears to be a misconception. Lubarsky and colleagues demonstrated no increased risk of either prolonged labor or operative delivery, confirming the results of two earlier studies (Brown et al, 1991, Tuimala and coworkers, 1987).

IMPACT OF PREGNANCY ON TEENAGERS

Klein described adolescent childbearing as initiating a syndrome of failure: failure to complete one's education, failure in limiting family size, failure to establish vocation and become independent.

CAUSES OF TEENAGE PREGNANCY

- Adolescent sexual behavior
- Lack of education about contraception
- Dating and domestic violence
- Sexual abuse (Studies have found that between 11-20% pregnancy is direct result of rape)
- Socioeconomic factors
- Lack of parental guidance
- Early marriage.

COMPLICATIONS OF TEENAGE PREGNANCY (TABLE 13.1)

Teenage pregnancy is considered high risk pregnancy as complications are more common and more severe among teenagers. Adolescents are less likely to seek prenatal care, often only in third trimester. The important maternal and perinatal complications of teenage pregnancy are listed in Table 13.1.

Antepartum

Pregnancy Induced Hypertension, Pre-eclampsia and Eclampsia

Several studies suggest that there is increased risk of PIH, pre-eclampsia and eclampsia in young teenagers than older age group. More likely to occur among unbooked cases with no antenatal care.

Anemia

Anemia is common in pregnancy but even more common in adolescent girls. According to RCH survey 2002, there are 171,644 girls aged 10-19 years with anemia, 28% mild, 43% moderate and 24% severe anemia.

Table 13.1: Complications of teenage pregnancy	
Maternal	
Antepartum:	PIH Anemia STIs and HIV APH Preterm delivery IUGR
Intrapartum:	Obstructed labor Birth injuries
Postpartum:	PPH Anemia Depression Sepsis
Perinatal:	LBW Prematurity High Perinatal and neonatal mortality Inadequate childcare and breastfeeding

Nutritional Deficiency

This results from poor eating habits, attempt to loose weight, snacking, fast food which is prevalent in urbanized areas.

Sexually Transmitted Diseases and HIV

There is increased risk of STIs in adolescents because of biological and social factors. The risk of parent to child transmission is also greater in adolescents.

Intrapartum

There is increased risk of preterm labor (due to increased incidence of genital tract infections) prolonged labor, obstructed labor and birth injuries.

Postpartum

Anemia if pre-existing, can be further worsened by blood loss during delivery.

Pre-eclampsia and eclampsia may worsen in postpartum period.

Puerperal sepsis is more common due to anemia and poor hygiene.

Depression: This can be serious as adolescents have to cope with the new life circumstances.

Risks to the Child

Low birth weight: Incidence of low birth weight and prematurity is high in adolescent pregnancy.

Perinatal and neonatal mortality: This is high due to prematurity, LBW babies, and infection.

Inadequate childcare and breastfeeding is a problem especially in single adolescent mothers. Adolescent parents are faced with excessive stress due to lack of adequate knowledge of child development. They are developmentally immature and possess inappropriate child rearing attitude.

Maternal Mortality

For numerous developing nations, maternal mortality remains among the three top causes of teenage deaths. Most deaths are due to embolism, hypertensive disorders or ectopic pregnancy. In developing countries, complications of pregnancy results in death of 70,000 teenage girls every year. Risk of death following pregnancy is twice as high as in 15-19 years as those between 20-24 years. Maternal mortality can be up to 5 times higher in girls below 14 years compared to those between 20-24 years. Unsafe abortions with its complications is also a a major contributor to teenage mortality.

TEENAGE PREGNANCY IN UNMARRIED GIRLS: THE PROBLEM OF UNSAFE ABORTION

Pregnancy in unmarried adolescent girl leads to unsafe abortion because of social stigmas and lack of safe abortion services. The use of health services by adolescent is limited because of poor knowledge and lack of awareness, lack of privacy and confidentiality, lack of counseling skills at service provider levels. Adolescents who are more vulnerable for pregnancy are engaged girls, street girls, sexually abused teenagers, sex workers, mental and physically disabled orphans.

The comparison of pregnancy and child birth is marreid and unmarried teenage girls is illustrated in Table 13.2.

Complications of Abortions in Adolescents

Immediate

- Hemorrhage and shock
- Sepsis

Table 13.2: Comparison of teenage pregnancy among married and unmarried adolescent girls

Married	*Unmarried*
Immediate	
• More likely to seek or receive ANC	• Less likely to seek ANC
• More likely to have access to safe MTP	• More likely to resort to illegal and unsafe abortions and associated complications
• Depression due to stress of child rearing	• Guilt and depression due to social stigma
Remote	
• Chronic ill health and depression due to complications during pregnancy childbirth and postpartum period	• Chronic ill health and infertility due to complications during abortions
• Marital discord and divorce due to impaired sexual life resulting from childbirth injuries	• Interruptions of education/career

- Injuries ranging from genital lacerations to fistula to perforations of uterus
- Bowel injuries
- Peritonitis.

Long-term

- Chronic pelvic pain and infection
- Secondary infertility
- Subsequent spontaneous abortion
- Increased likelihood of ectopic pregnancy.

Psychological

- Guilt and depression.

PREVENTING TEENAGE PREGNANCY

The problem of preventing unwanted pregnancies in teenagers needs to be urgently addressed.

In UK Teenage Pregnancy Strategy (TPS) works at several levels to decrease teenage pregnancy and increase the social inclusion of teenage pregnancy by:

- Joint action making the branches of government and health education services work together effectively
- Preventing teenage pregnancy through better sex education and improving contraception services for young people
- Better support for teenage mother and better childcare.

The Dutch approach to prevent teenage pregnancy is a model for many other countries. The curriculum focuses on values, attitudes, communication and negotiation skills as well as psychological aspects of reproduction.

In developing world, reproductive health program aimed at teenagers are often small scale and not centrally coordinated. Laws against child marriage have reduced but not eliminated this practice. "Growing up" program initiated by FOGSI in partnership with Johnson and Johnson educate the school girls on menstruation, its myths and hygiene, ovulation and function of reproduction, value of good nutrition and exercises. Over 12 lakhs girls in more than 50 schools have been addressed in past 5 years.

Teenage Contraception and Counseling (Figs 13.1 and 13.2)

Since, unprotected intercourse is main cause of teenage pregnancy, contraception counseling is important. Contraception for teenagers is a huge challenge for the clinicians. Adolescents may lack knowledge or access to conventional methods of preventing pregnancy as they may be too embarrassed by such information. Even if they use, failure rate is high due to incorrect and inconsistent use.

- **Oral contraceptive pills** is the most effective method for adolescents. Compliance, however, remains a problem. It has few side effects and some benefit like reduction in dysmenorrhea

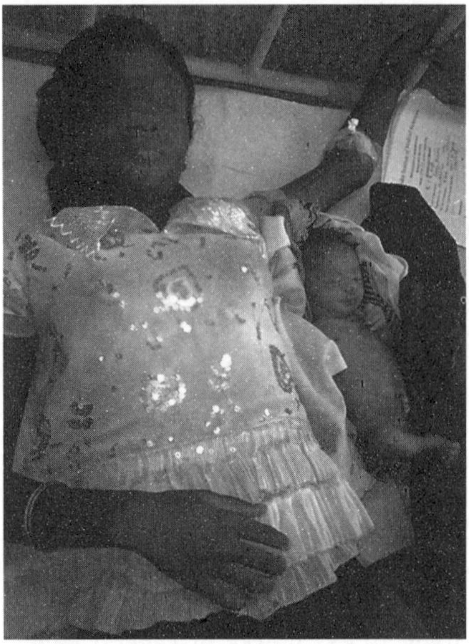

Fig. 13.1: Teenage mother with her newborn child

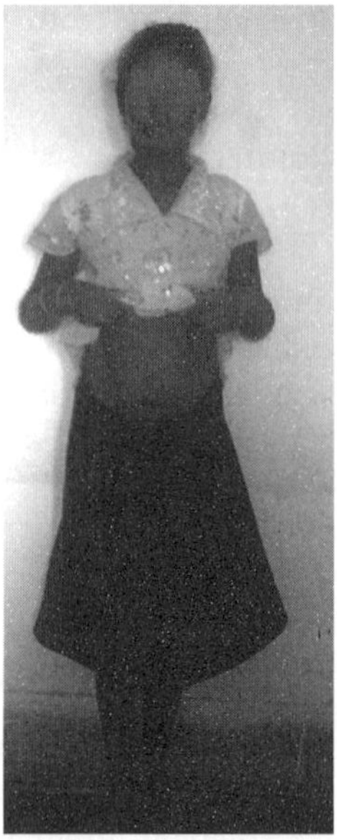

Fig. 13.2: Teenage girl with term pregnancy

- **Barrier methods:** As adolescents do not plan sexual encounters, barrier methods are not as effective in this population. They have high failure rates due to sporadic and improper use
- **Injectable contraception:** May be advised to some but menstrual irregularity and amenorrhea make it unacceptable to some
- **Emergency contraception:** Teenager should be made aware of option of EOC. Though this helps to avoid getting pregnant after unprotected intercourse, the best way is to educate them about importance of abstinence and safe sex.

CONCLUSION

Teenagers irrespective of their marital status, face potentially serious physical, psychological and social consequences from pregnancy and related complications. Information and counseling is the right of every pregnant woman. Adolescents especially needs to be dealt with sensitivity as they have special needs and concerns of their own. Health service providers need to be familiar with the issues and complications associated with teenage pregnancies. Counselers should develop a rapport with them to prevent early and repeat pregnancy, related problem, care of newborn and exclusive breastfeeding. Unmarried teenage pregnant should have access to safe abortion services and should have counseling regarding consequence of unsafe abortion. Adolescents coming to tertiary center after suffering complication of unsafe abortion should receive corrective counseling after prompt management. Teenagers should be aware of dangers of unprotected sex like risk of transmission of STIs especially HIV and unwanted pregnancy and should have knowledge of contraception as well as emergency contraception.

SUGGESTED READING

1. Berg CJ. Pregnancy related mortality in United States, 1987- 1990, Obstet gynecol 1996;88:161.
2. Boonstra H. Teen pregnancy: trends and lessons learned. Fam Plann Prospect 2002; 5.
3. Desilva MO. Teenage Sexual behaviour and pregnancy: Trends and determinants. Progress in obstetrics and gynaecology, vol 15 John Studd (Ed) Churchill Livingstone, chapter 8, 2003;123-33.
4. Gertzak-Uzan L, Hallack M, Press F Teenage pregnancy: Risk factors for adverse perinatal outcome. J Matern Fetal Med 2001;10:393-97.
5. Guttmacher A. Eleven million teenagers: what can be done about epidemic of adolescent pregnancy in United States ? New York, Alan Guttmacher Institute, 1976.
6. Klein L. Antecedents of teenage pregnancy. Clin obstet gynaecol 1978;21:115.
7. Lubarsky SL, Schif E, Friedman SA, Mercer BM, Sibai BM. Obstetric characteristics amongs.
8. McAnarney ER, et al. Obstetric, neonatal and psychological outcomes of pregnant adolescents, Pediatrics 1978;61:199.
9. Roza Olyai, Prabuddh S Mittal. Teenage pregnancy (Case Studies): Gynaecological manual on adolescent girls and young women. Ashwini Bhalerao Gandhi, Parag Biniwale, Fogsi Publication, Jaypee 2009, Chapter 16, section 4: 132-37.
10. Sheil O, Turner M. Adolescent gynaecology. Progress in Obstetric and gynaecology, vol 12, John Studd (Ed) 1996, Churchill Livingstone, chapter 12, 215-32.
11. UNFPA World population Report 1999. Geneva : UNFPA, 1999.

14

Fertility Preservation in Adolescent Girls

Alka Kriplani, Divya Awasthi

INTRODUCTION

There has been worldwide concern for preservation of fertility in adolescent girls at risk of ovarian damage. In prepubertal and adolescent girls, fertility may be impaired by gonadotoxic treatments, repeat ovarian surgery or genetic disorders. Recently various possible options have emerged like cryopreservation of embryos, mature and immature oocytes and ovarian cortex prior to gonadotoxic therapy and doing conservative surgery in the form of ovarian cystectomy for benign conditions.

INDICATIONS OF FERTILITY PRESERVATION IN GIRLS

Gynecologic Oncological Conditions

Ovarian tumors are the most common neoplasm of the gynecologic tract of childhood. They represent approximately 1% of childhood cancer. Tumors of the fallopian tubes, uterus, and cervix are extremely rare in pediatrics. In children as in adults, ovarian tumors are classified histologically into epithelial tumors, sex-cord stromal tumors, and germ cell tumors. In children, germ cell tumors outnumber epithelial tumors and this difference persists until approximately 20 years of age. Germ-cell tumors of the ovary (e.g. dysgerminomas, teratomas, embryonal carcinomas) are treated primarily with surgery for staging and debulking.

Nongynecologic Oncological Conditions

Childhood cancers are estimated to occur in ~13 of 100,000 children under 15 years of age (Belgian Society of Paediatric Haematology and Oncology, unpublished data), with 45% being cases of leukemia and lymphoma, 20% craniospinal tumors, 8% neuroblastomas, 8% soft tissue tumors, 7% nephroblastomas, 3% retinoblastomas and 9% other rare tumors. Cancer treatment is the most frequent cause of ovarian damage in girls. In a recent study, the relative likelihood of female childhood cancer survivors ever conceiving was 0.81 (95% confidence interval 0.73-0.90; P , 0.001) compared with their female siblings.[1] Gonadal failure in these girls is caused by the accelerated and premature depletion of germ cells in the gonads as a result of the toxic effect of chemotherapy and radiotherapy. Between 1974/1976 and 1989/1996, the 5-year relative survival rate for childhood cancers at all sites combined improved from 56 to 75%.[2] It has been estimated that approximately one in 250 young adults will be childhood cancer survivors by 2010.[3] Furthermore, the number of young women diagnosed with cancer has been increasing, hence the importance of preservation of fertility in these young girls.

In girls exposed to radiotherapy, the degree of impairment depends on the radiation dose, radiation field, fractionation schedule and age at the time of treatment.[4,5] Effective total sterilization doses are 20.3 Gy at birth, 18.4 Gy at 10 years and 16.5 Gy at 20 years. Wallace et al were able to calculate 95% confidence limits for age at which Premature Ovarian Failure (POF) occurs for estimated radiation doses to the ovary, from 1 Gy to the effective sterilization dose and from birth to 50 years. For example, irradiation of the ovaries at the age of 10 years, with 3, 6, 9 and 12 Gy, would result in POF at the age of 36.7, 26.5, 19.7 and 15.3 years, respectively.[6] As far as chemotherapy is concerned, the nature and extent of ovarian damage depends on the drug given, the dose received and the age of the patient. Many drugs are gonadotoxic,[7] with alkylating agents posing the greatest threat. The relative contribution of every individual drug can be difficult to determine, because most treatments are given in the form of multidrug regimens. The risk of subfertility after cancer treatment can be classified according to malignant disease type and its associated treatment.[8]

Gynecologic Non-oncological Conditions

Repeat ovarian surgery may also be associated with POF. Ovarian cysts in girls are often diagnosed as a result of ovarian torsion. Diagnosis of torsion is not always easy and late diagnosis may increase the risk of irreversible necrosis and the need for aggressive surgery, such as oophorectomy. Moreover, mature teratomas, the most frequently encountered ovarian cysts in prepubertal girls, can recur in 15% of cases, requiring repeat surgery. Ovarian torsion may also occur without underlying cysts, with an increased risk of recurrence. Endometriosis is a common condition with high recurrence rate that may require repeat ovarian surgery. Ovarian cryopreservation could therefore be discussed in case of repeat ovarian surgery in young girls, especially if only one ovary remains, or when there is an increased risk of ovarian torsion, in this case, ovariopexy should be performed during the same procedure. POF may also be related to endocrine or genetic diseases, such as galactosemia and Turner's syndrome. Ovarian function appears to be preserved for longer in patients with mosaic Turner's syndrome. Cryopreservation of ovarian tissue has therefore been proposed for girls with Turner's syndrome, especially the mosaic type.

Nongynecologic Benign Conditions

Certain benign conditions such as myelodysplasia, aplastic anemia, thalassemia, drepanocytosis and multiple sclerosis, as well as severe rheumatic diseases, such as Wegener's syndrome, polyarthritis and systemic lupus erythematosus, may also necessitate administration of high doses of chemotherapy with or without bone-marrow transplantation. In these patients too, fertility preservation options should be contemplated.

OPTIONS FOR FERTILITY PRESERVATION IN GIRLS

The theoretical strategies to preserve fertility in women with cancer include: (1) frozen storage of embryos, (2) frozen storage of oocytes for future IVF, (3) frozen storage of ovarian tissue or the whole ovary for future transplantation, (4) frozen storage of ovarian tissue or isolated follicles for *in vitro* growth and maturation, (5) ovarian transposition before radiotherapy, (6) hormonal protection with GnRH analogs, and (7) pharmacological protection with anti-apoptotic agents (e.g. sphingosine-1-phosphate).

Embryo Cryopreservation

Cryopreservation of embryos is a clinically well-established technique but requires ovarian stimulation, oocyte retrieval, and IVF, which normally takes 2-5 weeks. However, delaying cancer treatment for embryo storage is not practical for many cancer patients and could be risky for a certain type of cancer. It is definitely not an option for prepubertal girls and is often unacceptable to women who do not have a partner or do not want to use donor sperm to fertilize their eggs. Embryo cryopreservation should be considered as a primary option for fertility preservation in women who have a partner and enough time to undergo at least one IVF cycle.

Oocyte Cryopreservation

This strategy has less ethical problems and does not require a male partner but will also delay cancer therapy because it requires ovarian stimulation before harvesting oocytes. The current pregnancy rates are significantly lower than those seen with embryo cryopreservation. Human oocytes can be cryopreserved at the metaphase II stage or at the germinal vesicle (GV) stage, although its efficacy and safety are unknown. For oocyte cryopreservation in some adolescent patients, gonadotropins must be administered at low doses to avoid ovarian hyperstimulation in these young girls with a large ovarian reserve.[9] However, oocyte retrieval may be difficult in these usually sexually immature subjects and therefore not applicable in the case of younger patients. Cryopreservation of oocytes has been described in prepubertal girls in association with ovarian cortex cryopreservation. At the time of surgical biopsy, antral follicles observed on the ovarian surface are aspirated and the retrieved immature oocytes are then matured *in vitro* and cryopreserved.

Using this method, Revel et al were able to cryopreserve 11 mature oocytes from three prepubertal girls aged 5, 8 and 10 years.[10]

Ovariopexy and Ovarian Transposition

Pelvic irradiation can result in the loss of ovarian function if the dose of radiation delivered to the ovaries is more than 300 cGy.[11] In the case of

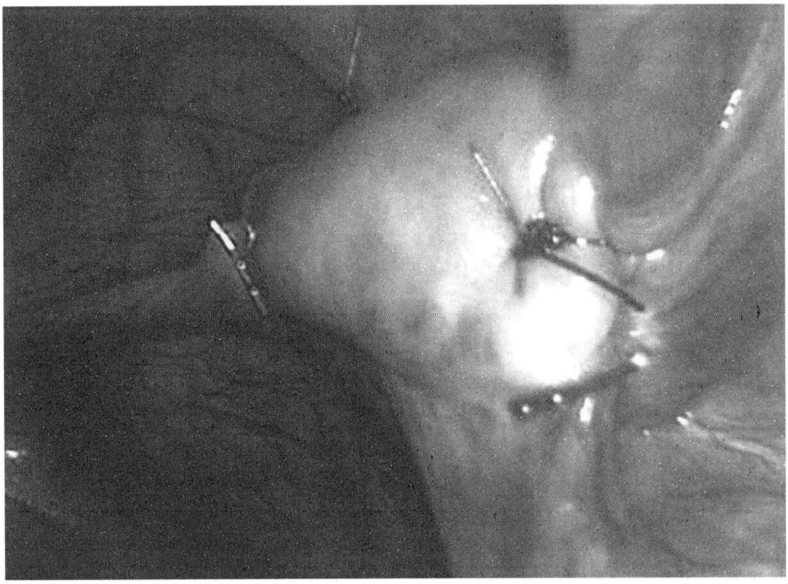

Fig. 14.1: Ovariopexy-ovary is fixed as far as possible from the midline. Clips are placed to allow ovary localization during radiotherapy *(For color version, see Plate 1)*

pelvic irradiation, the ovary could be moved outside the pelvis, which may require section of the utero-ovarian ligament and fallopian tube. The ovary is anchored, as high as possible, to the anterior abdominal wall, laterally in the paracolic gutter. Titanium clips are placed on the two opposite borders of the ovary to allow radiological identification prior to radiotherapy (Fig. 14.1). The success of ovarian function preservation by means of ovarian transposition prior to radiotherapy ranges from 16 to 90%.[12,13]

When the ovaries are transposed to an abdominal position, spontaneous pregnancy may not be possible, unless a second procedure is performed to relocate the ovaries back to the pelvis. Furthermore, should these patients need IVF in the future, oocyte retrieval may be technically more challenging. Candidates for ovarian transposition should therefore be selected carefully, taking into account all variables that may affect its success rate. It should also be borne in mind that when gonadotoxic chemotherapy is associated with radiation there is no strong rationale for this procedure.

Ovarian Cortex Cryopreservation

Ovarian cortex cryopreservation was initiated more than 10 years ago and performed with a view to either future reimplantation or follicular isolation and *in vitro* maturation (IVM). IVM of follicles isolated from cryopreserved ovarian cortex has not yet resulted in pregnancy, but the reimplantation technique has yielded pregnancies and live births. At least ten children have been born after orthotopic reimplantation of frozen-thawed ovarian cortex.[14,15]

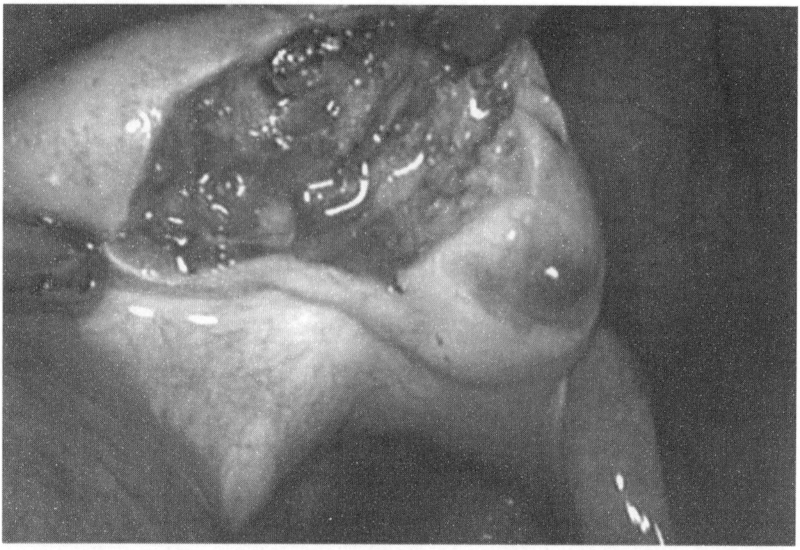

Fig. 14.2: Cortical ovarian biopsy from a 12-year-old girl. The posterior part of the left ovarian cortex (2.5 × 1.5 cm) is removed *(For color version, see Plate 1)*

Conservative Surgery (Fig. 14.2)

It is prudent to perform conservative surgery in young girls in the form of cystectomy and avoid ovariotomy as much as possible. In cases of large ovarian cysts (endometriotic cysts, dermoid cyst), even when no ovarian tissue can be recognized there remains healthy ovarian tissue near the ovarian ligament which should be left. The cystectomy can be done laparoscopically or after laparotomy. The elliptical incision is given over the most prominent part of ovarian cyst away from infundibulopelvic and ovarian ligament (Fig.14.3). The cyst wall is separated and removed. Ovary may be reconstructed after cystectomy with Vicryl 20. However, in large ovarian cyst, one should always try to salvage as much ovary as possible and avoid ovariotomy in young girls.

Cyst Wall

In cases of germ cell tumors, the other healthy ovary should be preserved and if in doubt, tissue should be sent for frozen section. If torsion is suspected, an emergency laparoscopy should be performed to establish the diagnosis and avoid ovarian damage. Several studies have shown that estimation of the degree of necrosis during surgery is inaccurate. Color, size, and edema of the twisted ischemic adnexa usually do not reflect the true damage to ovarian tissue. Despite the "necrotic" appearance of the twisted ischemic ovary, detorsion is the only procedure which should be performed (Figs 14.4A and B). Adnexectomy should be avoided as ovarian function is preserved in 88 to 100% of cases.[16]

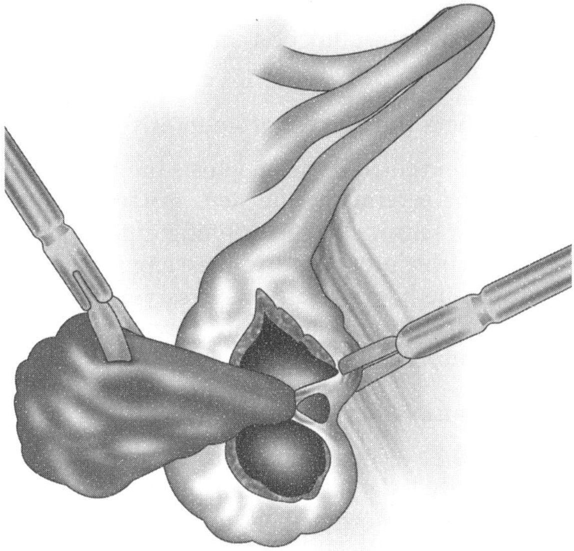

Fig. 14.3: The lining is separated easily from the ovarian capsule and stroma except where adjacent to the areas of endometriosis

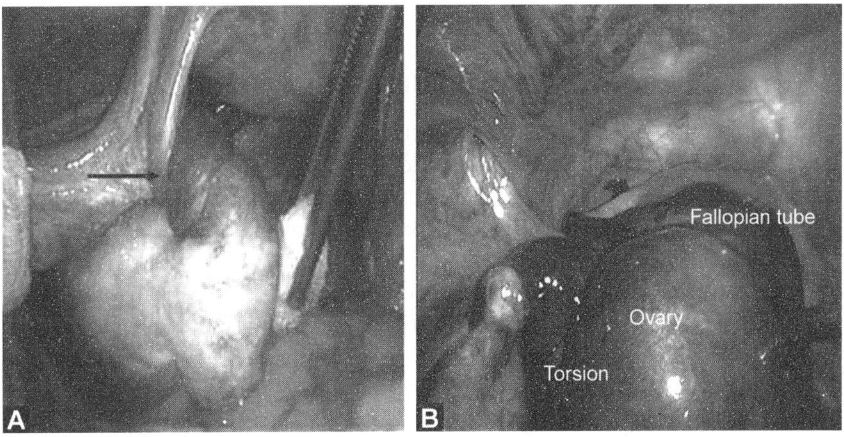

Figs 14.4A and B: (A) Ovarian torsion without gangrene, (B) Ovarian torsion with gangrene *(For color version, see Plate 2)*

Gonadotropin-Releasing Hormone (GnRH) Analogs

The efficacy of GnRH analog treatment to protect gonads from cytotoxic cancer therapy is controversial. Most animal and human studies have shown that GnRH agonist can protect primordial follicles from chemotherapy because prepubertal ovaries were found to be more resistant to alkylating agents. The results of the prospective clinical study done by Blumenfeld and his colleagues[17] were convincing: in the GnRH-treated group, 15 of 16 patients (94%) resumed spontaneous menstruation within 3-8 months after termination of chemotherapy, whereas in the control group only seven of 18 patients (39%) regained ovarian function and 11 patients (61%) experienced premature ovarian failure.

Sphingosine-1-Phosphate (Antagonist of Apoptosis)

Oocyte death can be prevented if the apoptosis program of oocytes can be inactivated. One of the several specific steps in the apoptosis program is generation of the stress sensor ceramide. Sphingosine-1-phosphate (S1P), a potent antagonist of the proapoptotic messenger ceramide, can be a potentially promising method as a fertility-preserving therapy. However, its efficacy and practicality to protect human oocytes from the toxicities of cancer therapy have not been investigated.

Risk of Cancer Cell Transmission

One of the major concerns related to autotransplantation is the risk of cancer cell transmission. For the safety of autotransplantation of ovarian tissue in cancer patients, reliable screening methods to detect minimal residual disease in ovarian tissue should be developed. In fact, it may be feasible to screen metastatic cancer cells harbored in the stored tissue before transplantation using immunohistochemistry, flow cytometry, or molecular genetic techniques such as reverse transcriptase–polymerase chain reaction and fluorescence *in situ* hybridization.

ETHICAL ISSUES IN FERTILITY PRESERVATION

Although nobody can deny the importance and priority of cancer therapy, the efforts to preserve fertility should not be ignored. At present, most strategies to preserve fertility in women are still experimental and do not guarantee the recovery of fertility. Oocyte and ovarian tissue cryobanking before cancer therapy appear to be promising options for fertility preservation. The primary ethical consideration is the safety of the procedure. Oocyte cryopreservation requires ovarian stimulation and oocyte retrieval, which can delay cancer treatment and increase the chance of cancer growth and metastasis. Ovarian stimulation with gonadotropin increases the E2 concentration, which may aggravate estrogen-sensitive tumors such as breast cancer. It is not ethical to offer oocyte cryopreservation to preserve fertility in estrogen receptor-positive breast cancer patients since the risk is clear. Ovarian tissue cryopreservation is also ethically challenging. The more serious concern is the risk of cancer cell reintroduction to the patient with autotransplantation of ovarian tissue. If cancer recurs after transplantation of stored ovarian tissue, it may not be ethically acceptable.

CONCLUSION

Fertility preservation research offers hope for future childbearing for many cancer patients who may otherwise be faced with infertility in later life. As cancer survival rates increase, the need to address quality-of-life issues such as fertility preservation becomes even more pressing. The ethical issues encountered in this research are unique from other areas of medical research and should be addressed after assessing risk benefit ratio.

REFERENCES

1. Green DM, Kawashima T, Stovall M, Leisenring W, Sklar CA, Mertens AC, Donaldson SS, Byrne J, Robison LL. Fertility of female survivors of childhood cancer: A report from the childhood cancer survivor study. J Clin Oncol 2009; 27:2677-85.
2. Greenlee RT, Hill-Harmon MB, Murray T, Thun M. Cancer statistics, 2001. CA Cancer J Clin 2001;51:15-36.
3. Blatt J. Pregnancy outcome in long-term survivors of childhood cancer. Med Pediatr Oncol 1999;33:29-33.
4. Wallace WH, Shalet SM, Hendry JH, Morris-Jones PH, Gattamaneni HR. Ovarian failure following abdominal irradiation in childhood: The radiosensitivity of the human oocyte. Br J Radiol 1989;62:995-98.
5. Bath LE, Critchley HO, Chambers SE, Anderson RA, Kelnar CJ, Wallace WH. Ovarian and uterine characteristics after total body irradiation in childhood and adolescence: Response to sex steroid replacement. Br J Obstet Gynaecol 1999;106:1265-72.
6. Wallace WH, Thomson AB, Saran F, Kelsey TW. Predicting age of ovarian failure after radiation to a field that includes the ovaries. Int J Radiat Oncol Biol Phys 2005a;62:738-44.
7. Donnez J, Martinez-Madrid B, Jadoul P, Van Langendonckt A, Demylle D, Dolmans MM. Ovarian tissue cryopreservation and transplantation: A review. Hum Reprod Update 2006;12:519-35.
8. Wallace WH, Anderson RA, Irvine DS. Fertility preservation for young patients with cancer: Who is at risk and what can be offered? Lancet Oncol 2005b;6:209-18.
9. Oktay K, Oktem O. Fertility preservation medicine: A new field in the care of young cancer survivors. Pediatr Blood Cancer 2009;53:267-73.
10. Revel A, Revel-Vilk S, Aizenman E, Porat-Katz A, Safran A, Ben-Meir A, Weintraub M, Shapira M, Achache H, Laufer N. At what age can human oocytes be obtained? Fertil Steril 2009;92:458-63.
11. Husseinzadeh N, Nahhas WA, Velkley DE, Whitney CW, Mortel R. The preservation of ovarian function in young women undergoing pelvic radiation therapy. Gynecol Oncol 1984;18:373-9.
12. Aubard Y, Piver P, Pech JC, Galinat S, Teissier MP. Ovarian tissue cryopreservation and gynecologic oncology: a review. Eur J Obstet Gynecol Reprod Biol 2001;97: 5-14.
13. Scott SM, Schlaff W. Laparoscopic medial oophoropexy prior to radiation therapy in an adolescent with Hodgkin's disease. J Pediatr Adol Gynecol 2005;18:355-57.
14. Donnez J, Dolmans MM, Demylle D, Jadoul P, Pirard C, Squifflet J, Martinez-Madrid B, Van Langendonckt A. Livebirth after orthotopic transplantation of cryopreserved ovarian tissue. Lancet 2004;364:1405-10.
15. Andersen CY, Rosendahl M, Byskov AG, Loft A, Ottosen C, Dueholm M, Schmidt KL, Andersen AN, Ernst E. Two successful pregnancies following autotransplantation of frozen/thawed ovarian tissue. Hum Reprod 2008;23:2266-72
16. Oelsner G, Cohen SB, Soriano D, et al. Minimal surgery for the twisted ischaemic adnexa can preserve ovarian function. Hum Reprod 2003;18:2599-602.
17. Blumenfeld Z, Avivi I, Linn S, Epelbaum R, Ben-Shahar M, Haim N. Prevention of irreversible chemotherapy-induced ovarian damage in young women with lymphoma by a gonadotrophin-releasing hormone agonist in parallel to chemotherapy. Hum Reprod 1996;11:1620-6.

15 Sexually Transmitted Diseases including HIV and AIDS

Basab Mukherjee

INTRODUCTION

Adolescents comprise nearly one-fifth of the total population (22%). There are 225 million adolescents in the age group 10-14 years who contribute more than half of the adolescent population (Census 2001). Female adolescents comprise almost 47 percent of the total population.

Sexually transmitted illnesses, as a group, are among the most common diseases of the world. The incidence and prevalence of STIs among adolescents is increasing in both the developing and developed countries. This has far-reaching health, social and economic consequences for millions of teenagers.

Adolescence is a critical time of rapid and diverse transition. Through this period of growth, exploration of opportunities, and development of identity, girls and boys will face different sets of challenges and pressures, and adolescence may be viewed differently from one community or culture to the next. Despite these and other disparities, a common thread is that young people need the tools and education to become sexually healthy adults.

Most young people become sexually active during adolescence. In the absence of right guidance and information at this stage they are more likely to have multi-partner unprotected sex with high-risk behavior groups.[1]

AWARENESS OF STIs AND HIV IN ADOLESCENTS IN INDIA

A cross-sectional study of urban adolescent school girls in South Delhi revealed one-third having no accurate understanding of signs and symptoms of STIs. 49% thought condoms should not be available to the youth and a third believed OCPs were only for married women.[2] A similar survey was conducted among high school girls in Amritsar with added intervention. The poor knowledge about various STDs, their symptoms, complications and prevention improved considerably after the educational intervention.[3] According to the NFHS III, 64.3% of adolescent girls of age 15-19 years in the rural area have heard about AIDS.[4]

Over 35% of all reported AIDS cases in India occur among the young people in the age group of 15-24 years, indicating that young people are highly vulnerable. Majority of people are infected through unprotected sex.

A national study by NACO/UNICEF (National Behavioral Surveillance Survey, 2001) among young people (15-24 years) found that there is a high level of awareness about HIV especially among urban males. 83% respondents knew at least two correct modes of transmission of HIV/AIDS. However awareness was low in Jharkhand, Gujarat, Chattisgarh, UP and West Bengal.

PROBLEMS SPECIFIC TO ADOLESCENTS (BOX 15.1)

Most adolescents enter their reproductive years with no knowledge of how to protect and safeguard their reproductive and sexual health.

Physiologically, young people are more vulnerable to STIs than adults, girls more than boys. Gender imbalances, societal norms and economic dependence contribute to this risk. Lack of access to correct information, tendency to experiment and an environment that makes discussing issues around sexuality taboo adds to their vulnerability.

Social Factors

Early sexual activity occurs due to greater exposure to sexual content at an early age and increasing liberalization of the society. Sexual relations are often sporadic and unplanned and sometimes as a result of coercion. Often there are multiple sexual partners involved, making contact tracing difficult. Sexual activity is started before experience or skills in self-protection. There is also inadequate information or knowledge about STIs and protecting oneself.

Biological Factors

Girls specifically are more susceptible to STIs due to inadequate mucosal defense mechanisms, immature cervical lining and low levels of vaginal acidity.

Psychological Factors

Adolescents may lack knowledge of services available for treatment. Even if they have the information they may not want to avail the same due to embarrassment and fear of apathy from the health care providers. Often financial limitations and anticipation of being victimized in an unfamiliar atmosphere prevent them from getting the appropriate medication. Incorrect or inadequate treatment may sometimes be obtained from traditional healers or pharmacy stores.

Box 15.1: Problems specific to adolescents

- Social factors
- Biological factors
- Psychological factors
- Special attention groups

Special Attention Groups

These include street adolescents, sexually abused adolescents, commercial sex workers, adolescents with mental and physical disabilities, working adolescents. Box 15.2 lists the objectives of STI management services.

Box 15.2: Objectives of STI management services

- Network of public health, private sector providers and clinics
- Universal access
- Standardized treatment protocols
- Contact tracing
- Promoting barrier contraceptives
- Emphasizing on treatment compliance and prevention strategies by behavior modification and improved knowledge

SYMPTOMS OF STIs

A large number of infected individuals are carriers and do not cause any symptoms. Lower abdominal pain, itchy vaginal discharge and changes in menstrual flow may be noticed. Genital ulcers, a burning sensation while passing urine and pain during intercourse are some of the other complaints. Boxes 15.3 and 15.4 give information on the various aspects of STIs such as history and examination.

Box 15.3: History

- *Genital symptoms:* Abnormal vaginal discharge (associated foul odor, itching or abnormal color); genital ulcers and rash; pain—lower abdomen; urinary frequency
- *Sexual activity:* Initiation, use of barrier contraception, sexual orientation, number of partners, high-risk sexual activity (anal sex)
- *Past history of STIs:* History of infection in self/partner; treatment completion for self and partner for diagnosed STI/genital symptoms;
- *Personal history:* Substance abuse
- *Menstrual History*
- *Obstetric History*

Box 15.4: Examination

- *General examination:* Vital signs and inspection of the skin for patches/rash or plaques
- *Local examination:* External genitalia for ulcers, discharge, lumps, swellings, tears and scars (also inspect the perianal region)
- *Speculum examination:* Cervix for discharge, redness, erosions, easy bleed; vaginal walls for redness, discharge, ulcerations, warts, etc.
- *Vaginal examination:* Painful movement of cervix, tender fornices, uterine size, adnexal masses
- *Proctoscopic examination:* Ulcerations

DIAGNOSIS AND MANAGEMENT OF STIs

1. Educate and counsel patients regarding STIs and HIV, safer sex practices and compliance of treatment.
2. Treat partner when indicated and advice abstinence during treatment.
3. Encourage correct and consistent use of barrier contraceptives.

4. Discuss voluntary testing for HIV and hepatitis B.
5. Follow-up for persistent symptoms or future similar infections.

Table 15.1 list the treatment regimens for STDs.

Table 15.1: STD treatment regimens

Genital Herpes	Acyclovir 400 mg three times daily/200 mg five times daily for 7-10 days
Gonococci	Inj. Ceftriaxone 125 mg IM/ Tab. Cefixime 400 mg—single dose
Chlamydia	Azithromycin 1 gm oral—single dose/Doxycycline 100 mg twice daily for 7 days
Chancroid	Azithromycin 1 gm oral/Inj. Ceftriaxone 250 mg IM—single dose
Syphilis	Inj. Benzathine Penicillin G 24 L IM—single dose
	Doxycycline 100 mg twice daily for 14 days (Penicillin allergy)
HPV warts	Cryotherapy/Podophyllin resin 10-25%

CDC Upgraded Guidelines 2007

CONSEQUENCES OF STIs

PID from *Chlamydia* and gonorrhea has long-term consequences. Chronic pelvic pain and future subfertility are the principal concerns. HPV exposure during adolescence increases the risk of cervical neoplasia and genital warts. Persistent syphilis results in multiorgan damage in its tertiary stage.

The stigma and embarrassment of having a STI can affect psychological development and adverse attitudes towards sexuality later in life.

Vertical infections from HIV, hepatitis B and syphilis in childbearing adolescents may have adverse effects on the fetus.

PREVENTION (BOX 15.5)

Maintaining proper genital hygiene is important. Practicing responsible and safe sexual practices need to be followed. Partners should be faithful to one another and protection in the form of barrier contraceptives should always be used. Intercourse should be avoided if either partner has an STI. Any symptom of disease such as vaginal discharge, lower abdominal pain and itchy genitalia should not be ignored and promptly treated. Tracing of contacts should be attempted and partners should be treated.

Teenagers should be counseled that sex is not the only way to show affection. Other ways of showing intimacy should also be discussed.

A School-based Teenage Education Program (STEP) has shown that an HIV/AIDS and alcohol abuse educational program built with specific cultural, linguistic and community-specific characteristics could be effective.[5] School-based intervention and prevention programs have been appreciated by higher secondary adolescents of both sexes in an Indian survey in Coimbatore. In traditional countries like India, formulating a program that is consistent with parental and community values is a true challenge.[6]

Box 15.5: Prevention

- Genital hygiene
- Safe sexual practices
- Barrier contraceptive use
- Education and intervention programs

Access to appropriate information and services with confidentiality is absolutely necessary for all adolescents. To help ensure contraceptive use among sexually active adolescents, information and services must be made easily available through community-based facilities and outreach services. Providing the contraceptive services that respect adolescents' rights and respond to their needs, the community and society at large will benefit immensely.

A multi-disciplinary approach combining targeted interventions like early identification and treatment of STDs, condom promotion, blood safety, drug de-addiction programs and expanding and strengthening VCTCs and long-term strategies like awareness oriented to behavioral change especially among vulnerable populations, young people and women, steps towards improvement of literacy, status of women and overall development, reduction in poverty and development of primary prevention interventions like vaccines and microbicides will have to be considered for effective prevention and control of AIDS in India.[7]

Reaching youngsters at an impressionable age before they become sexually active; can lay the foundations for a responsible lifestyle, including sex and marriage.

CONCLUSION

- Adolescents are at a high risk of STDs and AIDS due to social, biological and psychological factors.
- Early recognition and prompt intervention is paramount to minimize long-term effects in women.
- Adolescents should have easy access to ARSH, which should be integrated into primary health care services.
- Prevention would essentially consist of education and awareness programs, which should be initiated at schools and colleges.

REFERENCES

1. Orientation Programme for ANMs/LHVs to provide adolescent-friendly reproductive and sexual health services – Hand Outs.
2. BMC Women's Health 2008;8:12.
3. Indian J Dermat Venerol Leprol 2009;75(5).
4. www.nfhsindia.org.
5. AIDS Behav, 2010; 14 (Suppl 1): S177-S184.
6. Health Administrator Vol: XVII, Number 1: 43-49.
7. Godbole S, Mehendale S. HIV/AIDS epidemic in India: Risk factors, Risk behavior and strategies for prevention and control. Indian J Med Res 2005;121 (4):356-68.

Section 4

ADOLESCENT GYNECOLOGICAL ISSUES

16 Diagnosis and Management of Endometriosis in the Adolescents

Prashanth K Adiga, Roza Olyai

INTRODUCTION

Endometriosis is defined as the presence of endometrial glands and stroma outside the normal anatomical lining of the uterus. The adolescent patient usually presents with chronic pelvic pain. It is estimated that 4-17% of postmenarcheal women may be suffering from endometriosis.[1] In this article, an outline on the diagnosis and management of endometriosis will be discussed.

The diagnosis of endometriosis is based on: (a) symptoms, (b) signs and (c) investigations.

Symptoms

It should also be noted that the symptoms of endometriosis can be diverse. The presentation of the disease in adolescent patient is different from that of an adult patient. One significant difference that adolescents primarily seek medical attention is because of pain rather than a concern for infertility.

The most common symptom noted is acquired or progressive dysmenorrhea, which was encountered in 64-94% of patients.[2] Menstrual pain often begins at or soon after the menarche and may initially be typical of severe primary spasmodic dysmenorrhea (beginning on about day one of menses and then gradually developing the more typical combinations of endometriosis symptoms[3]). Endometriosis should be considered in girls who do not respond to simple NSAIDs and Oral Contraceptive Pills. Other symptoms included acyclic pain (36-91%), dyspareunia (14-25%), and gastrointestinal complaints (2-46%).[4]

Signs

When evaluating an adolescent for suspected endometriosis or dysmenorrhea, the clinician should aim to rule out a pelvic mass or a congenital anomaly of the reproductive tract.[5] The pelvic examination in the adolescent patient with pelvic pain may be limited. A bimanual examination may not be necessary to evaluate pelvic pain, especially in adolescents who are virgins.[5]

If appropriate, a pelvic examination for:

1. Signs of uterosacral nodularity and levator tenderness
2. Presence of both diffuse and local pelvic tenderness and
3. Displaced uterus or an adnexal mass.

A rectoabdominal examination in the dorsal lithotomy position may be helpful to determine if a pelvic mass is present. To rule out vaginal obstructive anomaly such as a transverse vaginal septum, inserting a Q-tip into the vaginal vault and ensuring that it goes to an adequate length.[6]

The symptoms and the signs of endometriosis are put up in a nutshell in the Box 16.1 below:

Box 16.1: Symptoms and signs of endometriosis

Symptoms
- Progressive dysmenorrhea 64-94%
- Acyclic pain 36-91%
- Dyspareunia 14-25%
- Gastrointestinal symptoms 02-46%.

Signs
- Bimanual/rectoabdominal examination—to rule out pelvic mass or congenital anomaly of the reproductive tract
- Q tip test—to rule out vaginal obstructive anomaly.

Investigations

1. ***Imaging studies***
   - *Ultrasound:* Pelvic ultrasound can be used to help rule out the possibility of an ovarian mass or congenital anomaly of the reproductive tract. In a study by Umaria and Olliff, the sensitivity of ultrasound in detecting focal endometriotic implants was poor, but it detects endometriomas with 83% sensitivity and 98% specificity.[7]
   - *MRI:* MRI can detect endometrial implants with a sensitivity as high as 60%. MRI may be used as a noninvasive method for monitoring a patient's response to treatment, but cost and availability of MRI may prohibit this.[8]
2. ***Tumor markers***
   - *CA-125:* CA-125 is not helpful in the diagnosis of adolescent endometriosis, as these patients have early stage disease.
3. ***Laparoscopy:*** The definitive diagnosis of endometriosis is best established by laparoscopy, which can be performed safely in adolescents.[5,8] If the adolescent has persistent pain despite intervention with medical therapy, she should be offered laparoscopy for a definitive diagnosis. Surgical management may be required if a Müllerian anomaly is suspected or the endometriosis is of advanced stage.

   It is important to recognize the wide range of types and colors of lesions that can be observed in this disease. Most patients have stage 1 disease, as classified by the American Society for Reproductive Medicine.[9]

MANAGEMENT

Medical Management

The following drugs are used in the management of endometriosis as shown in the Box 16.2:

Box 16.2: Drugs used in the management of endometriosis

Drugs used in medical management of endometriosis

1. NSAIDs
2. Combined oral contraceptive pills
3. Progestins
   - Gestrinone
   - Medroxyprogesterone acetate
   - Norethindrone acetate
   - Megestrel
   - Depot medroxyprogesterone acetate
4. GnRH analogs

1. *NSAIDs and combined OC pills:* First-line treatment modalities should involve the use of NSAIDs and hormone therapy. The red lesions of endometriosis are known to be active producers of prostaglandins and leukotrienes and produce dysmenorrhea. NSAIDs suppress these lesions and produce relief. The combined oral contraceptive pills, when given continuously, causes anovulation, decidualization of the endometrium and suppresses the endometriotic implants. Use of OCs is not associated with a concomitant loss of bone mineral density (BMD)[10,11] and is effective in treating pain.
2. *Progestin-only preparations:* Progestin-only preparations produce symptomatic improvement in about 80% of the patients and disease improvement in about 60%.[12,13] When injectable progestins are being used, the possible side-effects on the bone density in the adolescents should be considered in the adolescent population and the need for add-back therapy in long-term treatment.

   The commonly used progestin is medroxyprogesterone acetate which has the following side-effects, i.e. weight gain (60%), bloating and edema (60%), anxiety or irritability (20%) and dysfunctional bleeding (20%).[12]
3. *GnRH analogs:* Gonadotropin-releasing hormone agonists create a hypoestrogenic state by downregulating the hypothalamic-pituitary axis.[5] These drugs are greatly effective in reducing the pain due to endometriosis in the adolescents. They alone, cannot be used beyond 6 months because of the side-effects on the bone mineralization. It has been suggested that this therapy is not be offered as a first-line treatment for adolescents younger than 16 years.[14] To minimize the side-effects of GnRH analogs, hormonal add-back therapy with norethindrone acetate 5 mg/day, vitamin D, calcium along with appropriate monitoring of bone mineral density.[5,6] It should be noted that adolescents who are initiated on GnRH analogs should always take adequate calcium and vitamin D supplementation.[15]

SURGICAL MANAGEMENT

Laparoscopy

This is typically performed in adolescents who have pain symptoms refractory to medical treatment or if there is concern about a Müllerian anomaly.

Flow chart 16.1: Algorithm for the management of endometriosis in adolescents

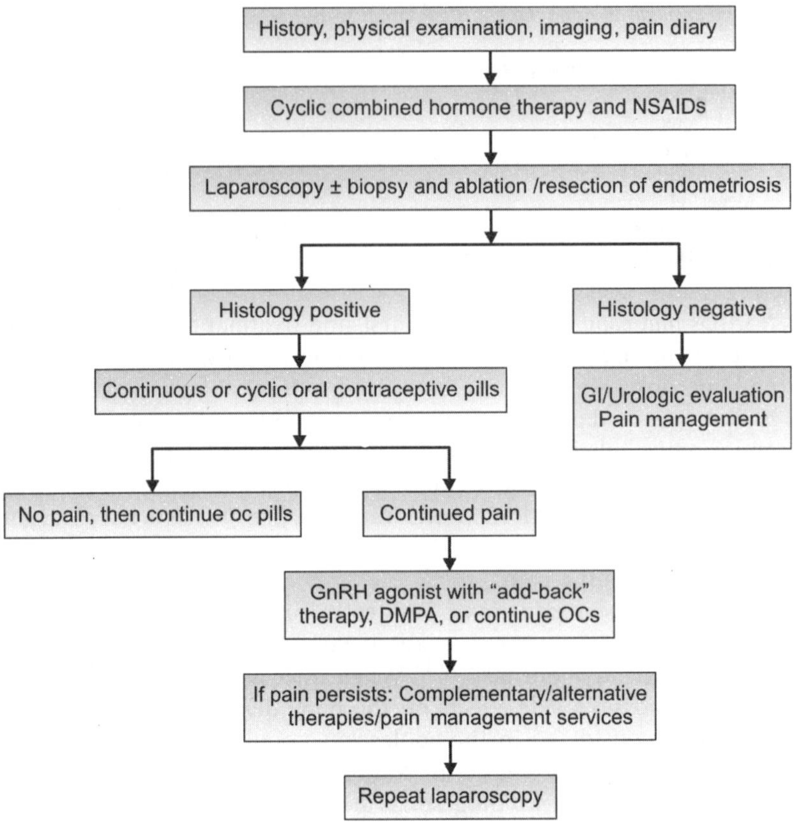

The purpose of surgical treatment is to remove the visible areas of endometriosis and restore normal anatomy by adhesiolysis.[15]

The standard technique and systemic investigation during laparoscopy includes a panoramic view and assessment of the:

- Vesicouterine peritoneum
- Anterior and posterior uterus
- Cul-de-sac and sigmoid
- Left ovarian fossa, ovary, and tube
- Right ovarian fossa, ovary, and tube
- Appendix and upper abdomen.

The algorithm for the management of endometriosis in adolescents is given in Flow chart 16.1.[5,16]

CONCLUSION

- Symptom of endometriosis in adolescents is mainly progressive dysmenorrhea.

- Acyclic pain, dyspareunia and gastrointestinal symptoms are the other symptoms of adolescent endometriosis.
- Aim of physical examination is to rule out a pelvic mass or a congenital anomaly of the reproductive tract.
- Ultrasound has a poor sensitivity in imaging for endometriotic implants.
- Definitive diagnosis of endometriosis is made by laparoscopy.
- NSAIDs and hormones are the first line of drugs in the management of adolescent endometriosis.
- Laparoscopy is intended in those who have pain symptoms refractory to medical treatment or if there is concern about a Müllerian anomaly.

REFERENCES

1. Laufer MR, Goitein L, Bush M, Cramer DW, et al. Prevalence of endometriosis in adolescent women with chronic pelvic pain not responding to conventional therapy. J Pediatr Adolesc Gynecol 1997;10:199-202.
2. Reese KA, Reddy S, Rock JA. Endometriosis in an adolescent population: the Emory experience. J Pediatr Adolesc Gynecol 1996;9:125-28.
3. Fraser IS. Recognising, understanding and managing endometriosis. J Hum Reprod Sci 2008;1:56-64.
4. Laufer MR. Identification of clear vesicular lesions of atypical endometriosis: A new technique. Fertil Steril 1997;68:739-40.
5. American College of Obstetricians and Gynecologists. Endometriosis in adolescents. ACOG Committee Opinion No. 310. Obstet Gynecol 2005;105:921-27.
6. Laufer MR. Current approaches to optimizing the treatment of endometriosis in the adolescents. Gynecol Obstet Invest 2008;66(suppl 1):19-27.
7. Umaria N, Olliff JF. Imaging features of pelvic endometriosis. Br J Radiol 2001; 74:556-62.
8. Black AY, Jamieson MA. Adolescent endometriosis. Curr. Opin. Obstet Gynecol 2002;14:467-74.
9. American Society for Reproductive Medicine: Revised American Society for Reproductive Medicine classification of endometriosis 1996. Fertil Steril 1997;67: 817-21.
10. Cromer BA, Blair JM, Mahan JD, Zibners L, Naumovski Z. A prospective comparison of bone density in adolescent girls receiving depot medroxyprogesterone acetate (Depo-Provera), levonorgestrel (Norplant), or oral contraceptives. J Pediatr 1996; 129:671-76.
11. Lara-Torre E, Edwards CP, Perlman S, Hertweck SP. Bone mineral density in adolescent females using depot medroxyprogesterone acetate. J Pediatr Adolesc Gynecol 2004;17:17-21.
12. Luciano AA, Turksoy RN, Carleo J. Evaluation of oral medroxyprogesterone acetate in the treatment of endometriosis. Obstet Gynecol 1988;72:323-27.
13. Schlaff WD, Dugoff L, Damewood MD, Rock JA. Megestrol acetate for treatment of endometriosis. Obstet Gynecol 1990;75:646-48.
14. Laufer MR, Sanfilippo J, Rose G. Adolescent endometriosis: Diagnosis and treatment approaches. J Pediatr Adolesc Gynecol 2003;16(suppl):S3-11.
15. Dovey S, SanFillipo J. Endometriosis and the adolescent. Clin Obstet Gynecol 2010; 53:420-28.
16. Bandera CA, Brown LR, Laufer MR. Adolescents and endometriosis. Clin Consult Obstet Gynecol 1995;7:200-08.

17 Fibroid Uterus in the Adolescent Girls

Gita Guin, Shashi Khare

Fibroid or fibromyoma of the uterus is the most common benign tumor of the uterus occurring in 20-50% of women over 30 years of age. Since the tumor depends on ovarian steroid hormones for its growth, in girls who are predisposed, ovarian activation at adolescence may trigger the growth of a tumor that is diagnosed later in life when it becomes symptomatic. The first report is by Wisot et al in 1969 of a myoma in a 13-year-old girl. Since then, there have been few reports of myoma in adolescent girls, most of them presenting as abdominal tumors.

PREDISPOSING FACTORS

1. *Race:* Fibroids are diagnosed at a younger age in black women as compared to white women; in them, the fibroids are more likely to be larger, multiple and symptomatic at an earlier age. Indians too have a genetic predisposition to developing fibroids.
2. Family history of fibroid in first or second degree relatives.
3. Anovulatory cycles which are common in girls at menarche result in unopposed estrogen stimulation of a susceptible myometrium.
4. *Obesity:* Poor dietary habit and sedentary lifestyle of the young girls is seeing obesity emerging as a major public health issue. Circulating androgens are converted to estrogens in the adipose tissues. There is also a reduction in the hepatic production of hepatic sex hormone binding globulin resulting in increased levels of circulating estrogens. A case controlled Thai study has reported a 6% increase in the risk of fibroids with each unit increase in BMI. Polycystic ovarian disease which is a common accompaniment of obesity can further worsen existing hormonal imbalances.
5. *Oral contraceptive pills:* With young girls becoming sexually active, it is not unusual, particularly in the more permissive societies, to come across an adolescent girl on oral contraceptives.

Besides these, there are unsubstantiated reports that consumption of soy (isoflavones) contributes to the growth of fibroids. Similarly, chemical pesticides and human growth hormone present in vegetables, fruits and dairy products can mimic estrogen in the body.

Clinical Features and Diagnosis

Majority of the fibroids in adolescent girls are asymptomatic as in the adult population and are discovered incidentally during an ultrasound examination to investigate puberty menorrhagia, pelvic pain or dysmenorrhea. Only rarely will the girl present with a palpable abdominal mass with or without pressure symptoms.

A young girl reporting to a busy gynecology OPD with any of the above symptoms is presumed more often than not as a young girl unable to cope with her menarche; considering that the girl and her guardian are equally reluctant for a per rectal examination, a gynecologist is often tempted into prescribing symptomatic treatment. However, if the girl happens to report repeatedly for the same complaints, it is prudent to subject her to a thorough clinical examination.

DIFFERENTIAL DIAGNOSIS

1. DUB and primary dysmenorrhea.
2. Adenexal masses: Infective (tubercular TO mass) and neoplastic ovarian masses.
3. Full bladder.
4. Pregnancy and its complications.

Associated Pathologies

Associated pathologies must be diligently looked for in all girls diagnosed with fibroid uterus as it may modify the treatment plan.

1. Endometriosis.
2. Polycystic ovarian syndrome.
3. Benign breast tumors.

INVESTIGATIONS

1. Complete blood count, ESR, bleeding profile and thyroid profile to rule out all the causes of menorrhagia and dysmenorrhea.
2. *USG:* High frequency abdominal ultrasonography will establish the diagnosis with certainty in as many as 73% of the cases.
3. *MRI:* Owing to its precision for identification of the nature, number and location, MRI is used in doubtful cases and is superior to USG in differentiating an adenexal mass.
4. *CT-scan:* Limited role as fibroids cannot be distinguished from normal myometrium, and degeneration and calcification in a young girl is extremely rare.

MANAGEMENT

Counseling and Follow-up

The very word "Fibroid Uterus", even though incidentally diagnosed and of little or no significance, will stir up a storm of anxieties, more so in a young girl who is just starting her reproductive life. With information being only click of a button away (and most of it not being applicable to adolescents), a practitioner must put in an earnest effort to counsel both the girl and her guardians. Small asymptomatic fibroids are to be left as such with the advice to follow-up periodically. Though debatable, this girl will possibly do well in not postponing her marriage and reproduction for the more pressing reason of her career.

Medical Management

Considering the age of the patient, ease of administration, safety and easy acceptability in young girls, medical management forms the mainstay of treating these patients.

Symptomatic Treatment

Symptom causing of big fibroids will put to test the clinicians knowledge and patience. As far as possible they are best managed conservatively for reasons of fertility preservation.

1. Iron and folic acid, calcium and other micronutrients.
2. *Nonsteroidal anti-inflammatory agents:* These are not very effective in controlling the menorrhagia due to fibroids (except indomethacin) but may significantly reduce the pain and dysmenorrhea in girls with fibroid uteri.
3. *Antifibrinolytics:* Tranexamic acid 2-4 gm daily in divided doses significantly reduces the blood loss (by as much as 40%) associated with fibroids but has no effect on dysmenorrhea. A Cochrane Review has found this to be more effective with less or equal side-effects as compared to ethamsylate, oral luteal phase progesterone, NSAIDs or placebo in reducing the blood loss.

Definitive Treatment

1. *Low dose OC pills:* The fibroids have a higher concentration of estrogen and progesterone receptors as compared to the surrounding myometrium. However, studies have shown that the low dose estrogen containing pills with a higher amount of progesterone reduce its size, along with a control of menorrhagia and dysmenorrhea. Low dose estrogen does not influence linear growth unlike high dose estrogen which causes early epiphysial closure.
2. *Progestogens:* Though progesterones have been implicated as promoters of fibroid growth, they are useful in treating anovular menorrhagia that is the most common presenting symptom in adolescent girls with fibroid. Norethisterone acetate given in doses of 5-10 mg two to three times a day from day 5 of the cycle for 20 days effectively reduces the bleeding. In young obese girls with PCOS, didrogesterone may be a lipid friendly alternative, although it is costly, less effective in reducing blood loss, and sedation may be problematic in a young school going girl. As a last resort, depot medroxyprogesterone acetate may help in achieving reduction in blood loss as well as reduction in uterine and fibroid volume. Osteopenia associated with long-term use is unacceptable during the period of maximum growth in bone density.

LNG-IUD (when the cavity is undistorted) will be reserved for the rare situation where all other measures to control the menstrual blood loss have failed. A low-dose levonorgestrel releasing intrauterine system (FIBROPLANT) reduces the side-effects of progesterone further while alleviating the anxiety associated with amenorrhea in a young girl.

3. *Antiprogesterones:* Mifepristone (RU 486) is an antiprogesterone drug with weak antiestrogenic activity. Different studies have used doses of 5-30 mg daily for 3 to 6 months with reported 50% reduction in size at half the cost of GnRH analogs over the treatment period. It causes less intense hot flushes much later in the course of treatment. Its effect on bone mineral density, which is a major concern, is also lesser. Once its safety in adolescents with yet maturing reproductive system and growing height is established, in its lowest effective dose, mifepristone will be a safe and cheap option in treating these girls with fibroid uterus.
4. *Danazol:* Danazol acts by inhibiting steroidogenesis and when used in doses of 100-200 mg for 3 months, it reduces the size of fibroids by 20-25% with reduced menstrual flow by 80%. However, because of its androgenic side-effects such as weight gain, dysphoria, acne, headache, unwanted hair growth and deepening of voice, it should be used with caution.
5. *Gestrinone:* It is a tri-enic steroid with antiestrogenic and weak antiprogestogenic activity. In few trials, when used in higher than recommended dose of 2.5 mg, it caused reduction in the size of the fibroid with fewer androgenic side-effects than progesterone. There is however no documentation of its use in adolescent girls.
6. *GnRH agonists and antagonists:* Besides its cost being a limiting factor, most studies have used it to postpone or avoid hysterectomy in near menopausal women. Its role in an adolescent girl with an immature hypothalamic-pituitary-ovarian axis who is gaining height and increasing bone density is debatable. Further, if a young girl with a fibroid uterus is as bad as to require these drugs, then she will require definitive treatment sooner or later. These drugs will only make surgical enucleation difficult and are followed by higher recurrence rates.
7. *Ormiloxifene/Centchroman:* This is a synthetic estrogen receptor modulator which suppresses the estrogen receptors in the reproductive organs like the ovaries, uterus and breasts while stimulating the estrogen receptors in other organs like the bones. It is cheap, easy to administer (60 mg twice weekly × 3 months, then once weekly for 3 months) and is advocated for the treatment of puberty menorrhagia. Its exact effect on the volume of uterine fibroids is unclear. While few studies claim a reduction in size, others have reported an increase in the size of the fibroids. Given under careful supervision, it can be used to treat the menorrhagia associated with fibroid uterus.

Newer drugs like Growth factor blocking agents and Synthetic Progesterone Receptor Modulators (SPRMs) like Asoprisnil and CDB-2914 and Pirfenidone (Aromatic inhibitor used in pulmonary fibrosis/

nonsteroidal) are under development. Serracor-NK, a combination of Serrapeptase and Nattokinase is claimed to help dissolve fibroids in the uterus.

Surgical Management

Very rarely will a young girl present with a myoma that can be managed by surgery alone. In this highly precarious situation, myomectomy, conventional, laparoscopic or hysteroscopic surgeries, need to be performed with utmost care to preserve integrity of the reproductive organs.

The safety of uterine artery embolization in a young girl is yet to be established considering that it may be followed by ovarian failure and its effect on future fecundity and recurrence is unclear. First generation thermal ablation (laparoscopic myolysis) has the risk of uterine rupture in labor and may not be used in an adolescent girl. Second generation ablation techniques like MR-guided laser ablation and MR-guided focused ultrasound surgery (MRgFUS) with or without pre treatment with GnRH analogs are newer avenues and may be the future treatment modality in a young girl with a large fibroid.

Hysterectomy as an option will be considered only in an adolescent girls with cerebral palsy or of unsound mind who is unable to cope with the symptoms of fibroid uterus and in whom fecundity is not an issue. Only in the rarest of rare circumstance will a conservative surgical procedure become complicated enough to warrant a hysterectomy.

CONCLUSION

1. The diagnosis of fibroid uterus in an adolescent girls will often be incidental and such patients are best managed by counseling, follow-up and symptomatic therapy.
2. Indomethacin (NSAID), tranexamic acid (antifibrinolytic) and progesterones are good for symptomatic control of excessive menstrual bleeding. The effect of ormiloxifene on the size of fibroids needs to be evaluated.
3. Mifepristone may emerge as the best option for definitive management.

SUGGESTED READING

1. Anderson J. Factors in fibroid growth. Bailliieres Clin Obstet Gynaecol 1998; 12(2):225-43.
2. Chiaffarino F, La Vecchia C, Marsico S, Surace M, Ricci E. Use of oral contraceptives and uterine fibroids: Results from a case control study. Br J Obstet Gynaecol 1999; 106(8)857-60.
3. Grigoreva V, Chen-mok M, Tarasova M, Mikhailov A. Use of a levonorgestrel-releasing intrauterine system to treat bleeding related to uterine leiomyomas. Fertil Steril 2003;79:1194-98.
4. Karim Tanweer, Patil Kundan, Panchal Anuradha, et al. Presentation and management of giant fibroid uterus in an adolescent girl. Dovpress Journal: 2010;3:13-15.
5. Kjerulff KH, Langenberg P, Seidman JD, et al. Uterine leiomyomas. Racial differences in severity, symptoms and age at diagnosis. J Reprod Med 1996;41(7):483-90.

6. Lethaby A, Vollhoven B, Sowter M. Preoperative GnRH analog therapy before hysterectomy or myomectomy for uterine fibroids. Cochrane Database Systematic Review 2000(2); CD 000547.
7. Lumbiganon P, Rugpao S, Phandu-fung S, Laopaiboon M, Vudhikamraksa N, Werawatakul Y. Protective effect of depot-medroxyprogesterone acetate on surgically treated uterine leiomyomas: A multicenter case-control study. Br J Obstet Gynaecol 1996;103:909-14.
8. Progress in Obstetrics and Gynaecology, Vol 17: Churchill Livingstone. Fibroid embolization; Aradhna Khaund, Mary Ann Lumsden; 333-342.
9. Recent Advances in Obstetrics and Gynaecology Vol 24: Jaypee Brothers Medical Publishers (P) Ltd. Magnetic Resonance Guided Thermal Ablation For Uterine Fibroids. Sue Zaher, Lesley Regan; 167-176.
10. Rein MS. Progesterone: A critical role in the pathogenesis in uterine myomas. Am J Obstet Gynecol 1995;172:14.
11. Ross RK, Pike MC, Vessey MP, Bull D, Yeates D, Casagrande JT. Risk factors for uterine fibroids: Reduced risk associated with oral contraceptives. Br Med Journal (Clin Res Ed) 1986;293:359-62.
12. Suchitra N Pandit, Sanjay B Rao, Ranjit Akolekar. Fibroids: National Series. The Federation of Obstetrics and Gynaecological Societies of India. The National Book Depot 2006.
13. Walker WJ, Pelage JP. Uterine artery embolization for symptomatic fibroids: Clinical results in 400 women with imaging follow-up. Br J Obstet Gynaecol 2002;109: 1262-72.

18 Non-Malignant Ovarian Lesions—A Cause of Concern and Caution in Adolescents

Aruna Kumar, Deepti Gupta

"It is the best thing in my opinion, for the physician to apply himself diligently to the art of foreknowing."

—Hippocrates

INTRODUCTION

Ovarian cysts/tumors in adolescents have always posed a dilemma to the treating physician. Dealing with ovarian tumors in adolescents is particularly a challenge because of their rarity, atypical symptoms, malignant potential and probable serious repercussions on the patient's reproductive life. Newer advents in imaging modalities, tumor markers and multimodal screening may help in early diagnosis, ruling out malignant neoplasm and thus, adopting more conservative approach to the management of these lesions in adolescents. Hence, it is empirical that gynecologists should be well versed with this topic.

INCIDENCE

Ovarian masses may be benign or malignant. Simple ovarian cysts are quite common with reported incidence of about 12-23%[1] in some studies. Endometriomas *per se* are rare in adolescents because endometriosis in adolescents usually presents early. The incidence of endometriosis in post-menarchal females is 4-17%. Incidence increases to 25-38%[2,3] in adolescents with pelvic pain and in adolescents in whom treatment with OCPs and NSAIDs has failed, the incidence is as high as 50-70%.[4,5] The incidence of PCOS is postulated to be around 20-30% and almost half of this group belongs to adolescent population.

As far as true ovarian tumors are concerned, they comprise 1.5% of all adolescent tumors with an absolute incidence of approximately 5.5%. Majority of ovarian tumors are germ cell tumors representing almost 60% of ovarian tumors in adolescents followed by yolk sac tumors and sex cord stromal tumors. The risk of ovarian malignancy varies inversely with age, highest incidence found in very young patients and lowest in adolescents.

Malignant neoplasms of the ovary have been discussed in detail elsewhere. This chapter will elaborate on the nonmalignant lesions of the ovary in adolescents.

CLASSIFICATION (TABLE 18.1)

Classification of ovarian tumors is done on **Histologic basis into Non-Neoplastic and Neoplastic lesions, as proposed by WHO** keeping the developmental embryology, endocrine activity and malignant potential in mind. Non-neoplastic lesions can be further divided as follows (Table 18.1):

Table 18.1: Classification of benign ovarian tumors[6]

Benign Ovarian Tumors	
Functional	Follicular
	Corpus Luteum
	Theca Lutein
Inflammatory	Tubo-Ovarian Abscess or Complex
Neoplastic	Germ Cell
	Benign Cystic Teratoma
	Others and Mixed
Epithelial	Serous Cystadenoma
	Mucinous Cystadenoma
	Fibroma
	Cystadenofibroma
	Brenner Tumor
	Mixed Tumor
Others	Endometrioma
	Polycystic Ovaries

SYMPTOMATOLOGY

Ovarian tumors are known for their silent presentation. Most commonly they present with complaints like pelvic pain which is usually a chronic discomfort, but may be acute and severe due to torsion, rupture or hemorrhage. Pelvic or abdominal mass is the next most common complaint. Other presenting complaints may be due to pressure symptoms on bladder or rectum, menstrual irregularities, abdominal fullness or bloating, abdominal distension, weight loss, etc. Endometriomas are rare in adolescents, because of early presentation of endometriosis with symptoms like dysmenorrhea, cyclic or noncyclic pain, gastrointestinal symptoms, abdominal pain, etc. Nevertheless it should still be kept in mind while dealing with any ovarian mass. Similarly adolescents with PCOS usually present to the gynecologist with concerns about obesity, hirsutism and oligomenorrhea /amenorrhea.

For a long time, it was assumed that ovarian neoplasm (benign/ malignant) did not cause any symptoms till it reached an advanced stage. However it has now become clear that ovarian neoplasms also cause particular symptoms at particular stages of disease progression. Keeping this fact in mind, **Symptom Index** has been developed for screening of ovarian cancer which is under trial in USA. Some of the symptoms that were

Table 18.2: Comparison of symptoms in benign and malignant tumors[7]

Symptom	Ovarian cancer (n = 44)	Benign Ovarian mass (n = 84)	IBS (n = 109)	Clinic (n = 1600)	P Value
	No. (%) of Women				
Type of pain					
Pelvic	16 (36)	13 (15)	10 (9)	160 (10)	< .001
Abdominal	10 (23)	9 (11)	22 (21)	121 (7)	< .001
Indigestion	4 (9)	4 (5)	16 (15)	111 (7)	.03
Bloating	20 (45)	12 (14)	19 (17)	123 (8)	< .001
Increased abdominal size	18 (41)	12 (14)	15 (14)	86 (5)	.001
Fatigue	10 (23)	12 (14)	30 (27)	269 (17)	.02
Urinary tract	11 (25)	6 (7)	21 (19)	192 (12)	< .001
Constipation	9 (20)	6 (7)	19 (17)	106 (7)	< .001
Diarrhea	2 (5)	6 (7)	26 (24)	93 (6)	< .001

Abbreviation: IBS, irritable bowel syndrome.

* Symptom severity scale is rated on a scale of 1 to 5, with 1 being minimal and 5 being severe.

associated significantly with malignant ovarian neoplasm are pelvic/ abdominal pain, urinary urgency/frequency, increased abdominal size/ bloating, difficulty in eating/feeling of fullness (Table 18.2) especially if they were present in last one year and for > 12 days per month. Patients were considered positive for symptom index if any 6 symptoms were present for > 12 times per month over the last 1 year. This symptom index may be of help in ruling out malignancy prior to taking a decision about surgical intervention.

It is important to note that many of these symptoms like bloating, constipation, diarrhea, etc. are considered nonspecific and insignificant by the adolescent patients and their caretakers. This causes delay in seeking treatment and by the time the patients report, a benign mass could have turned malignant or reached advanced stage.

ETIOLOGY

Most simple cysts are a result of natural phenomena of folliculogenesis and ovulation. Amongst all age groups, adolescents have the highest rates of PID which predisposes them to develop tubo-ovarian abscess.[8] Endometriosis and PCOS show some familial clustering. Many candidate genes like CYP 11A, CYP 17, CYP 21, androgen receptor, SHBG gene, insulin receptor gene have been implicated in the development of PCOS. The strongest evidence so far is in support of region near insulin receptor gene.[9] The risk of developing this syndrome in first degree relatives is 24% of mothers and 32% of sisters.[10] With an affected first degree relative, the incidence of endometriosis is also increased 10-fold.[11]

OVARIAN CYSTS

Functional ovarian cysts are the most common benign ovarian masses detected in adolescents.

Follicular cysts (50% of benign cysts)[1] develop due to nonrupture or non atresia of developing follicle, usually unilocular, asymptomatic and grow to maximum size of 8 cm. Sometimes they may continue to secrete estrogen. These cysts are lined by a layer of granulosa cells and surrounded by a connective tissue capsule. They are uncommon in premenarchal girls and hence whenever found, abnormal source of gonadotropin should be looked for.

Corpus luteum cysts are formed by intracystic hemorrhages and may be associated with amenorrhea, irregular menses or DUB and sometimes present with hemoperitoneum due to cyst rupture. Thus, it can be mistaken for ectopic pregnancy. These cysts are generally hormonally inactive. Cyst lining is made up of luteinized granulosa and theca cells which impart a typical golden yellow color.

Theca lutein cysts are usually bilateral, multicystic and may grow to a size of 25 cm. Chronic hyperemia or active/passive congestion of ovaries as seen in pelvic infection is another very common cause of cystic changes in ovary.

Endometriomas (Fig. 18.1) though rare should be considered as differential diagnosis of benign cysts because the incidence of endometriosis is quite high in adolescents. 65% of all adolescent endometriosis presents between 19-21 years. In adolescents with pelvic pain, incidence ranges from 25-38% and in adolescents who do not respond to OCPs and NSAIDs, incidence of endometriosis is as high as 70%. Endometriotic masses may simulate malignancy because of tissue implantation on adjacent surfaces and secondary fixation. Early recognition of symptoms, diagnosis and initiation of treatment are essential in preventing its progression, worsening of symptoms and most importantly development of infertility.

Polycystic ovarian syndrome is another common cause of enlarged ovaries in adolescents. The overall incidence of PCOS is about 20-30% of which about half the patients belong to adolescent group. Diagnosis is made by

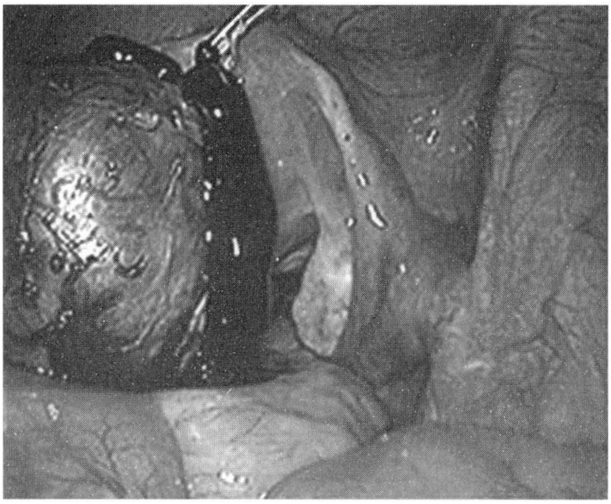

Fig. 18.1: Endoscopic view of ruptured chocolate cyst in the left ovary
(For color version, see Plate 2)

Rotterdam Criteria.[12] Traditionally it was believed that PCOS occurs because of aberrations in hypothalamo- pituitary- ovarian axis, high LH/ FSH ratios, increased androgen and peripheral estrones. Newer developments have shown the role of genetics, insulin resistance and inter-relationships between obesity and ghrelin. These patients present with oligo/ amenorrhea, hirsutism and obesity. Associated biochemical abnormalities include elevated free testosterone, LH/ FSH ratio > 3 and fasting glucose to insulin ratio < 4.5.

Mature cystic teratoma accounts for 10-15% of all benign ovarian lesions. It is the commonest ovarian germ cell tumor comprising about 2/3rd of ovarian germ cell tumors[1] and also the most common ovarian neoplasm in patients < 20 years. It is typically asymptomatic but may cause pressure symptoms or acute pain due to torsion (3-11%),[13] rupture (< 1%) or hemorrhage. Other complications include infection, hemolytic anemia and malignant degeneration. Mature teratomas are composed of well differentiated tissues arising from all three embryologic germ layers. These neoplasms are also referred to as **Benign Cystic Teratomas** or **Dermoid Cyst** of ovary (Fig. 18.2). They are bilateral in 12% and may coexist with mucinous cystadenoma. It is postulated that teratomas originate from primordial germ cells. Anatomical distribution of teratomas along the line of migration of germ cells supports this fact.[14,15] Sophisticated cytogenetic techniques have also shown that these tumors are of germ cell origin and arise from a single germ cell after the first meiotic division.[16]

Other benign neoplasms of the ovary include **Serous Cystadenomas** which account for 20-30% of benign ovarian neoplasms, may be cystic, papillary or adenofibromatous. They are usually thin walled, unilocular, cystic, 20-30 cm in size. Rarely some exophytic masses may be associated with ascites and implantation of fragments, giving a false impression of malignancy. **Mucinous cystadenomas** are bilateral in 10%, multilocular and grow to very big sizes. They are the largest tumors found in human body.

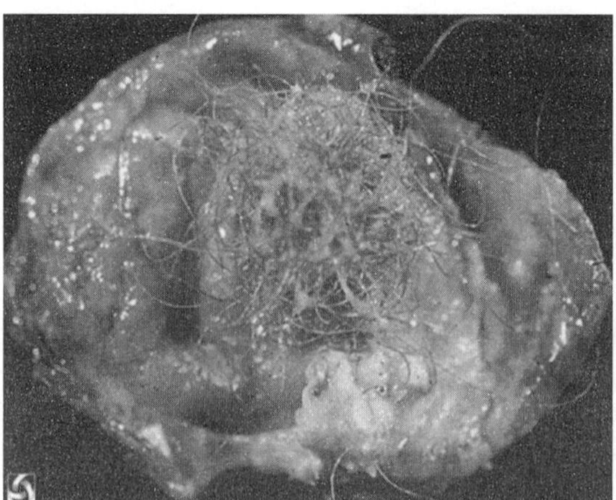

Fig. 18.2: Cut section of dermoid cyst showing pellet of hair *(For color version, see Plate 2)*

Other benign tumors like **Endometroid Adenofibroma, Clear Cell Adenofibroma, Androblastomas, Lipoid Cell Tumors, Thecoma and Fibroma** are rare in adolescents.

DIAGNOSIS

Diagnosis should be aimed at avoiding unnecessary invasive procedures particularly in adolescents, yet not to miss any ovarian malignancy when present (Fig. 18.3).

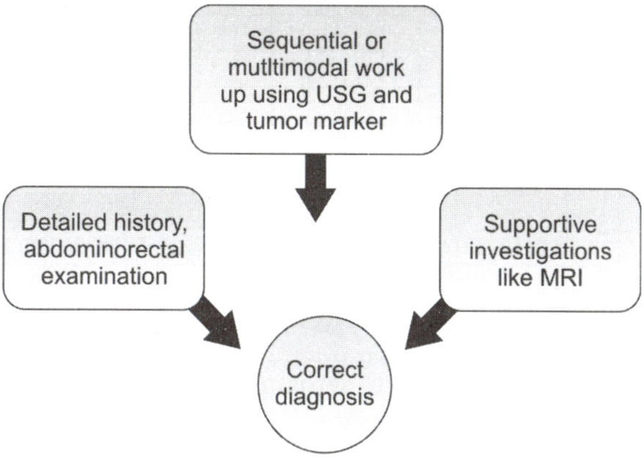

Fig. 18.3: Important steps to arrive at correct diagnosis

Nothing can replace a well taken detailed history, especially about symptoms, etiological factors and any affected relatives. Since bimanual pelvic examination may not be possible in adolescent patients, thorough **bimanual abdomino-rectal and abdominal examination** should be done to pick up any ovarian mass. Close attention must be paid to the physical characteristics like, size, shape, consistency, fixation, tenderness, etc. In all adolescents with ovarian mass, secondary sexual characters should be evaluated for any signs of hormonal effects. Importance of percussion in diagnosis of ovarian lesion should not be overlooked. Table 18.3 shows the difference in examination findings in benign and malignant ovarian neoplasms:

Table 18.3: Examination findings in benign and malignant ovarian neoplasms

Benign	*Malignant*
Unilateral	Bilateral
Cystic	Solid/complex
Mobile	Fixed
Smooth	Irregular
Unilocular	Multilocular
No ascites	Ascites
No growth	Rapid growth
Smooth rectovaginal septum	Nodularity of rectovaginal septum

In patients with symptoms suggestive of endometriosis, "**Benjamin Sign**", i.e. persistently high BBT or fluctuating BBT can be used for screening

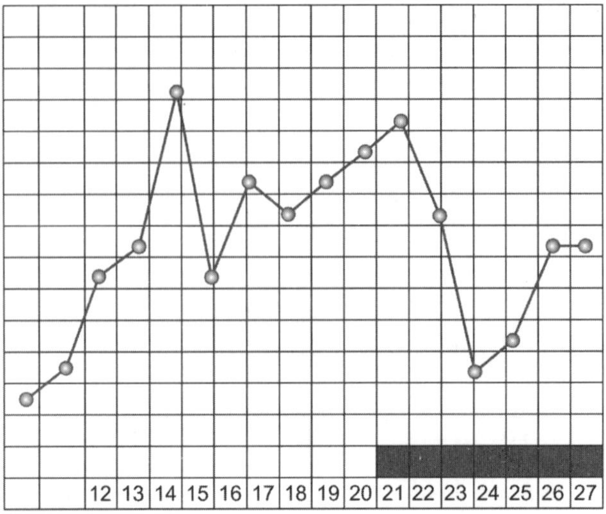

Fig. 18.4: Graph showing persistently elevated BBT, i.e. Positive Benjamin Sign

and patients who have positive Benjamin Sign should be subjected to laparoscopy to confirm the diagnosis.[17] This will help in preventing many unnecessary laparoscopies (Fig. 18.4).

Baseline investigations should always include a pregnancy test regardless of elicited sexual history. Chest radiograph should be done. Abdominal X-ray may show calcifications particularly in mature cystic teratoma.

Ultrasonography is an important diagnostic test which can provide good anatomic details. Simple cysts are seen as unilocular and anechoic cysts, usually < 10 cm (Fig. 18.5). Hemorrhagic/chocolate cysts typically show ground glass appearance or diffuse internal echoes (Fig. 18.6).[18] Hyperechoic wall foci and multilocularity are also pointers of endometriomas.[18] USG has

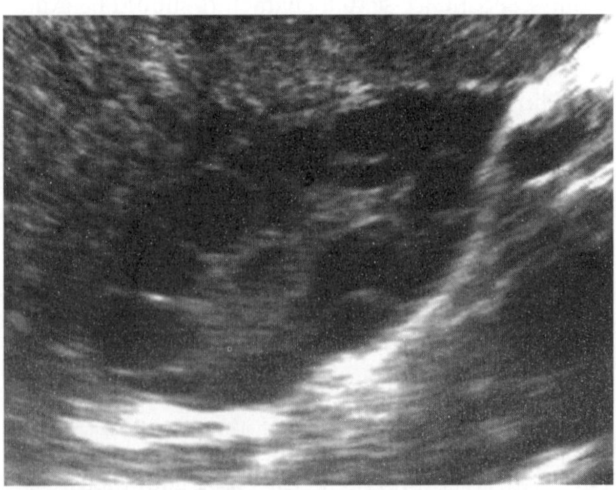

Fig. 18.5: Classical sonographic appearance of polycystic ovary

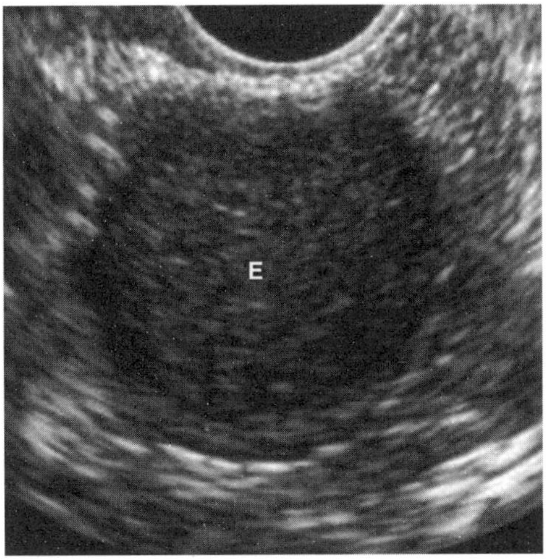

Fig. 18.6: USG appearance of endometrioma with diffuse internal echoes

a sensitivity of 83% and specificity of 98% in diagnosing endometriomas and this accuracy may be further increased by Doppler flow analysis which shows increased pericystic blood flow with RI > 0.45.[19] USG findings suggestive of polycystic ovaries are enlarged ovaries with > 12 small follicles 5-9 mm in size.

Ultrasonic findings of teratomas include echo densities, regionally bright echoes, hyperechoic lines and dots, and fluid-fluid levels.[20] In a study by Mais et al, transvaginal ultrasonography had a sensitivity and specificity of 84.6% and 98.2%, respectively, for differentiating cystic teratoma from other ovarian masses.[21] In another trial, Patel et al demonstrated a 98% positive predictive value and 85% sensitivity using ultrasound to diagnose and identify cystic teratomas.[22]

Ovarian volume > 20 cm should arouse strong suspicion of malignancy. Other USG findings suggestive of malignant ovarian mass include solid/complex components, multilocular/septate mass, evidence of surface nodularity or papillae and heterogeneous echotexture. **Doppler USG** may further help in confirming the diagnosis. Central vascularity in the mass, RI < 0.4 and PI < 1 are some findings suggestive of malignancy.

MRI gives the definite advantage of imaging entire pelvis in multiple planes in a single sitting, allows better evaluation of indeterminate masses and maximizes diagnostic accuracy. "Shading effect" seen on MRI is very characteristic of hemorrhagic/chocolate cyst and is seen as mixing of hypodense areas with hyperdensities because of presence of blood products. Endometriosis appears as hyperintense on T_1 weighted images and as hypointense on T_2 weighted images (Fig. 18.7).[19] CT scan usually reveals the complex appearance of ovarian teratomas, with dividing septa, internal debris, fat attenuation (93%), and distinct calcification (56%).[20] MRI can sufficiently differentiate lipid density from other fluid and blood and may be another useful adjunct for diagnosis of ovarian teratomas, with an accuracy of 99%.[23]

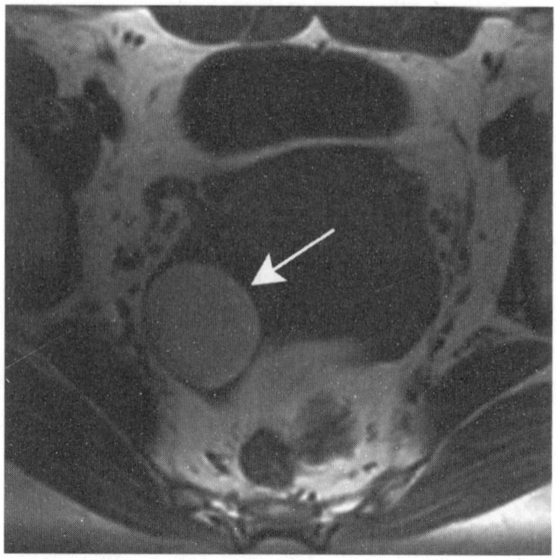

Fig. 18.7: T1-weighted magnetic resonance image of an endometrioma. The characteristic high signal intensity (similar to that of fat) shows right adnexal endometrioma (arrow).

MANAGEMENT

Management of ovarian tumors in adolescents should aim to conserve the reproductive potential without jeopardizing her life (Fig. 18.8). It is important to decide whether to keep the patient under observation or proceed with surgery and whether laparoscopic approach is justified for surgery.

Asymptomatic cystic adnexal masses should be followed as they are almost always benign and regress spontaneously in 3 to 6 months. They should be kept under close observation and the risk of ovarian torsion should be explained. These patients may be offered ultrasound guided or laparoscopic cyst aspiration, but the recurrence rate may be as high as 50%. Decision of surgical intervention for functional ovarian mass if taken prematurely can cause ovarian and tubal adhesions and thus have adverse affect on future fertility. Surgery is indicated in following situations:

- Ovarian cyst > 6 cm without regression for 6-8 weeks
- Any cystic structure > 10 cm
- Solid ovarian lesion
- Ovarian lesion with papillary excrescences in wall
- Ascites
- Bilaterality.

Management of **Endometriosis** in adolescents is primarily non- surgical and includes prolonged suppression of ovulation. Endometriotic lesions in adolescents are usually atypical and endoscopist can miss 7% lesions or underdiagnose 50% lesions.[24] Recently studies have shown 83.5% concordance between ultrasound staging and laparoscopic staging of endometriosis.[25] This fact can help in reducing many unnecessary laparoscopies as the anxiety associated with any surgical procedure is very

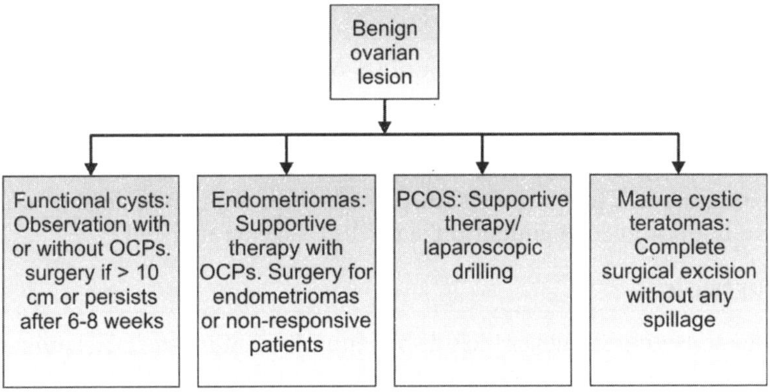

Fig. 18.8: Brief outline of management of benign ovarian lesions

high in adolescents. **Endometriomas** < 2 cm should be coagulated, laser ablated or excised, but if > 2 cm, they should be resected thoroughly. Goals of surgery in endometriosis should be to remove all apparent edometriosis and restore anatomical relations. There is no proven difference between efficacy of open and endoscopic surgery which has the advantages of shorter hospital stay, difficult to notice scar, decreased postoperative pain and recovery time.

The primary aim of treatment in **PCOS** now is improvement in insulin resistance. Lifestyle modification, weight loss of 2-7% and exercise significantly improves ovulatory function and hyperandrogenism. Patients who do not respond well to lifestyle modification alone, may be given supportive therapy with low dose combined OCP, antiandrogens and insulin sensitizing agents like metformin. If surgery is required, ovarian drilling should be preferred over wedge resection.

Surgical management of **mature cystic teratomas** includes only removal of the affected gonad with preservation of ipsilateral tube.

FOLLOW-UP

Adolescents treated for ovarian tumors need **strict vigilance and close follow-up**, particularly if ovarian preservation was attempted. Detailed history, thorough clinical examination, ultrasonography and specific tumor marker are all important integral parts of follow-up. Functional cysts have excellent prognosis. But Patients diagnosed and treated for endometriosis are prone to develop infertility. Hence they should be closely monitored. Likewise, patients of PCOS not only suffer from infertility but may develop potential long-term sequels like NIDDM, endometrial, ovarian and breast cancer. This risk is increased because of prolonged anovulation and continued unopposed estrogen. The relative risk of developing ovarian cancer in patients with PCOS is 4.1.

PROGNOSIS

Prognosis is good for most benign ovarian tumors. Patients with endometriosis or PCOS are likely to develop infertility. In its pure form, mature cystic teratoma of the ovary is always benign, but in approximately 0.2-2% of cases, it may undergo malignant transformation, mainly squamous cell carcinomas. The prognosis for patients with malignant degeneration is generally poor but dependent on stage and degenerated cell type.[13]

SCREENING

Various screening strategies include bimanual/ abdomino-rectal examination, tumor markers, USG. It is a known fact that early diagnosis of ovarian cancers dramatically improves survival, yet routine screening is not recommended for general population.

FERTILITY PRESERVATION

No matter how meticulous the surgery is, some of healthy ovarian follicles are unintentionally removed along with the cyst wall and blood supply jeopardized in some. Therefore while operating on non-malignant ovarian lesions, aim should be to preserve as much ovarian tissue as possible. Meticulous hemostasis and adhesion prevention strategies should be used to improve future fertility. Patients with PCOS should be offered ovarian drilling rather than ovarian wedge resection. Diagnosis of ovarian malignancy should be confirmed before embarking on more extensive surgery. Whenever malignancy is suspected intraoperatively, attempts should be made to preserve atleast one ovary. If there is high suspicion of malignancy preoperatively, prepubertal girls may be offered Gonadal shielding, Oophoropexy, Ovarian tissue cryopreservation or Hormonal gonadoprotection. Likewise postpubertal girls may be offered Embryo freezing with partner/ anonymous donor sperm or Oocyte cryopreservation.

CONCLUSION

Ovarian tumors in adolescents are still quite confusing both in terms of diagnosis and management because they lack early warning signals and management decision has to be made weighing malignant potential and endocrine and reproductive functions. Certainly over the last few decades, better diagnosis and more correct staging have improved peri- and post-operative care. There is still a strong need for a good screening test and novel approaches to treatment. Gynecologists have a serious responsibility because they have to consider the potential for preservation of both endocrine and procreative function while dealing with ovarian tumors in adolescents. Hence, wise decisions must be made based on foundation of accurate diagnosis, current classification, thorough understanding of natural history of various lesions and the opportunities for successful non-operative management.

ACKNOWLEDGMENT

Fig. 18.1 has been taken from the internet, article "Endometriosis", from Wikipedia.
Fig. 18.2 has been taken from the website The OvarianCystCure.com.
Fig. 18.5 has been taken from the website IVF-Infertility.com.
Figs 18.6 and 18.7 have been taken from the website emedicine. medscape.com.

REFERENCES

1. Huffman JW. Ovarian tumors in children and adolescents, in Huffman JW, et al (Eds): The gynecology of childhood and adolescence, 2nd edn Philadelphia: WB Saunders co. 1981.
2. Vercellini P, Fedele L, Arcaini L, Bianchi S, Rognoni MT, Candiani GB. Laparoscopy in the diagnosis of chronic pelvic pain in adolescent women. J Reprod Med 1989;34:827-30.
3. Kontoravdis A, Hassan E, Hassiakos D, Botsis D, Kontoravdis N, Creatsas G. Laparoscopic evaluation and management of chronic pelvic pain during adolescence. Clin Exp Obstet Gynecol 1999;26:76-7.
4. Reese KA, Reddy S, Rock JA. Endometriosis in an adolescent population: the Emory experience. J Pediatr Adolesc Gynecol 1996;9:125-28.
5. Laufer MR, Goitein L, Bush M, Cramer DW, Emans SJ. Prevalence of endometriosis in adolescent girls with chronic pelvic pain not responding to conventional therapy. J Pediatr Adolesc Gynecol 1997;10:199-202.
6. Paula J, Adams Hillard. In: Berek and Novak's Gynecology, 14th edition 2007.
7. JAMA 2004;291:24.
8. Lawson MA, Blythe MJ. Pelvic inflammatory disease in adolescents. Pediatr Clin North Am 1999;46:767-82.
9. Tucci S, Fullterweit W, Conupton ES, et al. Evidence for association of polycystic ovary syndrome in Caucasian women with marker at insulin receptor gene locus. J Clin Endocrinol Metab 2001;86:446-49.
10. Kahsar, Miller MD, Nixon C, Boots LR, Aziz R. The prevalence of polycystic ovaries in first degree relatives of polycystic ovarian syndrome. Fertil Steril 1996;66: 942-47.
11. Dharmesh Kapoor and Willy Davila. 'Endometriosis', eMedicine (2005).
12. Rotterdam ESHRE/ASRM sponsored PCOS consensus workshop group. Revised 2003 Consensus on diagnostic criteria and long term health risks related to Polycystic Ovarian Syndrome. Fertil Steril 2003;81:19-25.
13. Comerci JT Jr, Licciardi F, Bergh PA, Gregori C, Breen JL. Mature cystic teratoma: A clinicopathologic evaluation of 517 cases and review of the literature. Obstet Gynecol. Jul 1994;84(1):22-8.
14. Kumar V, Abbas AK, Fausto N. Robbins and Cotran Pathologic Basis of Disease. 7th ed. Philadelphia: Elsevier Saunders; 2005.
15. Ulbright TM. Gonadal teratomas: a review and speculation. Adv Anat Pathol. Jan 2004;11(1):10-23.
16. Linder D, McCaw BK, Hecht F. Parthenogenic origin of benign ovarian teratomas. N Engl J Med Jan 9 1975;292(2):63-6.
17. Onetto E. Rev. Chil. Soc. Chil. Obst. and Gin. Inf and Adols. 1977, 4(2):11.
18. Arrive L, Hricak H, Martin MC. Pelvic endometriosis: Magnetic Resonance Imaging. Radiology 1989;171:687-92.
19. Patel MD, Feldstein VA, Chen DC, Lipson SD, Filly RA. Endometriomas: Diagnostic performance of Ultrasound. Radiology 1999;210:739-45.

20. Outwater EK, Siegelman ES, Hunt JL. Ovarian teratomas: Tumor types and imaging characteristics. Radiographics Mar-Apr 2001;21(2):475-90.
21. Mais V, Guerriero S, Ajossa S, Angiolucci M, Paoletti AM, Melis GB. Transvaginal ultrasonography in the diagnosis of cystic teratoma. Obstet Gynecol Jan 1995;85(1):48-52.
22. Patel MD, Feldstein VA, Lipson SD, Chen DC, Filly RA. Cystic teratomas of the ovary: Diagnostic value of sonography. AJR Am J Roentgenol Oct 1998;171(4): 1061-5.
23. Scoutt LM, McCarthy SM, Lange R, Bourque A, Schwartz PE. MR evaluation of clinically suspected adnexal masses. J Comput Assist Tomogr Jul-Aug 1994;18(4): 609-18.
24. Martin DC, Hubert GD, Vander Zwaag R, El- Zeky FA. Laparoscopic appearance of peritoneal endometriosis. Fertil Steril 1989;51:63-7.
25. Exacoustos C, Zupi E, Carasotti C, et al. Staging of pelvic endometriosis: role of sonographic appearance in determining extension of disease and ,odulating surgical approach. J Am Assoc Gynecol Laparosc 2003;10:378-82.

19 Adolescent Gynecological Malignancies

Krishna Kavita Ramavath

INTRODUCTION

Adolescence, the developmental period between the childhood and adulthood is a unique stage of life during which rapid physical (biological), cognitive, intellectual (psychological) and emotional maturation occurs.

There are 1.2 billion adolescents worldwide and one in every 5 people in the world is an adolescent. Because of the relatively low cancer incidence, the adolescent and young adult population has not been the focus of attention in cancer control and prevention programs. However, not everybody is free from concerns in this age group. As their intellectual development takes shape, the adolescents (in a state of remission or cure) begin to realize, that there is a chance of recurrence of their past illness, even if it is dim in occurrence and this haunts the young minds. Psychologically these patients may suffer from a lifetime of poor body self image and depression.

Considering the high survival rates of these cancers, physical and psychological long term effects, as well as maintaining quality of life are now important focuses of clinical research.

Adolescent Cancers: Incidence and Magnitude of the Problem

Total incidence of cancer in adolescents ranges from 95 to 225 per million person years and highest rates are recorded in Australia and Israel, while India and Japan are credited with the lowest number.

As per United States, Surveillance Epidemiology and End Results (SEER) program data during 1975-1995, the incidence of cancer in adolescents increased by 30%. UK cancer registry indicates that cancer in 15-19 year old adolescents is 50% higher than in young persons. Therefore over the past 10 years, ever increasing attention has been paid to the needs of adolescents with cancer worldwide.

Beating cancer is possible through Research, Outreach, Education and Screening. They are powerful tools that give us real hope. But when a situation arises, where malignancies are seen in children and young adolescents, it is so disheartening and worrisome because they have greatest impact on those individuals who have most of their potential years of life ahead of them.

It is important to start management of gynecologic cancer with right team and a winning game plan in these adolescents.

PELVIC TUMORS IN ADOLESCENCE

Malignant pelvic tumors in adolescents are rare. Cancers most commonly associated with adolescent females are:

1. Ovarian germ cell tumors
2. Ovarian stromal tumors
3. Genital rhabdomyomas
4. Cervical clear cell adenocarcinomas
5. Gestational trophoblastic tumors
6. Cervical cancer.

With sexual activity among adolescent women increasing, the incidence of cervical cancer and Gestational trophoblastic tumors is rising.

OVARIAN TUMORS

According to National Cancer Institute's SEER program, cancer statistics review (1973-1988), the most common tumors in adolescent females (15-19 years) are germ cell tumors (15%).

Malignant tumors arising in the ovaries of young females (less than 16 years of age) constitute a special group of neoplasms. It is well understood that preservation of ovarian tissue in these patients is essential in order to ensure normal physical development and child bearing potential.

Ovarian tumors are unusual in adolescents and account for less than 1-2% of all neoplasms in females younger than 26 years of age. It is postulated that 5 to 10% of all ovarian tumors appear before the 20s and one-fifth of them precede menarche.

Classification

Based on histogenetic origin ovarian tumors are classified into three predominant classes:

a. Common epithelial tumors
b. Germ cell tumors
c. Sex-cord stromal tumors.

During childhood and adolescence, the incidence of germ cell tumors far exceeds that of the epithelial ones.

Screening/Prevention

There are no known screening and prevention measures for GCTs and Stromal cell cancers. Abnormal enlargement of an ovary might be noticed at the time of an annual pelvic examination, increasing the chance for an early diagnosis and treatment. Girls who have not started menstruating by age 15 should be evaluated and part of this evaluation should include an analysis of the chromosomal abnormality that could predispose to a germ cell cancer.

Germ Cell Tumors of the Ovary (GCT)

All the germ cell tumors share a common cell origin. GCTs are the most common ovarian histologic type diagnosed between the ages of 15-19 years:

a. Germ cell tumors account for 4% of all cancers in children and adolescents under the age of 20 years.
b. GCT of the ovary are aggressive tumors seen most often in young women of pre-teen and adolescent girls and are generally curable if found and treated early.
c. Ovarian GCT can be difficult to diagnose early, as there are no specific symptoms in the early stages. The only symptoms may be a swelling or hard distended abdomen without weight gain. Malignant GCT exhibits an extremely rapid growth pattern. Sudden onset of abdominal pain may be the sign of torsion or rupture.

Histological Typing of Ovarian Germ Cell Tumors: WHO Classification of Tumors

a. Primitive germ cell tumors:
   i. Dysgerminoma
   ii. Endodermal sinus tumor or Yolk sac tumor
   iii. Embryonal carcinoma
   iv. Polyembroma
   v. Non-gestational choriocarcinoma
   vi. Mixed germ cell tumor.
b. Biphasic or Triphasic teratoma:
   i. Immature teratoma
   ii. Mature teratoma
      1. Solid
      2. Cystic:
         a. Dermoid cyst
         b. Fetifom teratoma (homunculus).
c. Monodermal — Highly specialized:
   i. Thyroid Tumor:
      1. Struma ovarii
         a. Benign
         b. Malignant
         c. Neuroectodermal tumor
         d. Carinoma
         e. Melanocytic
         f. Sarcoma
         g. Sabaceous tumor
         h. Pituitary type tumor
         i. Others
   ii. Carcinoid.

Stages of Ovarian Germ Cell Tumors

a. *Stage-I*
   Stage 1A: Cancer is limited to one ovary.
   Stage 1B: Cancer is found in both ovaries.
   Stage 1C: Cancer is found in one or both ovaries and one of the following occurs:

- Cancer is spread to the outside surface of one or both ovaries
- The outer covering of the tumor has ruptured
- Cancer cells are present in the fluid of the peritoneal cavity or in the washings of the peritoneum.

b. *Stage-II*

Stage IIA: Cancer is found in one or both ovaries and has spread into pelvis and/or the uterus and/or the fallopian tubes.

Stage IIB: Cancer is found in one or both ovaries and has spread to other tissues within the pelvis.

Stage IIC: Cancer is found in one or both ovaries, has spread to the uterus, fallopian tubes, and/or other tissues in the pelvis and one of the following occurs:

- Cancer is found on the surface of one or both ovaries
- The outer covering of the tumor has ruptured
- Cancer cells are present in the fluid of the peritoneal cavity or in the washings of the peritoneum.

c. *Stage-III*

Stage IIIA: Cancer is found in one or both ovaries and in pelvis and microscopic cancer cells are found in the peritoneum.

Stage IIIB: Cancer is found in one or both ovaries and has spread to the peritoneum. Peritoneum tumors no longer than 2 cms across, are present in the abdomen. Cancer has not spread to the lymph nodes.

Stage IIIC: Cancer is found in one or both ovaries and has spread beyond pelvis into peritoneum. Peritoneal tumors larger than 2 cms, with lymph node involvement in pelvis and spread to the outer surface of the lever or spread to small bowel or omentum.

d. *Stage-IV*

Cancer is found in one or both ovaries and has metastasized not only in the pelvis and abdomen, but also to other parts of the body.

Dysgerminomas (Fig. 19.1)

They are the most common malignant germ cell tumors, which account for about 30-40% of all ovarian cancers of germ cell origin. They make up 5-10% of ovarian cancers in younger adolescents. They are found in both sexes and may arise in gonadal or extragonadal sites. They are the female equivalent of testicular seminomas.

The histologic characteristics are very distinctive. The large round cells with abundant, clear, pale-staining cytoplasm, conspicuous uniformity of the cell and nuclear size is the hallmark of dysgerminomas. About 65% of dysgerminomas are stage-1 at diagnosis. About 85-90% of stage-1 tumors are confined to one ovary. Dysgerminomas are bilateral in 10-15%.

The clinical presentation is usually of a rapidly growing tumor presenting as an increase in abdominal girth, palpable abdominal mass, with pain and ascites being a feature of advanced disease.

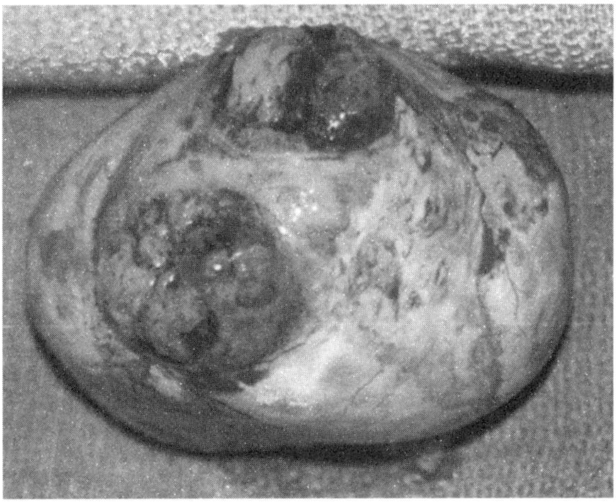

Fig. 19.1: Dysgerminoma (*Courtesy:* img.medscape.com/.jpg)
(For color version, see Plate 2)

5-10% occur in phenotypic females with abnormal gonads. They are associated with pure gonadal dysgenesis (46XY, bilateral streak gonads) or mixed gonadal dysgenesis (45X/46XY, unilateral streak gonad, contralateral testis) with Androgen Insensivity (46XY testicular feminization). It is mandatory that all premenarchal girls with a pelvic mass should undergo a preoperative karyotype because gonadoblastomas can occur in dysgenetic ovaries. Serum LDH is the tumor marker for dysgerminoma and can be used to monitor the response to the therapy.

Treatment

It is based on the degree of malignancy. It is primarily surgical with proper staging. Chemotherapy or radiotherapy is given to patients with metastatic disease. Treatment for these cancers in adolescence should be a **multi-disciplinary setting** and in most cases surgery should be conservative with the aim of preserving sexual and reproductive function. Prognosis for most malignant tumors that occur in adolescence is good.

When there is involvement of opposite ovary, peritoneal involvement and ascites, total abdominal hysterectomy with bilateral salpingo-oophorectomy is required, followed by postoperative radiation as the tumor is radiosensitive.

In less aggressive tumors, unilateral oophorectomy and lymphadenectomy of the affected side followed by chemotherapy may be sufficient, together with careful long-term follow-up.

Radiation Therapy

Dysgerminomas are very sensitive to radiotherapy and doses of 1500 to 3500 cGy may be curative for gross metastatic disease, but the major disadvantage is the loss of fertility.

Chemotherapy

Now regarded as a **treatment of choice** with obvious advantage of preservation of fertility. Combination chemotherapy information for GCT of the ovary is given in Table 19.1.

Table 19.1: Combination chemotherapy for GCT of the ovary

	Regimen and Drugs	*Dose and Schedule*
BEP	Bleomycin	15 units/m^2/wk × 5; then on day 1 of course 4
	Etopside	100 mg/m^2/wk × 5 days every 3 weeks
	Cisplatin	20 mg/m^2/wk × 5 days
		100 mg/m^2/day × 1 day, every 3 weeks
VBP	Vinblastine	0.15 mg/kg/days 1 or 2 every 3 weeks
	Bleomycin	15 units/m^2/wk × 5; then on day 1 of course 4
	Cisplatin	100 mg/m^2/day × 1 day, every 3 weeks
VAC	Vincristine	1-1.5 mg/m^2/day × 1 day, every 4 weeks
	Actinomycin	0.5 mg/m^2/day × 1 day, every 4 weeks
	Cyclophosphomide	150 mg/m^2/day × 1 day, every 4 weeks

Teratomas: Mature Cystic Teratoma, Dermoid Cyst

These are the most common benign neoplasms (38.6%) of the ovary in the adolescent age group. They may be unilateral or bilateral (10%). They are derived from totipotent primordial germ cells and contain ectodermal, mesodermal and endodermal tissue in varying amounts, with a preponderance of skin, sebum and hair (dermoid cyst) (Fig. 19.2), mature brain tissue and intestinal epithelium.

Mature differentiated teratomas are usually benign. Approximately 2% will undergo malignant transformation. Patients may present with abdominal pain or a mass as well as GI symptoms. The presence of a multicystic tumor

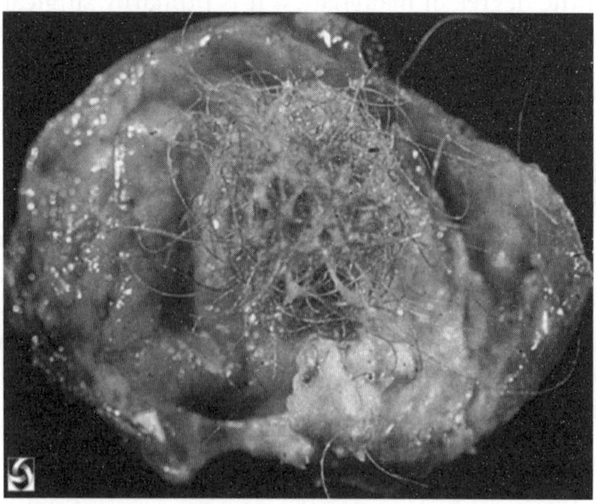

Fig. 19.2: Dermoid cyst (*Courtesy:* theovariancystcure.com) *(For color version, see Plate 2)*

with mixed solid and cystic areas is confirmed on an Ultrasound. X-ray examination may show areas of calcification and teeth like structures.

If thyroid tissue is greater than 50%, it is termed as struma ovarii. It is usually unilateral and very infrequently leads to thyrotoxicosis, upto one-third patients develop ascites and some may develop hydrothorax (Meig's syndrome). Ovarian torsion and also spontaneous rupture may be seen in 1-3%.

Treatment

Current **state of art** in the surgical treatment includes, resection of the cystic teratoma without spillage of tumor contents and taking care to preserve as much of the affected ovary as possible.

Close inspection of the contralateral ovary should be done for the evidence of bilateral disease.

The various options available for surgical approach must be considered in this age group. Traditionally, patients in these clinical situations have undergone open laparotomy. More recently with technological advances more surgical options are available. The use of **minimally invasive Surgical techniques** like **laparoscopy and Robotic surgeries** have shown to be generally safe and effective. This type of Robotic surgery is best performed by a surgeon experienced with ovarian cancer, such as **a gynecological oncologist.**

Compared with long instruments used in endoscopy, Robotic surgical systems use smaller instruments that provide increased range of motion. This can be very helpful when operating on children and adolescents.

Chemotherapy

It is the treatment of choice. The dosage schedule is same as described earlier.

Endodermal Sinus Tumors (EST) of the Ovary

They are the most common ovarian malignant GCT in pediatric and adolescent age group. As they are derived from primitive yolk sac, EST have also been referred to as yolk sac carcinomas.

EST occurs in patients with median age group of 16-18 years. One-third of the patients are premenarchal at the time of diagnosis. The EST are unilateral in 100% of cases; thus biopsy of the opposite ovary in such young patients is contraindicated. They are always large (> 15 cm). Cystic areas with hemorrhage and necrosis are seen in these rapidly growing tumors. The histological hallmark of EST is **Schiller-Duval Body** (Fig. 19.3).

Presenting Symptoms

Abdominal or pelvic pain or abdominal enlargement. Asymptomatic pelvic mass is seen in 100%. Many EST secrete AFP, as they are derived from primitive Gut and Liver.

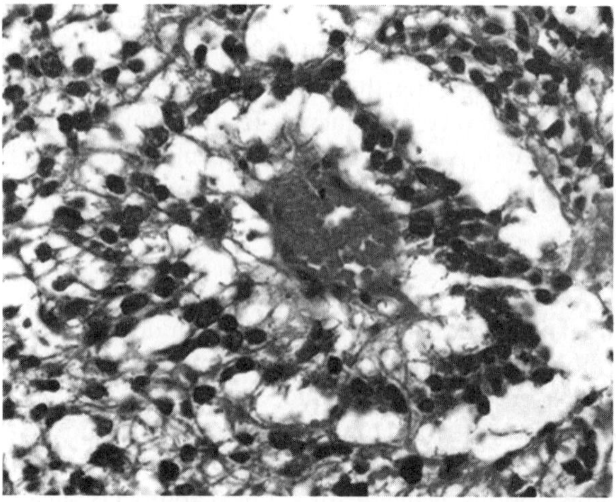

Fig. 19.3: Schiller-Duval body (*Courtesy*: web pathology-visual survey of surgical pathology) *(For color version, see Plate 3)*

Treatment

Surgery

The treatment of EST consists of surgical exploration, unilateral salpingo-oophorectomy and a frozen section for diagnosis.

Bilaterality is not seen in these lesions. Staging and tumor cytoreduction are not necessary as all points with EST are treated with adjuvant or therapeutic chemotherapy.

Chemotherapy

VPB (Vinblastine, Cisplatin, Bleomycin) is a more effective regimen than **VAC** (Vincristin, Actinomycin, Cyclophosphamide) in the treatment of these tumors. This protocol has improved survival rates and furthermore, with conservative surgery and adjuvant chemotherapy, fertility can be preserved in these adolescent girls. For high risk GCTs of any histological type, with massive metastatic disease, cisplatin containing combination chemotherapy, preferably **BEP** (Bleomycin, Etopside, Cisplatin) or **POMB-ACE** (Vincristine, Bleomycin, Cisplatin, Etopside, Actinomycin-D, Cyclophosphamide), should be used.

EMBRYONAL CARCINOMA OF THE OVARY (FIG. 19.4)

It is an extremely rare tumor which accounts for about 4% of all ovarian GCTs. It is a highly malignant tumor and diagnosed before puberty in 50% of patients. Presenting signs and symptoms include an abdominal mass (80%) abdominal pain (53%) or both.

Embryonal carcinomas secrete estrogens and many patients present with precocious pseudopuberty or irregular bleeding. Many of these tumors secrete β-hCG and AFP which are used as tumor markers.

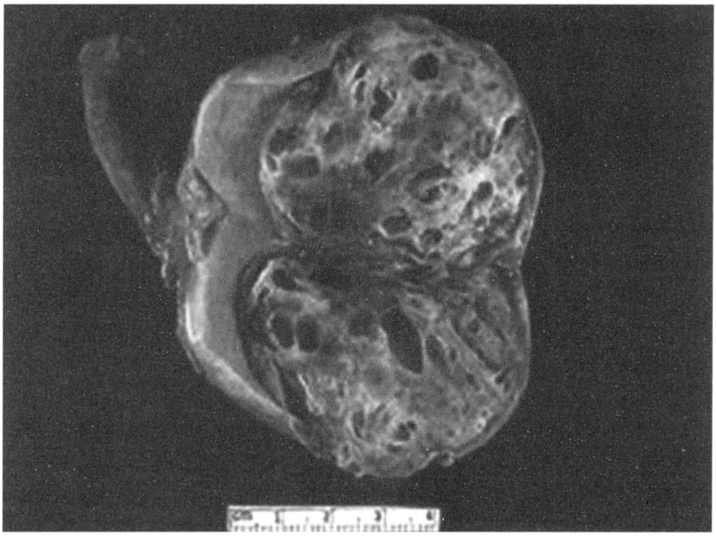

Fig. 19.4: Embryonal carcinoma of the ovary (*Courtesy*: Chad A Hamilton, MD, Walter Reed Army Medical Center emedicine:webmed) *(For color version, see Plate 3)*

Primary lesions are large and about two-thirds are confined to one ovary at the time of diagnosis. Sixty percent of patients present with Stage 1A disease. Treatment is similar to that of ESTs.

POLYEMBRYOMA

These are extremely rare tumors which are composed of "embryoid bodies" replicating the structures of early embryonic differentiation. Most polyembryomas occur before puberty with a median age of presentation at 12 years.

The symptoms may be precocious pseudopuberty, abdominal distention and vaginal bleeding. Elevated levels of tumor markers like Human Placental Lactogen (HPL), AFP and β-hCG may be seen. Treatment is anecdotal and may consist of surgery followed by combination chemotherapy.

CHORIOCARCINOMA OF THE OVARY (FIG. 19.5)

Non-gestational choriocarcinoma is again an extremely rare tumor of the ovary. It has same appearance as gestational choriocarcinoma.

Most patients are in the pediatric age group and younger than 20 years. Isosexual precocity occurs in 50%. After puberty, the patients may present with vaginal bleeding and elevated levels of β-hCG, mimicking an ectopic pregnancy.

Patients usually present at an advanced stage and prognosis is poor due to metatstasis.

Combination chemotherapy with BEP or MAC regimen (Methotrexate, Actinomycin-D and Cyclophosphamide) may offer complete responses.

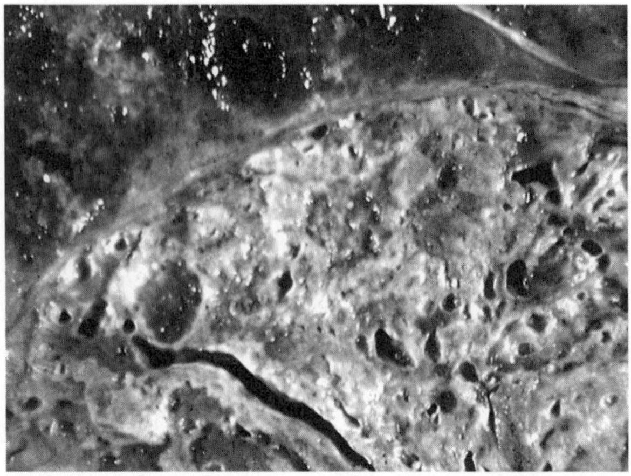

Fig. 19.5: Choriocarcinoma of the ovary (*Courtesy:* Cancercare)
(For color version, see Plate 3)

MIXED GERM CELL TUMORS

Mixed GCT of the ovary contains two or more elements of GCT and account for 8% of malignant ovarian GCTs. Commonest combination is dysgerminoma and Endodermal Sinus Tumor (EST). The mean age at the diagnosis is 16. These girls often present with precocious puberty, as the mixed lesions secrete either AFP, HCG, both or none, depending on the components. Presenting symptoms may be an abdominal mass or pain.

These lesions should be managed by appropriate fertility preserving staging operations and post-op chemotherapy with BEP regimen. Prognosis is dependent on the size of the primary tumor and also its most malignant component.

GONADOBLASTOMA

These tumors have both germ cell and sex-cord stromal component. They occur in girls in their teens. Eighty percent of these patients are phenotypical females with virilization and 20% are phenotypical males with cryptorchidism, hypospadias and female internal secondary sex organs. Over 95% have an abnormal karyotype with a Y chromosome. Most of the tumors are bilateral and in 50% of cases gonadoblastoma is overgrown by Dysgerminoma or Immature teratoma, Endodermal Sinus Tumor or Choriocarcinoma.

Treatment of these tumors in the presence of a Y chromosome requires bilateral oophorectomy with preservation of the uterus if desired.

SEX-CORD STROMAL TUMORS OF THE OVARY (SCST)

They comprise 5-8% of all ovarian malignancies. These tumors arise from sex cords and stroma (mesenchyme) of the embryonic ovary. They are made up of the granulosa and theca cells, the testicular components of Sertoli and Leydig cells and fibroblasts.

Patients often present with precocious puberty, abnormal vaginal bleeding due to excess estrogen and virilization, clitoromegaly or male-pattern hair distribution due to excess androgen production.

GRANULOSA – STROMAL CELL TUMORS

The granulosa cell tumors are rare, accounting to about 1-2% of all ovarian malignancies. They are seen in women of all ages and are found in prepubertal girls in 5% of cases. GCT often secrete **inhibin** which serves as a useful serum tumor marker.

Juvenile Germ Cell Tumors

Account for 5% of all ovarian tumors with more than 50% of tumors diagnosed in patients younger than 20 years and 5% occurring before puberty. They present with sexual pseudo precocity because of estrogen secretion. In post pubertal girls they are associated with menorrhagia or secondary amenorrhea.

Juvenile GCTs can be a component of various syndromes including **Potter's syndrome** when they occur with multiple congenital anomalies, **Ollier's disease**, when they occur with endochondromatosis and **Maffucci's syndrome**, when they occur with endochondromatosis and hemangiomatosis.

Treatment

Unilateral salpingo-oophorectomy with staging is appropriate. Advanced tumors are successfully treated with platinum based combination chemotherapy, i.e. BEP.

SERTOLI-LEYDIG CELL TUMORS

Extremely rare and account for less than 0.2% of ovarian cancer. Less than 5% of these tumors occur before puberty. Excess androgen secretion leads to virilization in 70 to 85% of patients. Rarely they are associated with isosexual precocity due to excess estrogen. These neoplasms may produce AFP. In patients who desire to preserve their fertility, unilateral salpingo-oophorectomy and staging is appropriate. Treatment of recurrent disease is done with pelvic irradiation and VAC regimen. The five years survival rate is 70-90%. Poorly differentiated tumor results in poor prognosis.

EPITHELIAL OVARIAN TUMORS

Epithelial ovarian tumors in pediatric and adolescent age group account for about 19% of all ovarian tumors. They occur almost exclusively after puberty with mean age of diagnosis around 14-19 years. Most common symptoms at presentation are dysmenorrhea, abdominal pain, abdominal distension, nausea, vomiting and vaginal discharge.

Borderline tumors are of low malignant potential and are mostly seen in adolescents and account for the prolonged survival. Unilateral salpingo-oophorectomy and staging leads to excellent survival and reproductive outcomes.

With sexual activity among adolescent women increasing, the statistics record an increase in the incidence of cervical cancer and Gestational trophoblastic tumors. This chapter focuses on the important considerations of these two malignancies.

GESTATIONAL TROPHOBLASTIC DISEASE (GTD) (FIG. 19.6)

Gestational trophoblastic disease (GTD) describes a group of interrelated neoplasms derived from the trophoblastic cells of the fetal chorion. They include trophoblastic lesions arising from the chorionic villi (hydatidiform mole—complete and partial) and those trophoblastic lesions without villi (placental site trophoblastic tumor and choriocarcinoma).

GTD is among the rare human tumors that can be cured even in the presence of wide spread dissemination. These tumors produce β-hCG, a clinically useful tumor marker. The most important microscopic features are enlarged edematous villi and abnormal trophoblastic proliferation. DNA flow and image cytometric analysis of nuclear DNA content are helpful in distinguishing a partial mole from a complete mole.

Only the salient points of the management of this tumor are considered here.

Any woman of reproductive age with vaginal bleeding should be evaluated with serum or urine β-hCG to exclude pregnancy as a contributing factor. When an abnormal pregnancy is diagnosed, the usual treatment is dilatation and curettage.

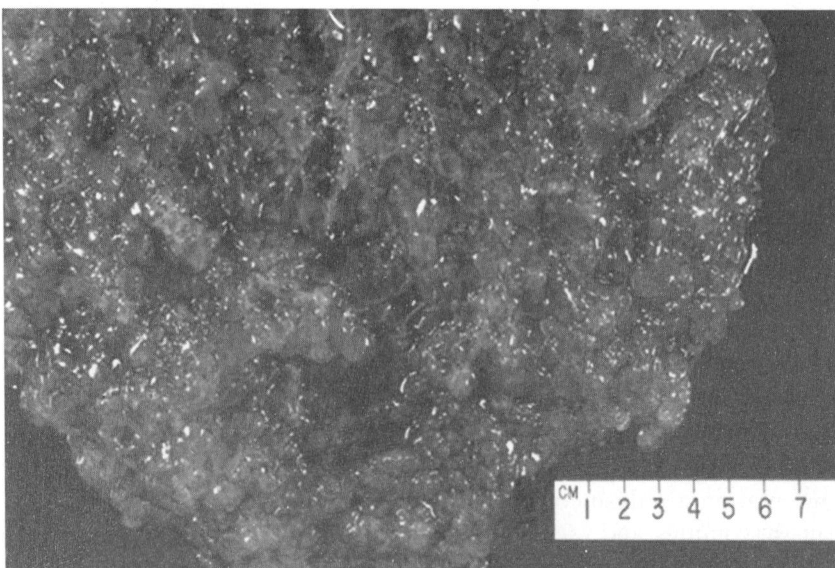

Fig. 19.6: GTD (*Courtesy:* cancer care) *(For color version, see Plate 4)*

SURVEILLANCE AFTER DIAGNOSIS OF GESTATIONAL TROPHOBLASTIC DISEASE

After evacuation of the GTD, surveillance with serial testing of β-hCG is mandatory.

The levels decrease within 48 hours after the surgical procedure, and then every week until three normal levels are recorded. Thereafter, β-hCG levels are evaluated monthly for 6 to 12 months. Effective contraception is necessary during the surveillance period to avoid misinterpretation of pregnancy or persistent or recurrent disease. In patients who demonstrate plateau or increase in β-hCG levels, malignant GTD is diagnosed, and additional therapy is required. These patients need CT of chest, abdomen and pelvis for establishing the anatomic distribution of the disease and for staging purposes.

Management

Therapy is individualized after identifying the high risk (poor prognosis), and low risk (good prognosis) disease. Recently International Federation of Gynecology and Obstetrics (FIGO) proposed a combined scoring and staging system based on the anatomic distribution of disease and risk factors.

In patients with low-risk disease, chemotherapy with either methotrexate or actinomycin D leads to cure in up to 90% of cases. In those who do not respond completely to this treatment, therapy with multi-agent chemotherapy with Etopside, Methotrexate, Actinomycin D, Cyclophosphamide, and Vincristine (EMA-CO) is required for cure.

Hysterectomy is required as a primary treatment in women who are not interested in further childbearing. Some may need thoracotomy or craniotomy for resection of metastasis not responding to chemotherapy.

Follow-up

For patients with malignant GTD after treatment, follow-up includes weekly β-hCG for 3 weeks, and then monthly until normal for 12 months. Contraception is imperative for 1 year following treatment.

UTERINE NEOPLASMS

Uterine neoplasms are rare and are often malignant when discovered in this population. Vaginal bleeding is the usual presenting symptom. Ultra radical surgery including total pelvic exenteration was done previously. Current Surgical practices are employing **minimally invasive surgeries and robotics** in this field and sometimes this may result in the ability to preserve reproductive function.

UTERINE SARCOMAS

These are typically diagnosed in postmenopausal women, but carcinosarcoma, one of the three main classifications of uterine sarcomas is commonly reported in adolescents.

These tumors are generally treated with hysterectomy and postoperative chemotherapy or radiotherapy or hormonal therapy. Recent reports of local resection with conservation of fertility have suggested good outcomes.

ENDOMETRIAL HYPERPLASIA AND CARCINOMA

This is the most common malignancy of the female genital tract which occurs typically in postmenopausal and obese women. This is exceedingly rare in adolescent population. It can be seen in pediatric age females associated with morbid obesity and also seen in patients with Turner's syndrome taking unopposed estrogen therapy, or with polycystic ovarian syndrome (PCOS). These patients generally present with irregular vaginal bleeding. Without treatment progression to invasive cancer occurs in 25% of the patients.

In adolescents since fertility preservation is important, the treatment with progestins (medroxyprogesterone Acetate 10 mg/day) often leads to regression of endometrial hyperplasia.

With well differentiated endometrial adenocarcinoma, these patients can be treated with high dose progestins, which successfully allows for fertility in 50% of them after treatment. They require a repeat biopsy in 3to 6 months to ensure normalization of hyperplasia or cancer. Persistent cancer or hyperplasia may require hysterectomy.

MALIGNANCIES OF CERVIX AND VAGINA

Malignancies of the external genitalia are extremely rare and uncommon, but some gynecological malignancies of vagina and cervix have greater incidence of the pediatric population. These include mullerian Rhabdomyosarcoma (RMS), Endodermal sinus tumors (EST), Diethyl-stilbesterol (DES) related vaginal and cervical cancers.

In addition, due to high incidence of sexual activity in adolescents it is observed that four out of five sexually active adolescent females were infected with Human Papilloma Virus (HPV), which is responsible for genital warts and carcinoma cervix later in life.

RHABDOMYOSARCOMA (RMS)

Also known as the sarcoma botryoides, rhabdomyosarcoma is the most commonly occurring soft tissue sarcoma in children younger than 15 years. Genitourinary sites comprise 20% of the primary locations of these tumors. They arise in perineum, vulva, uterus and cervix. Peak incidence has been reported to be in girls below 2 years of age with 90% occurring in girls below 5 years, although, it may occur in the cervix in older girls and adolescents.

The presenting features are usually of blood stained foul smelling vaginal discharge with frank bleeding or grape like mass protruding from the introitus (botrys in Greek is for grapes).

The tumor originates in the subepithelial layer of the cervical or vaginal epithelium and spreads within this layer producing a classical polypoid appearance before invading the vaginal wall. Later spread is via lymphatic and blood stream.

Treatment requires biopsy for histologic confirmation that is done at the time of Examination Under Anesthesia (EUA).

Treatment

Treatment options for RMS have undergone a significant change. In the past, radical pelvic exenteration (removal of bladder, colon, vagina, uterus and ovaries) was the primary therapy for these tumors. With this, there is poor survival and physical and psychological morbidity is more common. Current options include chemotherapy and local excision for certain cervical tumors.

Intergroup Rhabdomyosarcoma Study Group (IRSG) trail demonstrates, that less radical surgery (with preservation of pelvic organs when feasible) with chemotherapy consisting of Vincristine, Actinomycin-D, and Cyclophosphamide (VAC) with or without radiation leads to survival rates upto 90% for nonmetastatic disease.

The **novel approach** to treat this malignancy is with minimal invasive techniques. The reasons supporting this approach as the ideal one are:

- Shorter hospital stay, decreased postoperative pain and shorter recovery
- Wound infections are less common
- This is especially important in morbidly obese patients where seroma and hematoma formation are a common phenomenon.

The use of Robotic assisted laparoscopy offers further improvements. It achieves better visualization through use of a 3D image. Also the endowristed instrumentation allows for more precise anatomic dissection. In addition, there is increased surgeon comfort and decreased fatigue (Fig. 19.7).

The first Robotic surgery on embryonal RMS is done on an African adolescent female at 18 years of age with morbid obesity > 47 kg/m^2 in March 2007 by Jefferey M Fowler and others from The Ohio State University College of Medicine, USA.

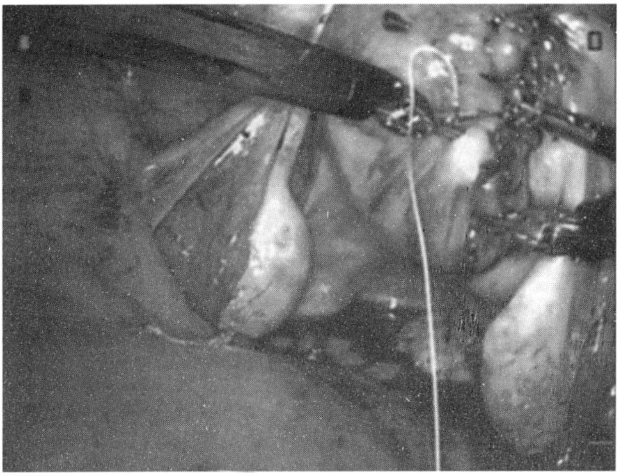

Fig. 19.7: Robotic surgery of RMS (*Courtesy*: Intuitive Surgical Systems, Sunnyvale, CA) *(For color version, see Plate 4)*

The authors have concluded saying that Robotic surgery can be safely and successfully applied to Radical hystercetomy and lymphadenectomy for uterine rhabdomyosarcoma.

This minimally invasive approach allows the patient a faster recovery and minimizes the time between surgery and initiation of adjuvant treatment.

CLEAR CELL ADENOCARCINOMA

Diethylstilbesterol was approved for use in the prevention of spontaneous abortion and preterm delivery from 1940s until 1971. Herbst and Scully reported primary vaginal clear cell adenocarcinoma in young women exposed to DES *in utero* and the drug was immediately withdrawn from the market. Approximately 3 million women were exposed to DES in the United States. Two-thirds of the girls exposed to DES have congenital abnormalities of the cervix like pseudopolyp formation, hypertrophy of endocervical tissue and vaginal abnormalities including incomplete septa, fibrous bands and vaginal adenosis.

The predominant symptom is vaginal bleeding and the risk of cancer is 0.14-1.4 per 1000 and therefore, merits colposcopy, follow-up from early teens.

Treatment

For early stage disease (90% of cases), radical hysterectomy and vaginectomy, lymphadenectomy with or without vaginal reconstruction are appropriate. For smaller, minimally invasive tumors, cervical cone biopsy or local vaginal resection with radiation may allow for uterine preservation and the potential for fertility.

SQUAMOUS CELL CARCINOMA OF THE CERVIX (FIG. 19.8)

With the increasing prevalence of HPV exposure in adolescent population, the higher incidence of cervical dysplasia is being diagnosed in these populations. The risk of cervix cancer is increasing. This group of population should undergo HPV vaccination (Fig. 19.9), and screening for early detection and prevention.

Vulvar malignancies in the adolescents are exceedingly rare. Literature shows only few documented cases of vulvar cancer in women younger than 20, the youngest being 13.

High grade vulvar intraepithelial neoplasia, a precursor lesion to squamous cell carcinoma of the vulva is being diagnosed with increased frequency on younger women because of sexual exposure to HPV.

Treatment

Optimizing chances for cure while minimizing disfiguring radical procedures, multi-modality therapy including limited resection of the tumor mass combined with chemotherapy and radiotherapy is the standard of care.

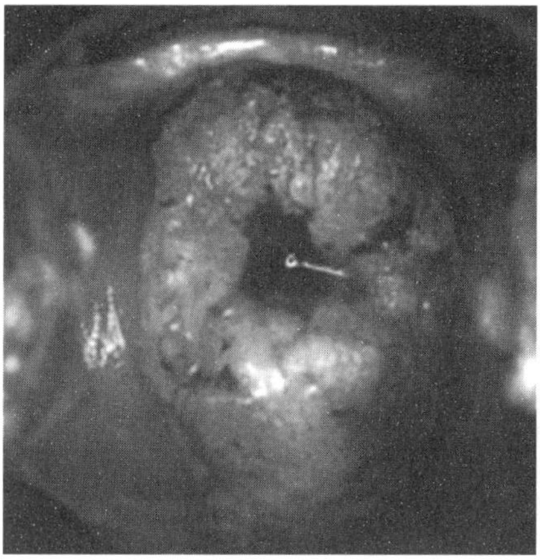

Fig. 19.8: Cervical cancer *(For color version, see Plate 4)*

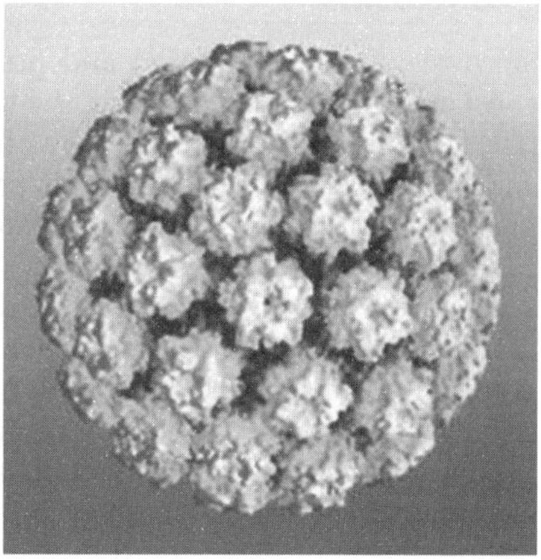

Fig. 19.9: HPV (*Courtesy*: Citizendium, citizens compendium) *(For color version, see Plate 4)*

With this pretext of adolescent gynecological malignancies, the challenges to a gynecological oncologist are obvious. In addition to the dreaded disease, the complexity of physical and mental health of these adolescents is a concern. So the approach to the management needs delicate skills and reasoning. Because they are not in the full adulthood but in the transitional state, the multidisciplinary approach of the management with balance and flexibility suits them most.

FERTILITY PRESERVATION AND FUTURE

Preservation of fertility is important to adolescent and young adult survivors of cancer. Many survivors will maintain their reproductive potential after the successful completion of treatment for cancer. However total-body irradiation, radiation to the gonads, and chemotherapy regimens containing high-dose alkylators can place women at risk for acute ovarian failure or premature menopause.

The risk of compromised fertility depends on multiple factors, including the age of the patient, type of therapy, dose and duration of therapy, and type of tumor. Fortunately, it is now possible for young people seeking to preserve their fertility to consider a range of therapeutic interventions. These include the use of gonadotrophin-releasing hormone (GnRH) analogs during chemotherapy in an attempt to protect the ovaries, gamete collection and freezing for subsequent artificial insemination or *in vitro* fertilization (IVF), freezing of ovarian tissue in the hope that oocyte harvest might be possible in the future, and surgical transposition of ovaries out of radiation treatment fields. However, many of these techniques remain experimental with, as yet, unproven benefits.

CONCLUSION

Survival rates of childhood and pre-pubertal female cancer patients are constantly increasing. However, the lifesaving treatments carry a significant risk for infertility. Chemotherapy and radiotherapy might induce oocyte and follicular loss, infertility and premature ovarian failure. In order to preserve the fertility potential, several options are currently available, many of those should be considered as experimental.

Ovarian transposition out of the radiation field may considerably reduce the radiation dose and should be considered for patients younger than 40 years of age. Embryo cryopreservation is a well established technique. Oocyte cryopreservation or vitrification can also be performed.

Ovarian tissue cryopreservation has the potential of preserving thousands of primordial follicles. The thawed ovarian tissue can be autotransplanted orthotopically or heterotopically.

Until now, only one human live birth has been reported. The strategy for preservation of fertility prior to cancer treatment should be tailored according to the patient's age.

ACKNOWLEDGMENTS

My special thanks to Prof. Magrina. F. Javier, Mayo Clinic, Dept. of Gynecology, Scottsdale, Arizona for his guidance in bringing out this article.

My sincere thanks to Intutive Surgical Systems, image.medscape.com, ovariancystcure center, emedicinewebMD, Citizendium Citizens Compendium, web pathology, visual survey of surgical pathology and patho doc for the image courtesy.

SUGGESTED READING

1. Rubin SC, Lewis Jr JL. Tumor antigens in ovarian malignancy. Clin Obstet Gynecol 1986;29:693-704.
2. Red Orbit:Gynecologic Malignancies in Adolescents.
3. Tsai JY, Saigo PE, Brown C, LaQuglia MP. Diagnosis, pathology, staging, treatment and outcome of epithelial ovarian neoplasia in patients age < 21 years. Cancer 2001;11:2065-70.
4. Young JL, Wu XC, Roffers SD, Howe HL, Correa C, Weinstein R. Ovarian cancer in children and young adults in the United States, 1992-1997. Cancer 2003;97:2694-700.
5. Elford KJ, Spence JH. The forgotten female: pediatric and adolescent gynecological cancers and their reproductive consequences. J Pediatr Adolesc Gynecol 2002;15:65-77.
6. Falcone T, Aharan M, Bedaiwy MA, Goldberg JM. Ovarian function preservation in the cancer patient. Fertil Steril 2004;81:243-57.
7. Chen VW, Ruiz B, Killeen JL, Cote TR, Wu XC, Correa CN. Pathology and classification of ovarian tumors. Cancer 2003;97:2631-42.
8. Zalel Y, Piura B, Elchalal U, Czernobilsky B, Antebi S, Dgani R. Diagnosis and management of malignant germ cell ovarian tumors in young females. Int J Gynaecol Obstet 1996;55:1-10.

9. Schneider DT, Calaminus G, Wessalowski R, Pothmanathan R, Selle B, Sternschulte W, et al. Ovarian sex-cord stromal tumors in children and adolescents. J Clin Oncol 2003;21:2357-63.
10. Massimi P and L Banks. Repression of p53 transcriptional activity by the HPV E7 proteins. Virology 1997;227(1):255-59.
11. McDonald C. Cancer statistics, 1999: Challenges in minority populations. CA Cancer J Clin 1999;49(1):6-7.
12. Mitchell MF, et al. A randomized clinical trial of cryotherapy, loop electrosurgical excision and laser vaporization for treatment of squamous intraepithelial lesions of the cervix. Am J Obstet Gynecol 92:737-44.
13. Moscicke AB, et al. Risk factors for abnormal anal cytology in young heterosexual women. J Cancer Epidemiol Biomarkers Prev 1999;8(2):173-78.
14. Olatunbosun OA, Okonofua FE, Ayangade SO. Outcome of cryosurgery for cervical intraepithelial neoplasia in a developing country. Int J Gynaec Obst 1992;38: 305-10.
15. Palank C. An introduction to colposcopy concepts, controversies and guidelines. ADVANCE for Nurse Practitioners 1998;6(10):45-50,91.
16. Roden RB, DR Lowy and JT Schiller. Papillomavirus is resistant to desiccation. J Infect Dis 1997;176(4):1076-79.

20 Anemia in Adolescents

Jayam Kannan, Malathi G Prasad

INTRODUCTION

Anemia afflicts an estimated two billion people worldwide, mostly due to iron deficiency. It primarily affects women. Yet among adolescents, prevalence rates of anemia are closer for males and females in some parts of the world. The prevalence of anemia is disproportionately high in developing countries, due to poverty, inadequate diet, certain diseases, pregnancy and lactation, and poor access to health services. Young people are particularly susceptible because of their rapid growth and associated high iron requirements.

Anemia is a critical health concern because it affects growth and energy levels. In pregnancy it is associated with premature births, low birth weight, and perinatal and maternal mortality.

Adolescence is an opportune time for interventions to address anemia. In addition to growth needs, girls need to improve iron status before pregnancy. And both boys and girls are more accessible to information about anemia through schools, recreational activities and via the mass media than they will be later in their lives.

About 27% of adolescents are estimated to be anemic in developing countries compared to 6% in developed countries. Regional figures although varying by country and the region, WHO estimates that over 1/3 of the world's population suffers from anemia. India continues to be one of the countries with the highest prevalence of anemia. National family health survey estimates reveal the prevalence of anemia to be around 70 to 80% in children. Prevalence of anemia in India is high because of low dietary intake, poor availability of iron and chronic blood loss due to hook worm infestation and malaria.

CONSEQUENCES OF ANEMIA IN ADOLESCENTS

The health consequences of anemia in children and adolescents are well documented. In children, anemia affects physical growth and mental development. Other consequences including reduced levels of energy and productivity and impaired immune system functions develop as children mature. Boys and girls both need iron for growth during adolescence and girls have a continuing need to replace iron lost during menstruation.

RISK FACTORS

Risk factors for anemia in adolescents:

- Low intake of meat, fish, poultry or iron fortified foods
- Frequent dieting or restricted eating
- Vegan or vegetarian eating styles
- Meal skipping
- Chronic or significant weight loss
- Heavy menstrual periods
- Rapid growth, overweight and obese
- Participation in endurance sports
- Intensive physical training.

ANEMIA PREVENTION AND CONTROL

There are several national programs targeted at control and treatment of anemia during pregnancy. Indian Government started a National Anemia Prophylaxis Program in 1970 targeting pregnant and lactating women. Subsequently the program was modified and renamed the National Anemia Control Program (NACP) in 1991 for control and prevention of anemia in women of reproductive age and lactating women and pre-school children. These programs have been operational for over 35 years but have made a little difference on the overall prevalence of anemia during pregnancy. Several other programs focusing on issue of anemia include ICDS, Mid–day meal program, Kishori Swasthya Yojna, Matri Suraksha Abhiyan, IMA Anemia Free India, as a public-private partnership and Anemia Chale Jao, etc. 12 by 12 initiative is currently is being adopted to decrease the rate of anemia in adolescent population.

Appropriate anemia prevention and control program for adolescents do not exist in any country. UNICEF has initiated Adolescent Anemia Project in 11 states and has demonstrated significant improvement in hemoglobin level.

JUSTIFICATION FOR TARGETING ADOLESCENT ANEMIA

Adolescence is a period of rapid growth when iron requirement for both girls and boys increases. The incidence of iron deficiency amongst adolescents is rising. The awareness regarding anemia and appropriate diet is extremely poor in adolescents which is made worse by the lucrative promotional media.

Recommended Iron for School-Aged Children

Age (years)	Iron Intake (mg/day)
4-8	4
9-13	8
14-18	11 (boys)
	15 (girls)

Studies have shown that adolescents with anemia have decreased verbal learning and memory as well as lower standardized math scores. Even before anemia might develop, iron deficiency can cause shortened attention span, alertness and learning in adolescents.

There is evidence though that correcting the iron deficiency may improve learning. A study of adolescent girls with iron deficiency showed that their test scores improved after receiving iron supplements. Fortunately there are steps parents can take to prevent and treat iron deficiency and iron deficiency anemia in their kids.

Risk Groups

Adolescents with chronic illness, heavy menstrual blood loss (> 80 mL/month), or who are underweight or malnourished are at increased risk for iron deficiency. Overweight and obese children may also have iron deficiency and is also associated with low hemoglobin. Adolescents participating in endurance training and athletes are also at a higher risk for iron deficiency.

Iron Requirements

The minimum daily dietary iron requirement during adolescence is 12 to 15 mg/day. There is a misconception that only girls need iron during adolescence though requirement for growing boys also jumps up significantly. Iron requirements increase from approximately 1.0 mg/day of absorbed iron to approximately 2.5 mg/day during pubertal growth spurt in boys and by the end of adolescence decreases to the previous level of 1.0 mg/day. The peak requirement for absorbed iron in girls reaches a maximum of approximately 1.5 mg/day during puberty and remains at about 1.3 mg/day after puberty to replace menstrual blood loss. The deficiency gets further aggravated by not eating high iron containing foods (such as meat) as well as poor bioavailability of iron due to food habits. In early stages of iron deficiency, iron stores can be depleted without overt anemia but any further loss precipitates anemia.

Clinical Features

Adolescent anemia is like the tip of an iceberg, major part of iron deficiency is hidden as most adolescents with anemia are asymptomatic. A few may notice weakness, headache, irritability, fatigue, low physical performance, exercise intolerance and poor cognitive function. Pica or perverted appetite may occur in some adolescents. Pagophagia or pica for ice is considered quite specific for the iron deficiency state. The tragedy is that most of them are not even associated with anemia. Very few realize that just a few milligrams of iron can improve their memory or physical performance.

Adolescent girls performed significantly better on a test of verbal learning and memory after iron supplementation. In another study there was significant improvement in test scores following iron supplementation in both boys and girls. A study evaluating physical performance before and after iron supplementation showed significant improvement in treadmill endurance times in iron treated runners.

Diagnosis

Adolescent anemia is easy to diagnose and easy to treat. Yet it is rampant and not being identified as majority of the youth are not even aware of what is hemoglobin (Hb) or iron. Since iron deficiency is the most common cause of anemia in India, any one with significant pallor or hemoglobin less than 12 g% should be suspected to have iron deficiency anemia. Confirmatory tests include a complete blood count with red blood cell indices and serum ferritin. This will also help in identifying other causes of anemia.

Good food sources of iron include the following:

- Meat: Lamp, Liver and other organ meats
- Poultry: Chicken, duck, turkey, liver (especially dark meat)
- Fish: Shellfish including clams, mussels, oysters, sardines and anchovies
- Leafy greens of the cabbage family, such as broccoli, kale, turnip greens, and collards
- Legumes such as lima beans and green peas, dry beans and peas, such as pinto beans, black eyed peas, and canned baked beans
- Breads: Yeast leavened whole wheat bread and rolls, iron enriched white bread, pasta, rice and cereals.

Treatment

Treatments for anemia depend on severity and cause.

Iron deficiency from nutritional causes is rare in non-menstruating adults (men and post-menopausal women). The diagnosis of iron deficiency mandates a search for potential sources of loss such as gastrointestinal bleeding from ulcers or colon cancer. Mild to moderate iron deficiency anemia is treated by oral iron supplementation with ferrous sulfate, ferrous fumarate or ferrous gluconate. When taking iron supplements, it is very common to experience stomach upset and/or darkening of the feces. The stomach upset can be alleviated by taking the iron with food. However, this decreases the amount of iron absorbed. Vitamin C, aids in the body's ability to absorb iron, hence taking oral iron supplements with orange juice is of benefit.

Vitamin supplements given orally (folic acid) or subcutaneously (vitamin B_{12}) will replace specific deficiencies.

In anemia of chronic disease, anemia associated with chemotherapy, or anemia associated with renal disease, some clinicians prescribe recombinant erythropoietin, epoetin alfa to stimulate red blood cell production.

In severe cases of anemia or with ongoing blood loss, a blood transfusion may be necessary.

PRINCIPLES GOVERNING USE OF ORAL IRON

Iron is best absorbed from the duodenum and proximal jejunum. The expensive enteric coated or sustained release capsules which release iron further down to avoid gastric irritation are not absorbed well.

Iron tablet should not be taken with food as the phosphates, phytates, and tannates in food bind the iron and impair its absorption. Iron should preferably be taken two hours before or four hours after ingestion of antacids. Other inhibitors like tea, coffee, herbal drinks, calcium, etc. should not be consumed with iron tablets.

Iron is best absorbed in ferrous form in a mildly acidic medium. Adding a 250 mg ascorbic acid tablet at the time of iron administration enhances iron absorption.

The iron preparation used should be based upon cost and effectiveness with minimal side effects.

The cheapest preparation of iron is ferrous sulfate tablet with 300 mg of iron salt containing 60 mg elemental iron.

The gastric discomfort is directly related to the amount of elemental iron ingested. The preparations reported to have low incidence of side effects usually have low elemental iron content.

CONCLUSION

It is important to realize that anemia needs to be eradicated in the adolescent population as a part of adolescent health and well being. This can be achieved by active participation of all the practitioners with implementation of strategies to detect and treat anemia.

SUGGESTED READING

1. Alton I. Iron deficiency anemia. In: Stang M, Story M, eds. Guidelines for Adolescent Nutrition Services. Minneapolis, MN: Center for Leadership, Education and Training in Maternal and Child Nutrition, Division of Epidemiology and Community Health, School of Public Health, University of Minnesota; 2005:101-08.
2. Centers for Disease Control and Prevention. Recommendations to prevent and control iron deficiency in the United States. MWR 1998; 47(No. RR-3):25.
3. DiMeglio G. Nutrition in adolescence. Pediatr Rev. 2000 Jan;21(1):32-33.
4. Frith-Terhune AL, Cogswell ME, Khan LK, Will JC, Ramakrishnan U. Iron deficiency anemia: higher prevalence in Mexican American than in non-Hispanic white females in the third National Health and Nutrition Examination Survey, 1988-1994. Am J Clin Nutr 2000 Oct;72(4):963-68.
5. Looker AC, Dallman PR, Carroll MD, Gunter EW, Johnson CL. Prevalence of iron deficiency in the United States. JAMA 1997 Mar 26;277(12):973-76.
6. Zlotkin S. Clinical nutrition: 8. The role of nutrition in the prevention of iron deficiency anemia in infants, children and adolescents. CMAJ 2003 Jan 7;168(1): 59-63.

21 Management of Adolescent Genital Tract Abnormalities

Saria Tasnim

INTRODUCTION

Embryologically female urinary and genital tract are closely related and abnormalities of one system is often mirrored by abnormalities of other system.[1] About 10% of infants are born with some abnormalities of the genitourinary system.[1] Although many of the abnormalities are evident at birth like, ambiguous genitalia, hypospadias, some of the malformations are not diagnosed till adolescence. For example Müllerian duct anomalies may remain asymptomatic in 75% cases and in 25% cases they are present with primary amenorrhea, hematocolpos, and hematometra during adolescence.[2]

INCIDENCE

The incidence of congenital malformation of female genital tract is about 0.5% in female population.[3] Müllerian duct anomalies are estimated to occur in 0.1-0.5% of women. In a study from Bangladesh, it was found that among the congenital abnormalities of female genital tract, Müllerian agenesis with absent vagina was 13.5%, vaginal septum 13.5%, unicornuate uterus was 10.8%.[4] Acien et al reported incidence of Müllerian anomalies in 14.7% of women with recurrent pregnancy loss.[5] In a study among women with infertility and history of pregnancy wastage, incidence of Müllerian anomaly was 0.97% and bicornuate, septate and arcuate varieties were frequently observed.[6] Simon et al found that in the healthy fertile population, Müllerian duct anomalies have a prevalence of 3.2%.[7]

DEVELOPMENT OF THE GENITAL TRACT

The primordial germ cells migrate from the yolk sac to the urogenital ridge via the hindgut in both sexes about 3 weeks after fertilization. The mesothelium on the medial surface of the urogenital ridge forms the gonads. The testis determining factor gene is the SRY gene that must express before differentiation of the urogenital ridge to form a testis.[8] SRY cause undifferentiated cells to become Sertoli cells. The Sertoli cells express the SOX-9 and SF-1 genes, the latter is thought to activate Müllerian inhibitor substance (MIS) gene which cause regression of Müllerian structures.

If SRY does not express, the DAX gene expresses leading to ovarian development. With development of the ovary there is regression of the mesonephric ducts and development of the structures of paramesonephric ducts.[9] The reproductive organs that develop from the Müllerian ducts are fallopian tubes, uterus, cervix and upper three quarter of vagina. The lower part of the vagina is formed by the urogenital sinus which grows upwards and meets with the lowermost portion of the paired fused Müllerian ducts and canalization occurs.[9] Recent evidence shows that WNT4 gene is involved in the regulation of Müllerian duct development and ovarian androgen biosynthesis and a mutation of this gene may result in Müllerian abnormalities.[10]

TYPE OF ABNORMALITIES

Müllerian duct anomalies are categorized most commonly into 7 classes according to the American Fertility Society (AFS) Classification Scheme as follows (Table 21.1):[11]

Table 21.1: Classification of müllerian duct anomalies

Classification	*Anomaly*
Class I (Agenesis/Hypoplasia)	a. Vaginal
	b. Cervical
	c. Fundal
	d. Tubal
	e. Combined
Class II (Unicornuate)	a. Communicating
	b. Non-communicating
	c. No cavity
	d. No horn
Class III (Didelphys)	Didelphys
Class IV (Bicornuate)	a. Complete
	b. Partial
Class V (Septate)	a. Complete
	b. Partial
Class VI (Arcuate)	Arcuate
Class VII (DES-related)	DES-related

Reprinted by permission from the Amercian Society for Reproductive Medicine (Fertility and Sterility 1998; Vol. 49(6): page 944-945)

Class I (hypoplasia/agenesis): The most common form is the Mayer-Rokitansky-Kuster-Hauser syndrome, which is combined agenesis of the uterus, cervix, and upper portion of the vagina. Incomplete development sometimes affects lower parts of ducts only.

Class II (unicornuate uterus): A unicornuate uterus is the result of complete, or almost complete, arrest of development of 1 müllerian duct (Fig. 21.1). If the arrest is incomplete, as in 90% of patients, a rudimentary horn with or without functioning endometrium is present.

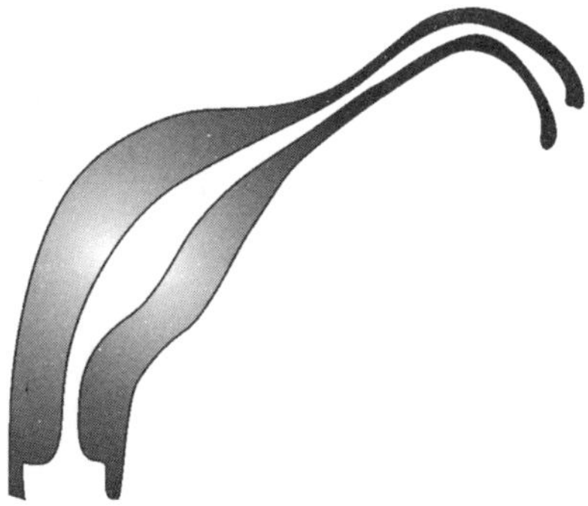

Fig. 21.1: Unicornuate uterus

Class III (didelphys uterus): This anomaly results from complete nonfusion of both Müllerian ducts. The individual horns are fully developed and almost normal in size. Two cervices are inevitably present. A longitudinal or transverse vaginal septum may be noted as well (Fig. 21.2).

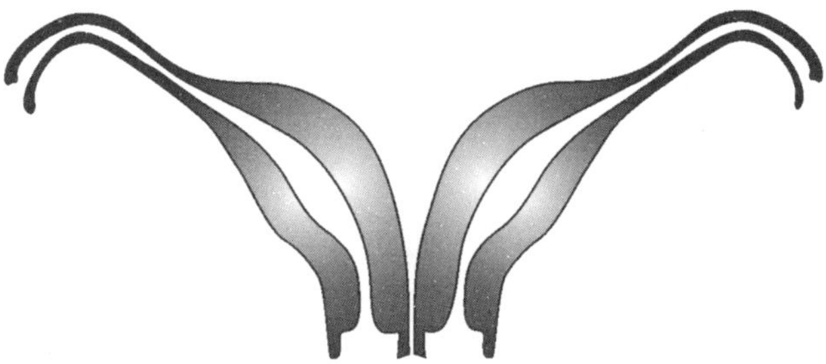

Fig. 21.2: Didelphys uterus

Class IV (bicornuate uterus): A bicornuate uterus results from partial nonfusion of the Müllerian ducts (Fig. 21.3). The central myometrium may extend to the level of the internal cervical os (bicornuate unicollis) or external cervical os (bicornuate bicollis). The latter is distinguished from didelphys uterus because it demonstrates some degree of fusion between the 2 horns, while in classic didelphys uterus, the 2 horns and cervices are separated completely.

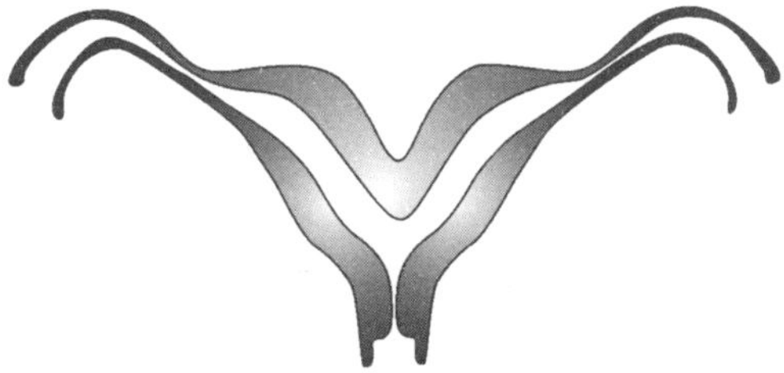

Fig. 21.3: Bicornuate uterus

Class V (septate uterus): A septate uterus results from failure of resorption of the septum between the 2 uterine horns. The septum can be partial or complete, in which case it extends to the internal cervical os. Histologically, the septum may be composed of myometrium or fibrous tissue. The uterine fundus is typically convex but may be flat or slightly concave (< 1 - cm fundal cleft) (Figs 21.4A and B).

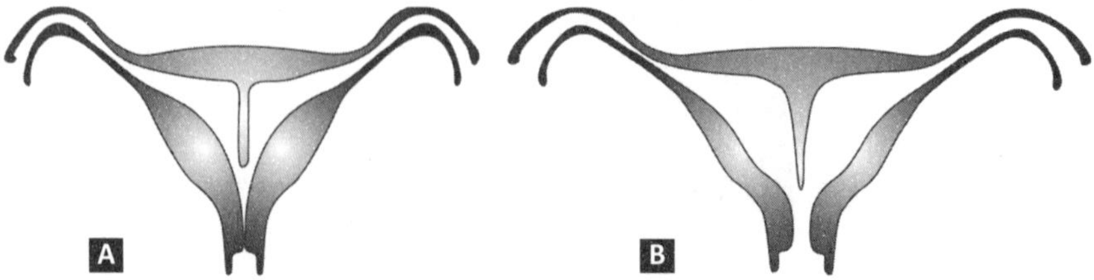

Figs 21.4A and B: Septate uterus

Class VI (arcuate uterus): An arcuate uterus has a single uterine cavity with a convex or flat uterine fundus, the endometrial cavity, which demonstrates a small fundal cleft or impression (1.5 cm). The outer contour of the uterus is convex or flat (Fig. 21.5).

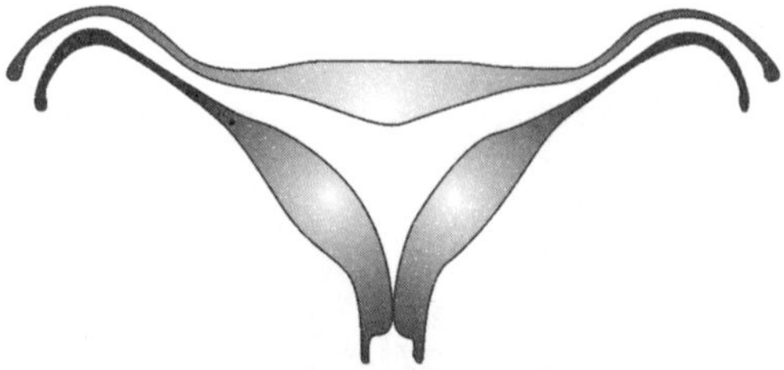

Fig. 21.5: Arcuate uterus

Class VII (diethylstilbestrol-related anomaly): Several million women were treated with diethylstilbestrol (DES), an estrogen analog prescribed to prevent miscarriage from 1945-1971. The drug was withdrawn once its teratogenic effects on the reproductive tracts of male and female fetuses were understood. The uterine anomaly is seen in the female offspring of as many as 15% of women exposed to DES during pregnancy (Fig. 21.6). Female fetuses that are affected have a variety of abnormal findings that include uterine hypoplasia and a T-shaped uterine cavity. Patients also may have abnormal transverse ridges, hoods, stenoses of the cervix, and adenosis of the vagina with increased risk of vaginal clear cell carcinoma. Imaging findings are pathognomonic for this anomaly.

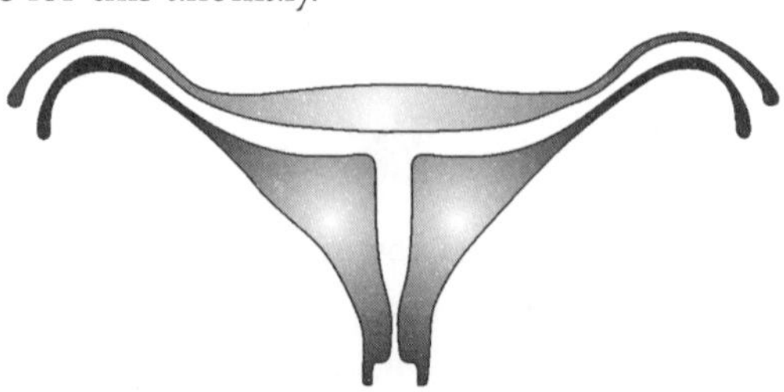

Fig. 21.6: Diethylstilbestrol exposed uterus

DIAGNOSIS

Clinical suspicion of genital abnormality can be investigated by a pelvic ultrasound with transabdominal and if feasible, transvaginal imaging. Müllerian duct anomalies may be suggested on transvaginal 2-dimensional (2D) sonographic imaging but newer 3-dimensional (3D) sonographic techniques offer relatively higher sensitivity and specificity.[12] Hysterosalpingography (HSG) performed under fluoroscopy, allows evaluation of the uterine cavity and tubal patency. MRI is considered the criterion standard for imaging uterine anomalies. MRI provides high-resolution images of the uterine body, fundus, and internal structure. In addition, it can help evaluate the urinary tract for concomitant anomalies.[13] Hysteroscopy is also a good diagnostic method to detect uterine anomaly. Final pathology is based on laparoscopy or surgical finding. Figures 21.7A and B show laparoscopic finding of an adolescent girl presenting at ICMH with primary amenorrhea and blind vagina showing full length of fallopian tubes and a strip of uterus. The girl had normal karyotype, height 150 cm and normal secondary sex characteristics.

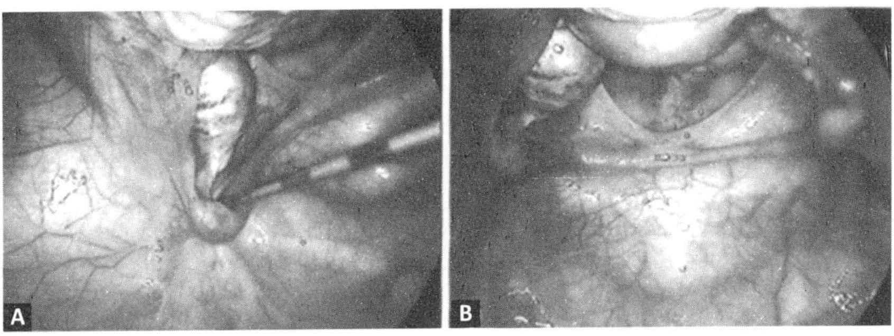

Figs 21.7A and B: Laparoscopic finding of an adolescent girl presenting with primary amenorrhea and blind vagina showing full length of fallopian tubes and a strip of uterus *(For color version, see Plate 5)*

MANAGEMENT

Management of abnormalities of lower genital tract include counseling to help cope up with the concerns about sexual activity and fertility. Specific management for absence of vagina include non surgical methods initially and then if necessary by surgical approach.[14] Nonsurgical method was pioneered by Frank and a review by Broadband and Wolf.[15,16] In this technique, the patient is instructed to use graduated glass which are placed against the introitus and blind vagina and gentle pressure is exerted in a posterior direction for approximately 10-20 minutes twice a day. Gradually the dilators will go further and further and it takes between 8 and 10 weeks of repeated use of the vaginal dilators to achieve successful results. If this fails, a vaginoplasty is done to create a neovagina artificially.[15,16] In McIndoe and Read technique, a cavity is created between the bladder and bowel at the site where the natural vagina would have been and this cavity is then opened by a split-thickness skin graft taken from the thigh and applied to the space on a plastic mould.[17] To avoid the scar of split thickness, skin graft amnion has been used to line the neovagina.[18]

The principle of vulvovaginoplasty pioneered by Williams include apposition of the labia majora in front of the neovagina to create a pouch into which the penis can be placed and sexual intercourse achieved.[19] Vechietti's operation involved use of a small olive which is placed in the dimple of the absent vagina. Laparoscopically wires can be brought out through the abdominal wall and then pressure exerted through spring device thereby creating a neovagina.[14]

Colpopoiesis-Adamyan's technique is a combined laparoscopic-perineal approach for absent uterus and vagina.[20] The perineal step consists of a transverse 3 cm incision between the rectum and urinary bladder at the level of the lower border of labia minora[20] (Fig. 21.8). Vaginal space is created by blunt and sharp dissection in the horizontal direction upto the pelvic peritoneum. The laparoscopic step consists of identification of the pelvic peritoneum[20] (Fig. 21.9). The fold is transected from below[20] (Fig. 21.10). The peritoneum is brought down into the created vaginal space using a grasper[20] (Fig. 21.11). The edges of the peritoneum are sutured to the edges of the skin incision with Vicryl stitches, forming the introitus (Fig. 21.12). A moist sponge or vaginal probe is then placed at the introitus to reestablish the pneumoperitoneum. Formation of the neovaginal vault is performed by laparoscopic placement of purse-string suture incorporating the bladder peritoneum, muscular uterine rudiments and peritoneal lining of pelvic side wall and sigmoid colon[20] (Fig. 21.13). The suture is tied with an extracorporeal knot without undue tension[20](Fig. 21.14).

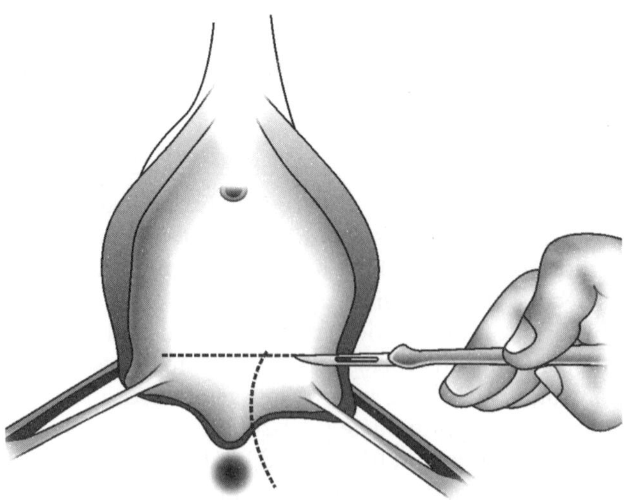

Fig. 21.8: Transverse incision

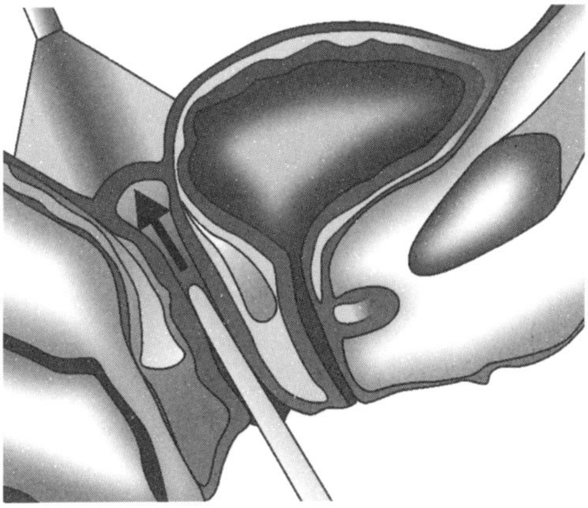

Fig. 21.9: Identification of pelvic peritoneum

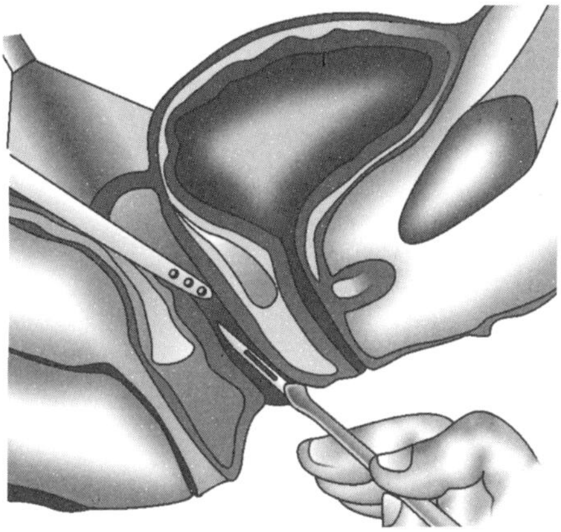

Fig. 21.10: Transection of fold

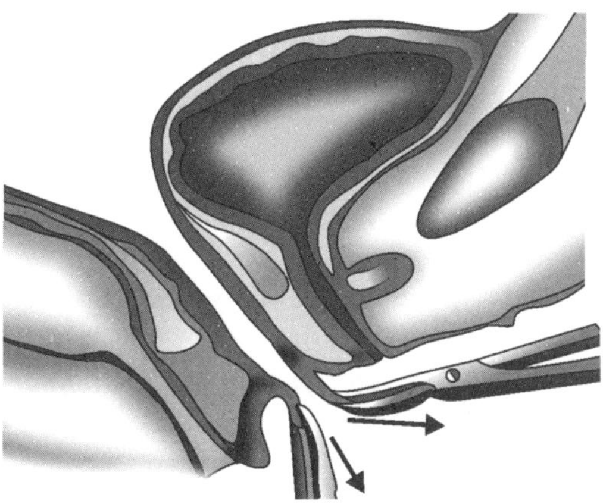

Fig. 21.11: Peritoneum is brought down

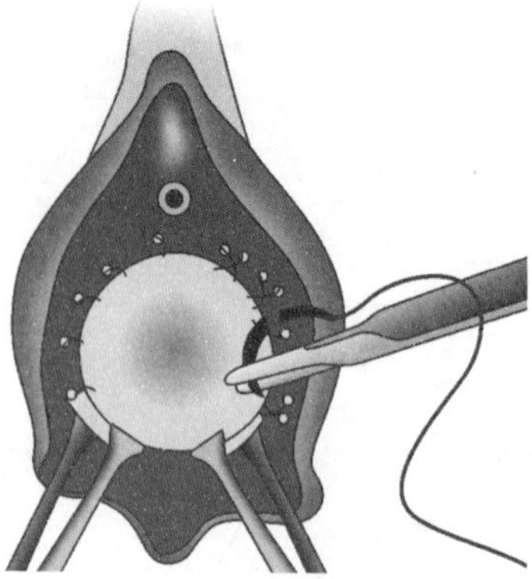

Fig. 21.12: Suturing the edge of peritoneum

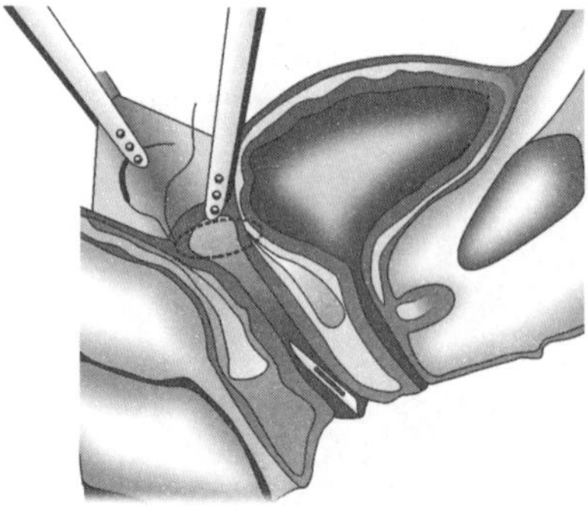

Fig. 21.13: Formation of neovaginal vault

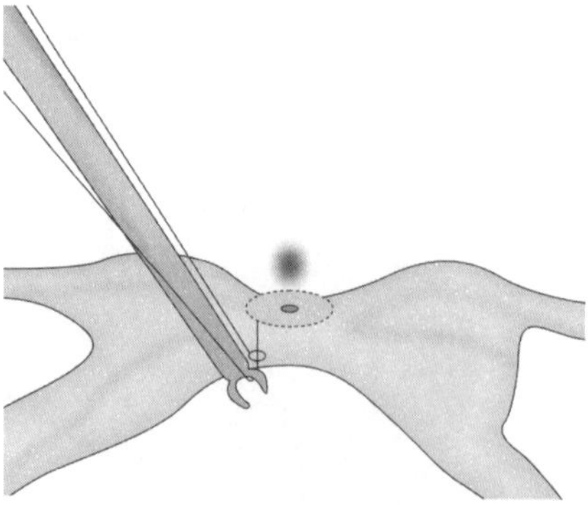

Fig. 21.14: Tying the suture with extracorporeal knot

Reconstructive Surgery in Different Types of Müllerian Anomalies

Didelphic and unicornuate uterus: Cerclage operation is favorably reported in cases of repeated miscarriage and premature labor.[21] Bicornuate uterus is usually not associated with reproductive problem hence surgical intervention is not essential.

Septate uterus: There are two routes of approach for surgical correction of septate uterus. These are Abdominal metroplasty and Hysteroscopic resection of septum and metroplasty. There are three approaches for abdominal metroplasty. These are Strassman, Tompkins and Jones approach. Strassman used to perform the surgery only in Bicornuate uterus. The incision line was horizontal and unification line was longitudinal (Figs 21.15A and B).[21]

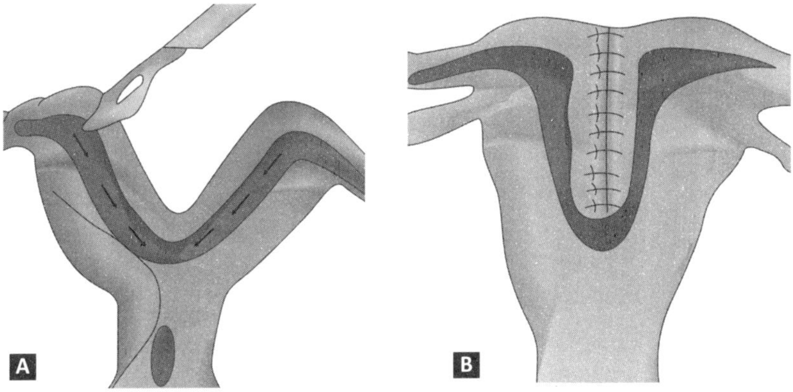

Figs 21.15A and B: Strassman procedure of metroplasty

In Tompkins' procedure, the incision is made precisely in the groove that can be palpated on the anterior fundal portion. The incision is then carried downward approximately 5 cm and at this point the knife enters into endometrial cavity[22] (Figs 21.16A and B). The uterine horns then separate spontaneously or by gentle pressure on the incision itself beginning at the point at which the endometrial cavity was first entered. The uterus is sutured into a complete single body.[22]

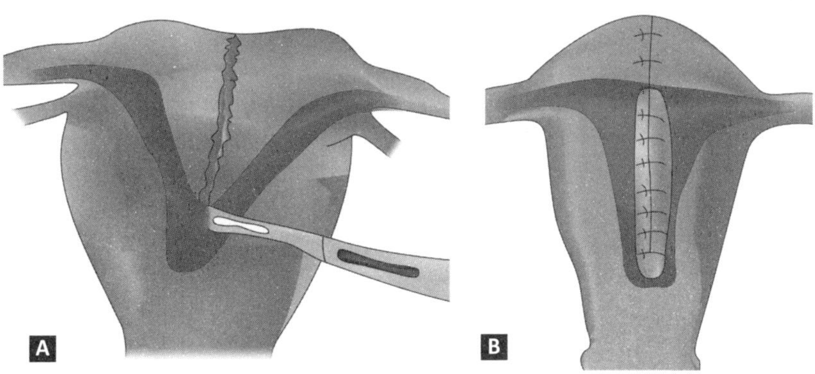

Figs 21.16A and B: Tompkins' procedure of metroplasty

In Jones' wedge metroplasty, a wedge shaped area is initially outlined by a suitable dye such as brilliant green. The fundal incision should be approximately 1 cm away from the tubal insertion and cut margins are approximated in three layers[22] (Figs 21.17A and B).

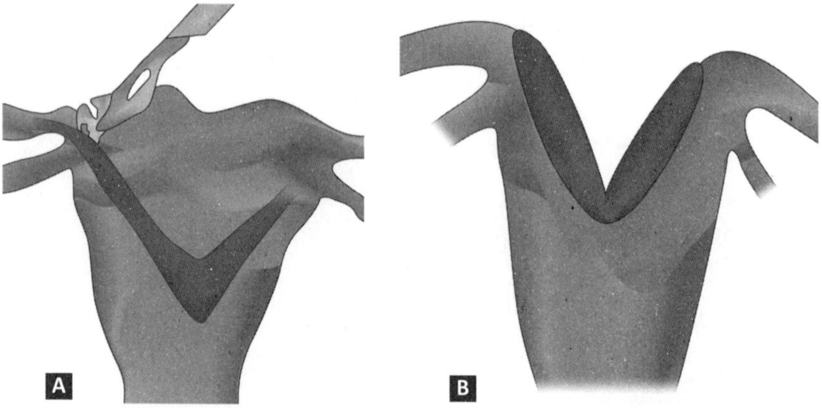

Figs 21.17A and B: Jones' wedge metroplasty

Hysteroscopic metroplasty is now the treatment of choice for septate uterus (Figs 21.18A and B). It is desirable that the endometrium is suppressed with Danazole or GnRH-analog for 2 months prior to surgery. A simple uterine septum without involving the cervix may be incised with scissors or the loop with cutting current under direct vision. The Nd-YAG laser may also be used. Postoperatively high dose of estrogen is administered to the patient to promote endometrial growth.[20, 22]

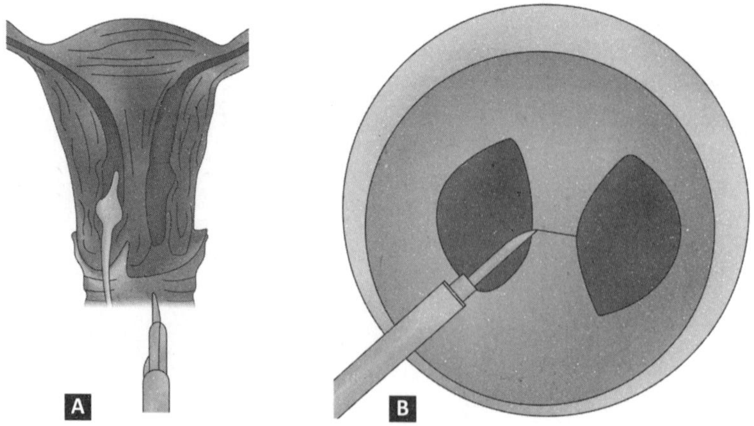

Figs 21.18A and B: Hysteroscopic septal incision

Importance of Timely Diagnosis and Social Issues Related during Adolescent Years

Patients with genital tract abnormalities should be thoroughly investigated to establish the exact nature of the abnormality and to diagnose any other associated malformation. Some 40% of patients with lower genital abnormalities will have renal abnormalities and 15% of them may have an absent kidney.[23] Obstructive lesions like imperforate hymen or imperforate vagina with a functional uterus should be diagnosed and treated as soon as the patient starts menstruating to prevent development of hematosalpinx which has more risk of interfering with future fertility. Psychological problems are usually profound and such patients generally are frightened and confused and express feeling of rejection.[23] Counseling is important for both the patient and parents to help them to accept the fact and to decide on how to cope up with the problem. Social impact depends on the age at which the diagnosis is made, nature of the abnormality, whether the girl is married or not, whether the girl has financial stability and self independence. In the existing social custom of early marriage and childbearing, social stigma of being single or childless, limited access to education and employment, the decision to choose an appropriate option is often more difficult. It is important that the patient herself and the parents understand the type of problem, the capability of maintaining sexual relation and fertility, the treatment options and threats.

CONCLUSION

Congenital malformation of genital organs is a critical problem that needs specialized care with psychological support. Reconstructive surgery is indicated for symptomatic cases. Social impact of the disease is also important to decide on the appropriate lifestyle for the girl.

ACKNOWLEDGMENT

I sincerely express my gratitude to Dr Ibrahim Syed, Dr Pranay Shah and Dr Chakrabarty B N for referring to the diagrams in the manuscript.

REFERENCES

1. Pratap Kumar and Narendra Malhotra (eds). Jeffcoate's Principle of Gynaecology. Seventh edition 2008. Jaypee Brothers Medical Publishers. New Delhi.
2. Golan A, Langer R, Bukovsky I, Capsi E. Congenital anomalies of the Müllerian system. Fertil Steril 1989; 51:747-55.
3. Nahun CG. Uterine anomalies. How common are they and what is there distribution among subtypes? J Reprod Med 1998;43:877-87.
4. HA Baby. Congenital abnormalities of female genital tract. Journal of Bangladesh College of Physician and Surgeons 2007;25(1):23-8.
5. Acien P. Incidence of Müllerian defects in fertile and infertile women. Human reprod 1997;12:1372-76.
6. Chakrabarty BN. Müllerian anomalies-infertility management. Bulletin of Reproductive Medicine 1999.

7. Simon C, Martinez L, Pardo F, et al. Müllerian defects in women with normal reproductive outcome. Fertil Steril. Dec 1991;56(6):1192-93. (Medline).
8. Berta P, Hawkins JB, Sinclair AH, et al. Genetic evidence equating SRY and the testis-determining factor. Nature 1990;348:448.
9. Debra S. Heller. Lower genital tract disease in children and adolescents—A review. J Pediatr Adolesc Gynecol 2005;18:75-83.
10. Pascal Philibert, Anna Biason-Lauber, Roman Rouzier, Catherine Pienkowski, Francoise Paris, Daniel Konrad, Eugene Schoenle, and Charles Sultan. Identification and functional analysis of a new WNT4 gene mutation among 28 adolescent girls with primary amenorrhea and Müllerian duct abnormalities: A French Collaborative Study J Clin Endocrinol Metab 2008;93:895-900.
11. AFS. The American Fertility Society classifications of adnexal adhesions, distal tubal occlusion, tubal occlusion secondary to tubal ligation, tubal pregnancies, Müllerian anomalies and intrauterine adhesions. Fertil Steril 1988;49(6):944-55. [Medline].
12. Raga F, Bonilla-Musoles F, Blanes J, Osborne NG. Congenital Müllerian anomalies: diagnostic accuracy of three-dimensional ultrasound. Fertil Steril 1996;65(3):523-8. [Medline].
13. Pellerito JS, McCarthy SM, Doyle MB. Diagnosis of uterine anomalies: relative accuracy of MR imaging, endovaginal sonography, and hysterosalpingography. Radiology 1992;183(3):795-800. [Medline].
14. Edmond DK. Congenital malformations of the genital tract and their management. Best Pract Res Clin Obstet Gynaecol 2003;17:19-40.
15. Frank RT. The formation of the artificial vagina without operation. Am J Obstet Gynecol 1938;35:1053-56.
16. Broadbent RT, Woolf RM. Nonoperative construction of the vagina. Plast Reconstr Surg 1984;73:117-22.
17. McIndoe AH and Bannister JB. An operation for the congenital absence of the vagina J Obstet Gynecol Br Commonwlth 1938;93:490-95.
18. Morton KE and Dewhurst CJ. Human amnion in the treatment of vaginal malformations. Br J Obstet Gynecol 1986;93:50-4.
19. Williams EA. Congenital absence of the vagina. A simple operation for its relief. J Obstet Gynecol Br Commonwlth 1964;71:511-17.
20. Pranay Shah (ed) In. Step by step Laparoscopy in infertility. 2007 Jaypee Brothers Medical Publishers. New Delhi.
21. Rock JA, Adam RA. Surgery to repair disorders of development. In: Nichols DH, Clarke-Pearson, eds. Gynecologic, Obstetric, and Related Surgery. 2nd ed. St. Louis, Mo:. Mosby-Year Book 2000:780-813.
22. Chakrabarty BN. Reconstructive surgery in infertility. In: Pankaj Desai, Narendra Malhotra, Duru Shah. Principles and practice of Obstetrics and Gynaecology for post graduates. Third edition. 2008 . Jaypee Brothers Medical Publishers. New Delhi.
23. Keith Edmond (ed). Dewhurt's Text book of Obstetrics and Gynaecology. Seventh edition. 2007. Blackwell Publishing.

Section 5

IMAGING, LAPAROSCOPY AND ROBOTICS

22 Imaging in the Adolescent Girls

Gita Guin, Shashi Khare

The present day practice of gynecology has moved generations ahead of an era when a diligent gynecologist would resort to one protocol of therapeutic evaluation and then another in an effort to pinpoint the problems in an adolescent girl. Further, in times of litigations, one must have a clear idea dictating the medical intervention and imaging modalities have helped the clinician to rationalize his actions.

X-RAY

A radiological estimation of bone age becomes essential in patients of precocious puberty and sexual assault and rape.

1. Puberty—Appearance of the epiphyses of the pelvis.
2. 16 yrs—Ossification centers of the transverse processes, spinous processes and upper and lower surface of the body of the vertebrae.
3. 15-18 yrs
   - Appearance of the epiphyses of the acromian processes.
   - Fusion of the olecranon process of the humerus.
4. 17-18 yrs
   - Fusion of the external and internal epicondyle of the lower end of the humerus.
   - Fusion of the lesser and greater trochanter of femur.
5. 18-20 yrs—Ossification of the wrist joint, elbow joint and bones of the foot.

ULTRASONOGRAPHY

Pelvis

Ultrasound has become an indispensible, cheap and easy way of peeping into the female pelvis. It is the investigation of choice in diseases of the female pelvis, particularly in an adolescent girl where it may not be possible to do a pelvic examination. In this age group, a trans-vesical, trans-abdominal (TAS) USG of the pelvis is the usual choice although it cannot duplicate the anatomic detail of the uterus, ovaries and adnexa as obtained by the trans-vaginal approach. It is done in various situations:

1. Precocious or delayed puberty.
2. Dysmenorrhea and pelvic pain.
3. Menstrual irregularities—Menorrhagia, Oligomenorrhea, amenorrhea, metrorrhagia, etc.

4. Evaluation of congenital anomalies (Figs 22.1A to C and 22.2).
5. Characterization and follow-up of an abnormality picked up on another examination, e.g. CT Scan or MRI.
6. Evaluation of a pelvic mass/screening for malignancy (Fig. 22.3).
7. Polycystic ovarian syndrome.
8. Suspected pregnancy or its complication.

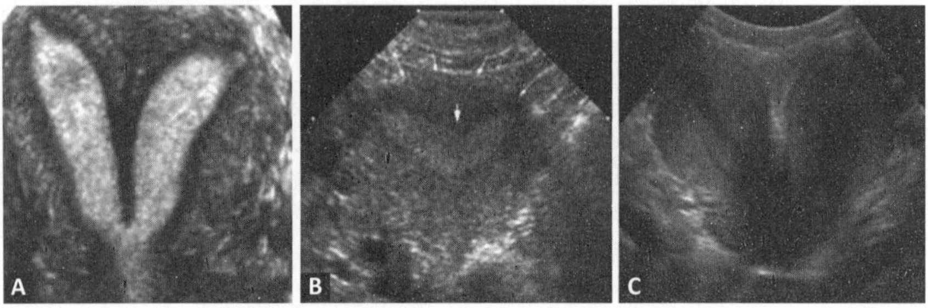

Figs 22.1A to C: Congenital malformations of the uterus: (A) Bicornuate uterus, (B) Arcuate uterus, (C) Uterus didelphys

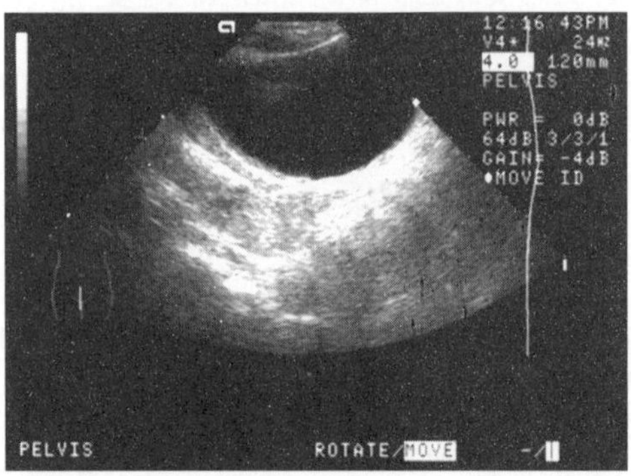

Fig. 22.2: Mayer-Rokitansky-Kushner-Hauser's syndrome

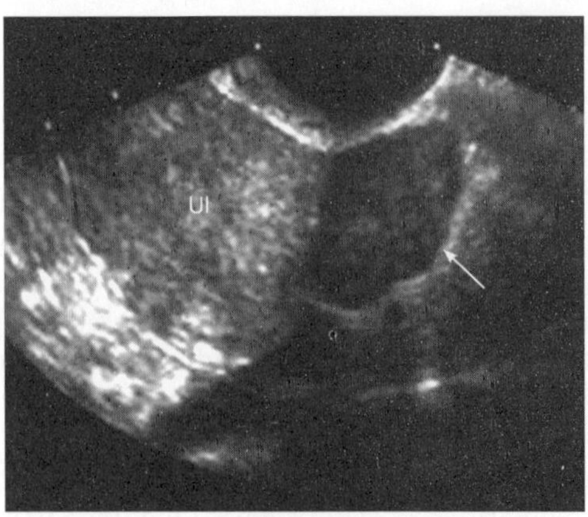

Fig. 22.3: Ovarian tumor

At the age of 2 years, the uterus measures 2.8 × 0.8 × 1.1 cm uterine growth begins at approximately 7-8 years of age, accelerates during puberty (4.0 × 1.2 × 1.6 cm at 13 years) and continues up to about 20 years of age, when it measures approximately 6-8.5 cm in length, the width of the corpus is 3-5 cm and the antero-posterior diameter is 2-4 cm.

The ovaries have marked variation in shape and orientation; therefore ovarian volume which is best measured by a three-dimensional USG is considered to be the most reproducible measure of ovarian size. The mean ovarian volume in pre-menarchal girls is about 3 ml which increases to 9.8 ml in menstruating girls.

With increasing prevalence of metabolic disorders in adolescent girls, polycystic ovaries (PCO) are becoming more common and may present in as many as 5-10% of adolescent girls. Two types of PCO are described on the basis of USG appearance: a *peripheral cystic pattern* in which small cysts are arranged in a necklace pattern in the subcapsular region and a *general cystic pattern* in which cysts are present in the subcapsular and stromal parts of the ovary. An increase in the amount and the echogenecity of the ovarian stroma distinguishes the PCO from the multifolicular ovary characteristic of normal puberty and hypothalamic anovulation.

Abdominal Cavity

USG of the abdominal cavity must always be done in children with suspected mullerian anomalies. Due to the closely related development of the mullerian and urinary systems, coexistent renal ectopia or agenesis is documented in 20-30% of these cases. It is also mandatory in GnRH independent precocious puberty suspected to be due to adrenal tumor. In complete androgen-insensitivity syndrome, an X-linked disorder, where the affected subject is phenotypically female but genotypically male, the testis will have to be located (abdominal cavity, inguinal canal or vulva) and removed to avoid future carcinoma.

CT SCAN AND MRI

These investigations are rarely requested as a first line imaging modality, but usually to resolve problems that may come up during an USG examination. In these cases, it can be tailored to the minimum required scanning planes thus avoiding claustrophobia, unnecessary exposure to radiation and expenditure in a young girl.

Pelvis and Abdominal Cavity

CT scan of the female pelvis is generally used for evaluation and characterization of pelvic masses and for staging of cancers. Magnetic resonance imaging is used for further evaluation in doubtful cases because of its excellent soft tissue detail. Some studies have shown that an MRI can differentiate a benign from a malignant neoplasm with fair amount of certainty.

Brain

In patients with GnRH dependent precocious puberty, a CT-MRI Scan of the brain is indicated to rule out hamartomas, craniopharyngiomas, meningitis, hydrocephalous or skull injury.

Similarly, in girls with delayed puberty and secondary amenorrhea with normal or low gonadotropic hormones, a CT-MRI Scan of the brain is indicated to exclude a pituitary micro or macroadenoma or rarely a hypothalamic space occupying lesion, which when absent indicates hypothalamic amenorrhea. As 10% of patients have macroadenomas (Fig. 22.4) which lead to subsequent optic nerve compression, an MRI early in the course of treatment is indicated.

NUCLEAR MEDICINE

Bone scanning, Positron Emission Tomography (PET) and Radioimmunotherapy help in the staging and follow-up of malignant tumors and may change outcome of malignant ovarian tumors and other tumors such as Sarcoma Botroides.

CONCLUSION(S)

1. Ultrasound has become an indispensable, cheap and easy way of investigation of diseases of the female pelvis in adolescents.
2. A trans-vesical, trans-abdominal (TAS) USG of the pelvis is the choice.
3. Ovarian volume by three-dimensional USG increases from 3 mL in premenarchal girls to 9.8 mL in menstruating girls.
4. An increase in the amount and the echogenecity of the ovarian stroma distinguishes the PCO from the multifollicular ovary characteristic of normal puberty and hypothalamic anovulation.
5. USG of the abdominal cavity must always be done in children with suspected mullerian anomalies to rule out coexistent renal anomalies.
6. CT scan and MRI must be reserved for doubtful cases.

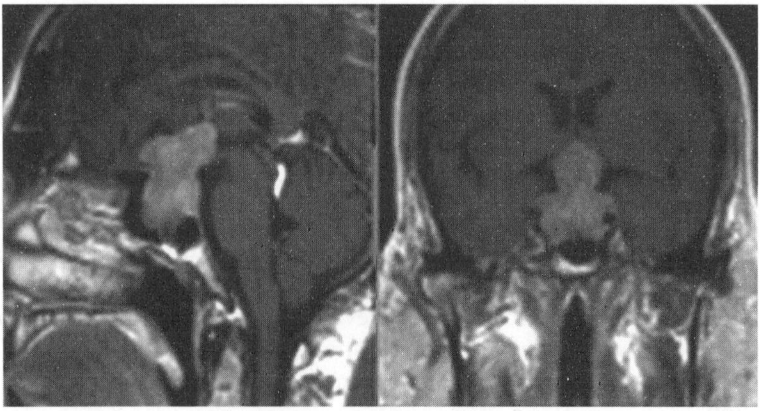

Fig. 22.4: Pituitary macroadenoma

SUGGESTED READING

1. Aubel S, Wozney P, Edwards RP. MRI of female uterine and juxta-uterine masses: clinical application in 25 patients. Magn Reson Imaging 1991;9:485-93.
2. David D, Stark et al. Magnetic Resonance Imaging, Mosby; 1992; second edition, volume-2.
3. Fundamentals of Diagnostic radiology 2007, 3rd Edition,William ES Brant. Genital Tract: Radiographic Imaging and MR. 909-23.
4. Haaga R, et al. Computerized Tomography and magnetic resonance imaging of the whole body. Mosby; 1994; third edition, volume-2.
5. Murase E, Sigelman ES, Outwater EK, et al. Uterine leiomyomas, histopathologic features, differential diagnosis and treatment. Radiographics 1999;19:1179-97.
6. Outwater EK, Sigelman ES, Hunt JL. Ovarian teratomas: Tumour types and imaging characteristics. Radiographics 2001;21:475-90.
7. Rha SE, Byun JY, Kim B, et al. Staging of early endometrial carcinoma: assessment with T2-weighted and Gadolinium enhanced T1-weighted MR imaging. Radiographics 1999;19:937-45.
8. Sam JW, Jacobs JE, Birnbaum BA. Spectrum of CT findings in acute pyogenic pelvic inflammatory disease. Radiographics 2002;22:1327-34.
9. Sharma SK. CT and MRI of the female pelvis. Imaging in Obstetrics and Gynaecology. 278-82.
10. Text Book of Radiology and Imaging, David Sutten, Churchill Livingstone 2003, Vol 1.
11. Troiano RN, McCarthy SM. Müllerian duct anomalies: imaging and clinical issues. Radiology 2004;233:19-34.
12. Ultrasonography in Obstetrics and Gynaecology. Callen: 2007: 5th edition, WB Saunders.
13. Woodward PJ, Sohaey R, O'Donoghue MJ, Green DE. Tumours and tumour like lesions of the testes: radiologic-pathologic co-relation. Radiographics 2002;22:189-216.

23 Endoscopic Surgery in Adolescent Girls

Prakash Trivedi, Anita Budania

INTRODUCTION

Endoscopic surgery has probably reached to all spaces of the human body and is done in a child and uptill a geriatric patient. Nearly 82% of pediatric surgeons in USA prefer Laparoscopic route with miniature optics and instruments. The Adolescent girls today have unique problems from lifestyle to pathology. Endoscopic surgery in adolescents have certain areas of concern, major advantage of avoiding open surgery and cosmetically it's the need and not an option alone. Some indications may be diagnostic, but many are therapeutic.

What special care is taken for endoscopic surgery in Adolescents?

1. Anesthesia: This is an important part as the peritoneal cavity may be smaller in many adolescents compared to adults, further the pressure at which the CO_2 is used for Insufflation in Laparoscopic would be lower at 12 to 10 mm Hg than 15 mm Hg as set for adults. Also the flow rate is less depending on the pathology.

   The maintenance of the body temperature, blood pressure, avoiding arrhythmia and may be LMA, i.e. Laryngeal mask anesthesia would be better than endotracheal intubation.
2. A thorough evaluation and investigation necessary for diagnosis prior to Endoscopic surgery is compulsory in adolescents.
3. The avoidance of a big scar in adolescents who are quite often unmarried is important to have small button-hole laparoscopy for long-term medical and social reasons.
4. Proper consent from parents/guardians is a must in addition to good counseling.

INDICATIONS OF ENDOSCOPIC SURGERY IN ADOLESCENTS

1. Severe or chronic pain in lower abdomen, dysmenorrhea not responding to NSAIds or OC. Specially in cases of endometriosis or endometrioma (Figs 23.1 to 23.4), hemorrhagic ovarian cyst or twisted ovarian cyst (Figs 23.5 and 23.6), pelvic inflammatory disease—tubo-ovarian mass, tuberculosis.
2. Polycystic ovarian syndrome in cases of delayed periods, amenorrhea, hirsutism, gross overweight.

3. Mullerian abnormalities with large hematometra, hematosalphinx or functionary rudimentary horn with pain (Figs 23.7 and 23.8).
4. Laparoscopic creation of neovagina in absent uterus (Figs 23.9A and B to 23.13).
5. Appendicectomy if is needed and heavily suspected (Figs 23.14 to 23.17).
6. Bariatric surgery in morbid obesity in adolescent teenager.
7. Excessive bleeding vaginally with fibroid or polyp or abnormal platelets like Glanzmann's thromboasthenia, etc.
8. Rare presacral neurectomy (Figs 23.18 and 23.19) in adolescents with repeat pelvic endometriosis-endometrioma-dysmenorrhea and uncontrollable pain.
9. Young adolescents with congenital uterocervical prolapse.
10. Debatable in laparoscopic hysterectomy in mentally retarded or adolescents who cannot take care of bleeding due to major medical reasons as certified by psychiatrist, gynecologist and physician.

Ovarian cyst in adolescents needs a special mention, they can present with pain, dysmenorrhea, irregular periods, urinary frequency, constipation,

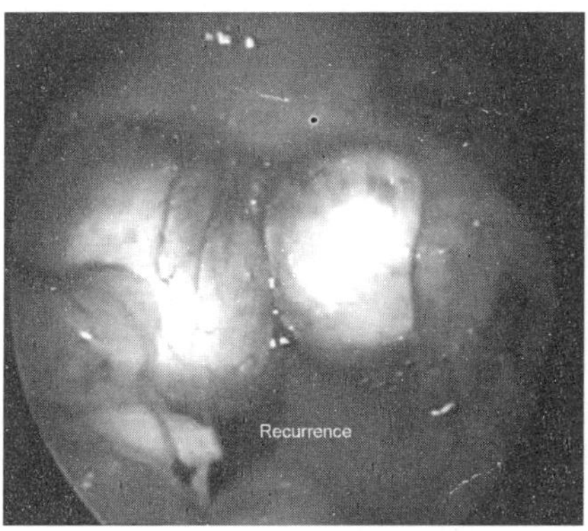

Fig. 23.1: Bilateral recurrent endometrioma
(For color version, see Plate 5)

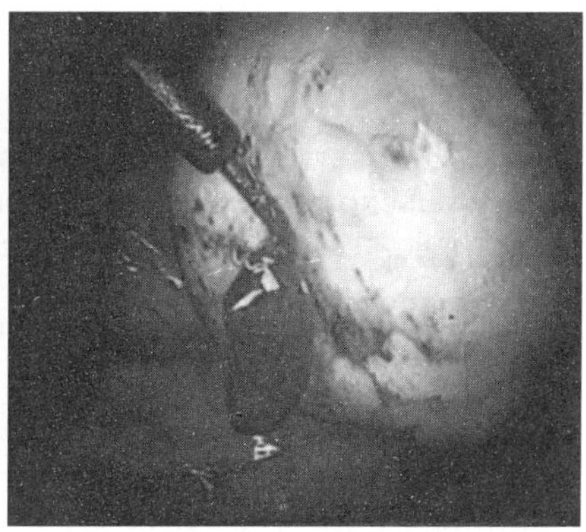

Fig. 23.2: Opening the endometrioma
(For color version, see Plate 5)

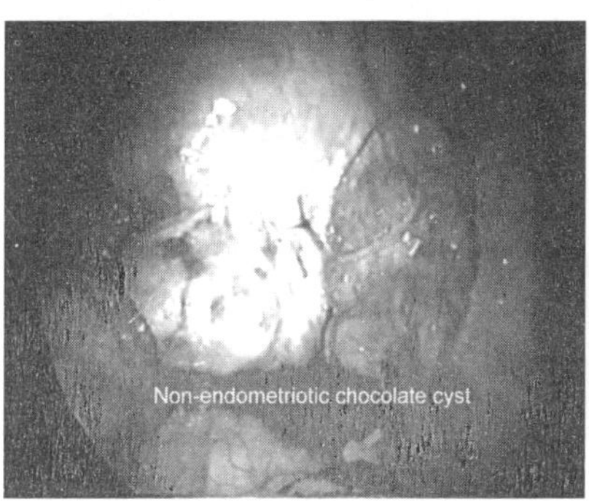

Fig. 23.3: Non-endometriotic chocolate cyst
(For color version, see Plate 5)

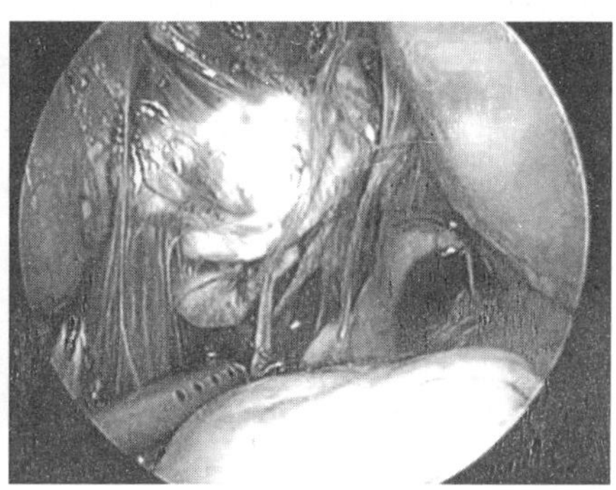

Fig. 23.4: Peritubal and peri-ovarian
(For color version, see Plate 5)

heaviness of pelvis, nausea and vomiting, etc.—if twisted or accidental detections on sonography. Despite of vastness of differential diagnosis, commonest are functional cyst ~ follicular or corpus luteal cyst (Spinelli et al[1]). If not worrisome for malignancy, follow-up by sonography after 2~3 menstrual cycles is enough (Strickland et al[2]). Though 45% are functional—follicular or corpus luteal cyst, 70% has spontaneous regression (Shapiro et al[3]). However persistent cyst of > 5 cm not responding to treatment should be considered for laparoscopic excision for diagnosis and relief of symptoms (Spinelli et al[1]) others consider 6~10 cm as a cut off. Cystectomy is better than aspiration as recurrence is less and we have a histopathology specimen (Laufer MR et al[4]). Laparoscopically it's better cosmetically, fast recovery and less intra-postoperative pain.[2,3] Even Dermoid cysts are common and can be bilateral in < 10%.

Around 4.4% of ovarian cysts between 15 to 21.5 years (Breen et al[5]) can be malignant having solid mass/septation/papillary projection/color Doppler indices showing free high flow, blood markers like HCG, CA125, PAP-14, alpha fetoprotein, carcino embryonic antigen, mullerian inhibiting substance, CT-MRI also can be useful.

We would like to briefly discuss each pathology with its endoscopic appearance and treatment avoiding exhaustive aspects of technique of endoscopic surgery.

Laparoscopic surgery in endometriosis/endometrioma—large in size, pain, severe dysmenorrhea followed by depot injection of GnRH agonist and later dydrogesterone10 mg for 25 days cyclically for 6-9 months.

ADHESIONS IN SEVERE ENDOMETRIOSIS (FIGS 23.5 AND 23.6)

Twisted Ovarian Cyst

Kindly note that even if the color Doppler shows twist and no blood supply in the ovary, untwisting laparoscopically, draining the cyst, rarely anchoring the ovary to round ligament may be considered.

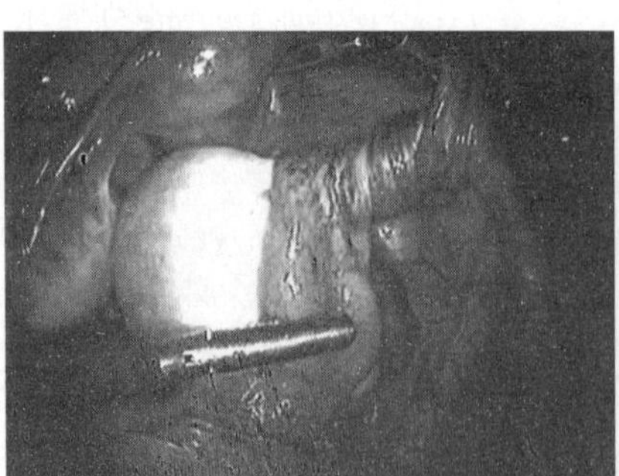

Fig. 23.5: Twisted ovarian cyst *(For color version, see Plate 6)*

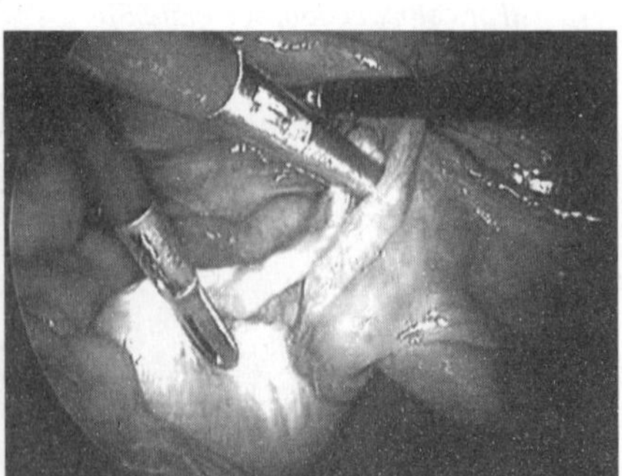

Fig. 23.6: Untwisted ovarian cyst *(For color version, see Plate 6)*

Cystic Adenomyosis

A rare case of juvenile cystic adenomyosis in a 19-year-old nulliparous patient presenting with secondary dysmenorrheal and non-cyclical pain whereas diffuse adenomyosis is a common finding in parous women. Laparoscopic resection and cystic adenomyosis in a teenager was done successfully (Elizabeth Ball et al[6]).

PCOS

Ideally after investigation first-line of treatment is lifestyle modification, reduction of weight; tablets like insulin sensitizer, anti-androgen are given first rarely close to the marriage a PCO drilling may be considered in selected patients.

Functioning Painful Rudimemtary Horn (Figs 23.7 and 23.8)

After identifying the horn, it is excised, with harmonic ace maintaining hemostasis. If the uterine wall is weakened, few endosutures are taken, horn is morcellated and removed.

Laparoscopic Creation of Neovagina in Cases of Absent Uterus, No Vagina (Figs 23.9A and B to 23.13)

In Rokitansky-Kustner-Hauser-Mayers syndrome of mullerian agenesis with no uterus, but presence of ovaries and tubes. A neovagina can be created by a 3~3.5 cm high density polymer ball with central holes to carry threads on both sides of the blind space between urethra and anal canal. The threads enter peritoneal cavity at the apparent apex of vagina.

The laparoscopic 5 mm trocars are placed higher through which threads are pulled retroperitoneallly so that the ball will get more horizontal pull, safe for bladder and rectosigmoid. The threads go through multiple holes in an orthopedic plate and finally rolled over the unidirectional tightening screws. These screws are moved clockwise only by half to one turn per day till 10~14 days, thus, slowly pulling the ball into an apparent vagina which is created automatically with growth of mucosal lining achieving a good depth till > 10 cm. The threads are now untied and the ball is easily removed from the vagina with threads and plate on the abdomen is free for removal.

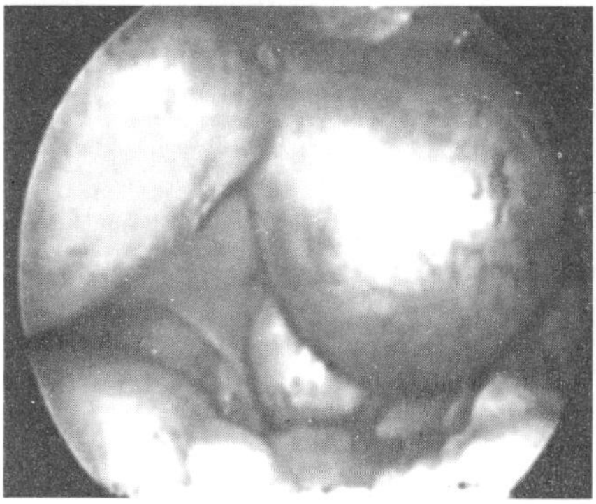

Fig. 23.7: Active rudimentary horn *(For color version, see Plate 6)*

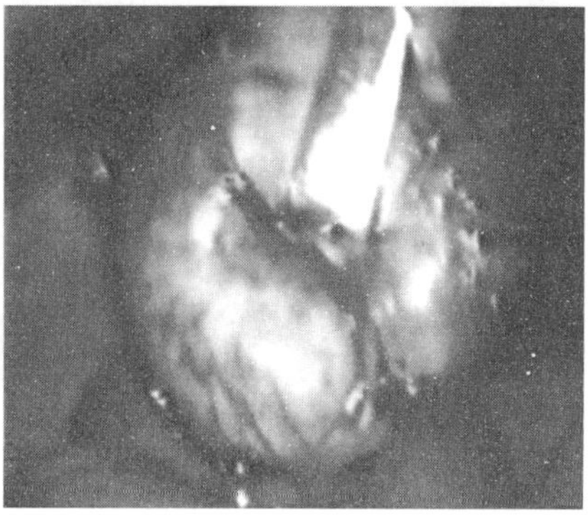

Fig. 23.8: Excision and removal *(For color version, see Plate 6)*

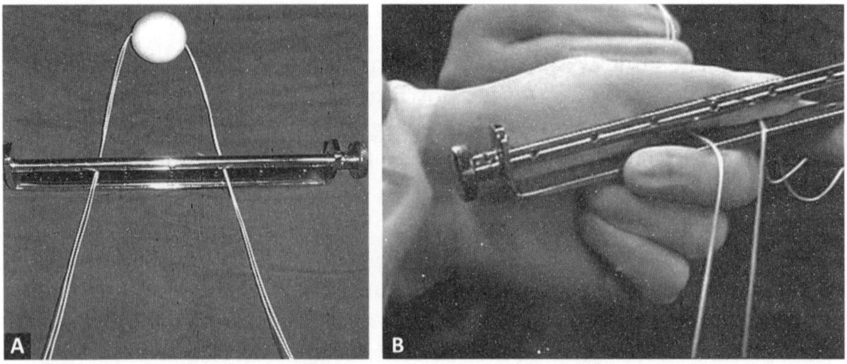

Figs 23.9 A and B: Trivedi's high density polymer ball device, central threads and the traction plate

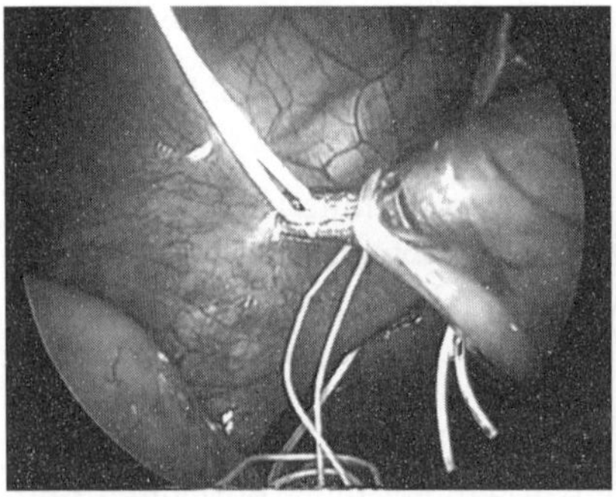

Fig. 23.10: Extraperitoneal traction *(For color version, see Plate 6)*

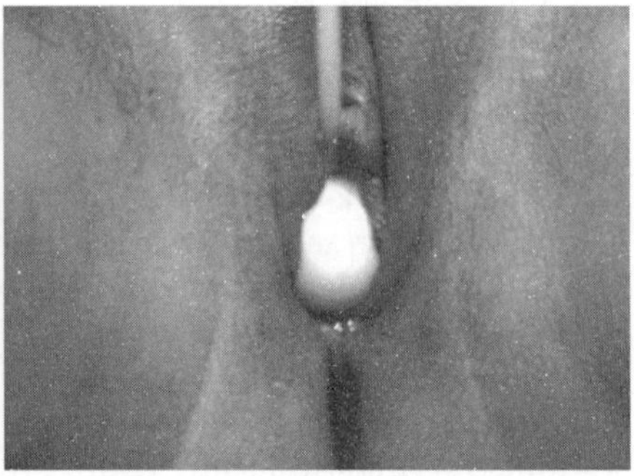

Fig. 23.11: Ball in the vaginal dimple. Suture pulled on the right side. Under traction from above *(For color version, see Plate 6)*

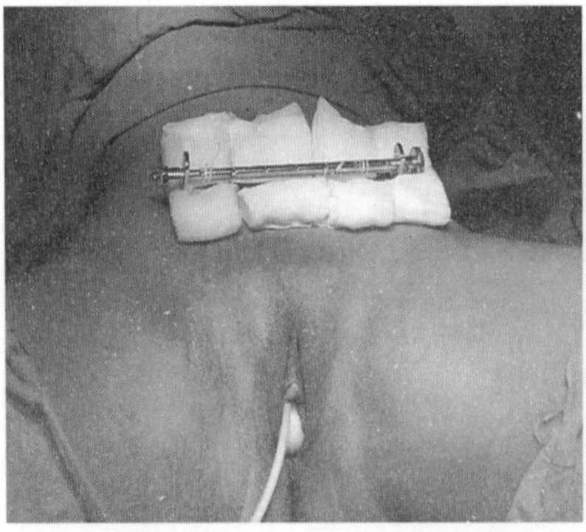

Fig. 23.12: Gradually escalating the traction *(For color version, see Plate 7)*

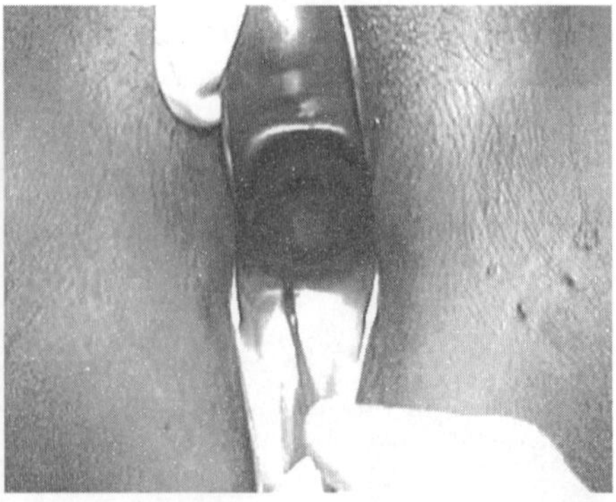

Fig. 23.13: Final result with good depth of vagina *(For color version, see Plate 7)*

LAPAROSCOPIC APPENDECTOMY IN ADOLESCENTS (FIGS 23.14 TO 23.17)

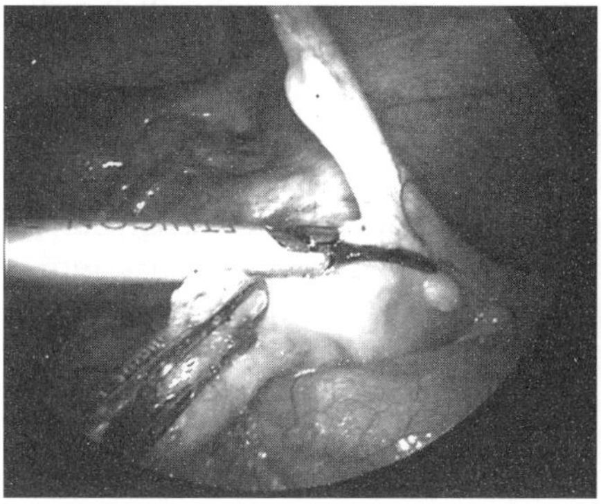

Fig. 23.14: Harmonic ace dissection *(For color version, see Plate 7)*

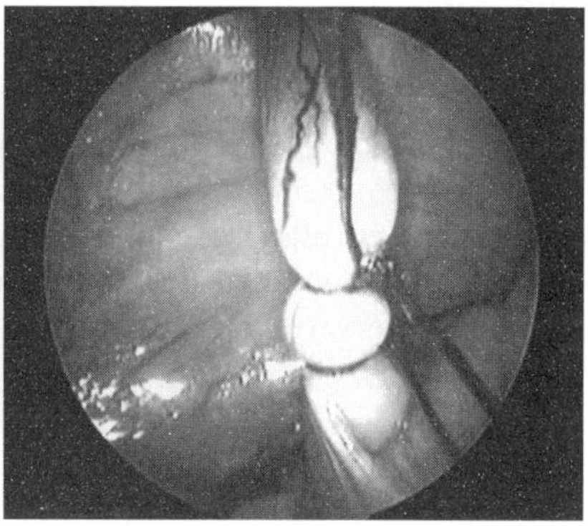

Fig. 23.15: Selfmade endoloops *(For color version, see Plate 7)*

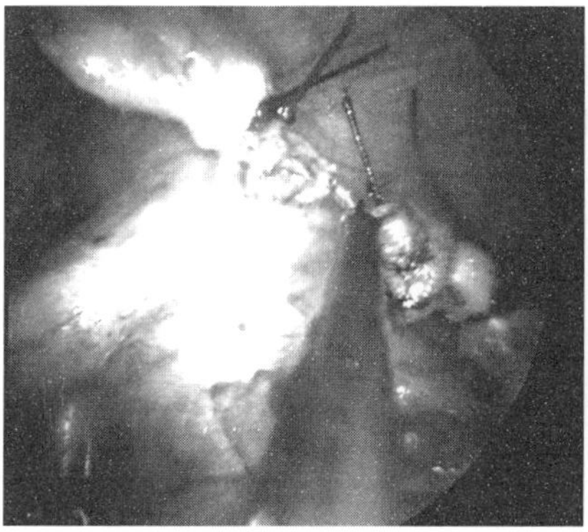

Fig. 23.16: Separation of appendix *(For color version, see Plate 7)*

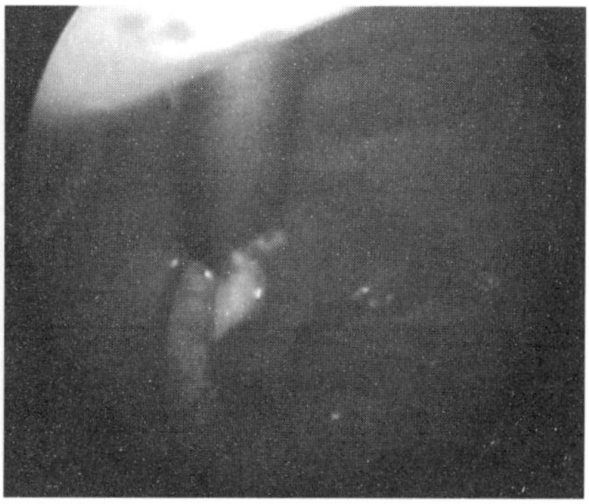

Fig. 23.17: Removal from 10 mm port *(For color version, see Plate 7)*

LAPAROSCOPIC PRESACRAL NEURECTOMY FOR SEVERE DYSMENORRHEA (FIGS 23.18 AND 23.19)

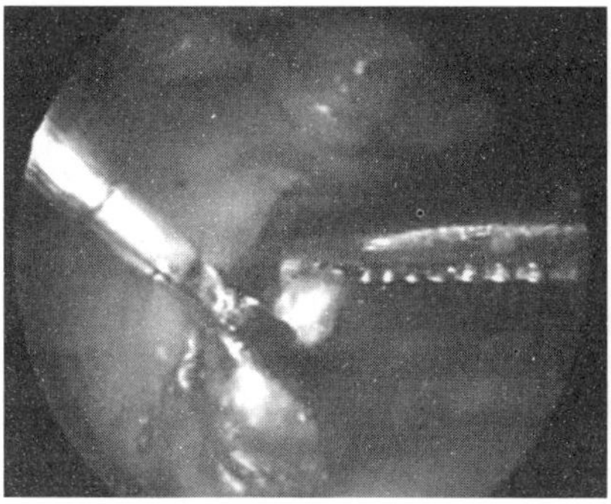

Fig. 23.18: Dissection of the presacral nerve *(For color version, see Plate 8)*

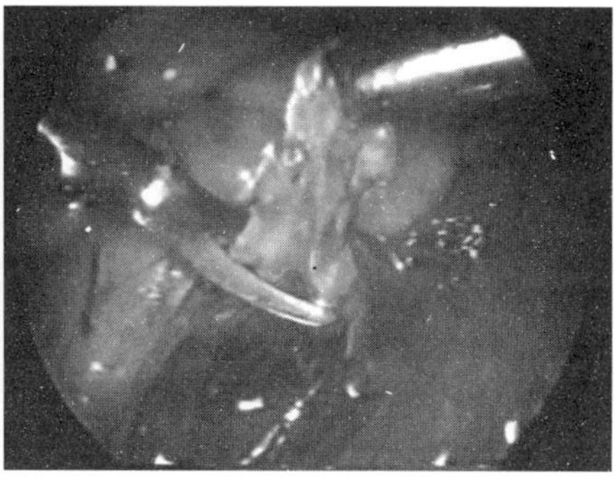

Fig. 23.19: Presacral neurectomy *(For color version, see Plate 8)*

CONCLUSION

Endoscopic surgery has an important role in adolescents, both diagnostic and therapeutic. The major benefit—cosmetically and fast recovery—is a boon with short hospital stay. Endoscopic surgery is useful for correction of multiple pathologies and anomalies as mentioned in indications.

Major requirements of endoscopic surgery in adolescents is an expert endoscopic with all necessary instruments, safe monitored anesthetist, proper OT set-up with facilities of documentation, profound respect to tissues, future fertility preservation, reducing recurrences and adhesions and minimal complications.

REFERENCES

1. Spinelli C, Di Giacomo M, Cei M, Mucci N. Functional ovarian lesions in children and adolescents: When to remove. Gynecol Endocrinol 2009;25(5):294-98.
2. Strickland JL. Ovarian cysts in neonates, children and adolescents. Opin Obstet Gynecol 2002;14(5):459-65.
3. Shapiro EY, Kaye JD, Palmer LS. Laparoscopic ovarian cystectomy in children. Urology 2009;73(3):526-28.
4. Laufer MR, Goldstein DP, Ovarian Cysts and neoplasms in children, and adolescents. Uptodate 2007.
5. Breen, JL, Maxson WS. Ovarian tumors in children and adolescents. Clin Obstet Gynecol 1977;20:607.
6. Elizabeth Ball, Masoud Ganji, Grace Janik, Charles Koh. Gynecol Surgery, 2009.

24 Robotic Surgery: Emergence of a New Gynecological Paradigm

Krishna Kavita Ramavath

INTRODUCTION

"Imagination is not unreal; it is the borderland of what is yet to be real. Everything you imagine can be created by a will that is guided by wisdom".

– Sri Sri Paramahamsa Yogananda, Author of 'Autobiography of a Yogi'.

Paramahamsa Yogananda's quotation summarizes well the state of art in Robotic surgery today. The Robo, which was once considered as fantasy, has now become a reality. It was in 1921 that Karel Capek introduced the term 'Robo' in his play "Rossom's Universal Robots". Since then the imposed limitations of the world are transcended through the process of imagination, creativity and willpower.

Over the past several decades, minimally invasive surgical techniques, instrumentation and technology have improved significantly. Their advantages are very popular among surgeons and patients. These techniques were successfully applied to adolescent gynecological tumors.

Laparoscopic technology has evolved since its early inception. A great advance was signified by the switch from a monocular direct vision through laparoscope to the indirect 2D image of the laparoscopic field projected onto a monitor screen. The introduction of fiber optics resulted in superior lighting system. Flexible scopes containing chips at their distal ends have allowed for visualization of structures over large organs. Incorporation of these technological advances at every step improved our surgical efficiency in the minimally invasive treatment procedures.

Many studies showed that laparoscopic procedures resulted in smaller incisions, decreased hospital stay, decreased risk of wound infection and quick return to work with decreased pain and better cosmetics.

But there are shortcomings and limitations to this conventional laparoscopy. Some of the prominent limitations are:

- Loss of tactile feedback
- Compromised hand-eye coordination
- Restricted degrees of motion
- Tissue manipulation is more dependent on visualization
- Physiologic tremors of the surgeon are transmitted through the instruments and delicate dissections and anastomoses are difficult to perform.

In order to overcome these limitations and to expand the benefits of minimally invasive surgeries, many scientists, doctors like general surgeons and endoscopists joined to become a team and strived hard to develop 'Robos'.

Today, Robos are developed in the field of surgery with the relentless professionalism and dedication of countless researchers and doctors. Their work and creativity have innovated the master slave manipulator, which works with high specificity and precision. Robotic surgery is the most important advancement of the millennium.

DEVELOPMENT OF ROBOTIC SURGICAL SYSTEMS—A BRIEF HISTORY

The history of Robotic surgery begins with PUMA 560, a robotic arm used to perform neurosurgical biopsy in 1985 by Kwoh et al.

Three years later, Davies et al performed a transurethral resection of the prostate using PUMA 560.

In 1988, Imperial College of London developed PROBOT for transurethral resection of the prostate (TURP).

ROBODOC, marketed by Integrated Surgical Systems (ISS) made history in 1992 as the first Robo assisting in Human total hip replacement surgeries. This is the first surgical Robo approved by US FDA (Food and Drug Administration).

In 1999, 'Orthopilot' with navigation system was developed.

The era of Robots in surgery commenced in 1994 and the use of robotics has evolved over the past twenty-five years. The ability to use robotic assisted surgery started with endoscopic surgery.

In 1993, the first AESOP (Automated Endoscope System for Optimal Positioning), a robot with voice controlled camera holder was used clinically and then marketed as the first surgical robot ever in 1994 by the USFDA. AESOP eliminated the need for a member of the surgical team to hold the endoscope in order for a surgeon to view his operative field.

Since then many robotic prototypes have been developed to add to the functions of the robot. A more active role for robotics was developed with an immerse environment that became known as robotic **telepresence technology.**

The most commonly used **master-slave manipulator** with 4 arms, one for camera and laparoscope and two for operating instruments is the **Da Vinci** surgical system. This system is evolved from the telepresence machines developed for NASA and US Army. It is approved by USFDA in 2005 for applying in gynecological procedures. This has proved to be a breakthrough technology and has stood the test of time.

With robotic surgery, surgeons do not move endoscopic instruments directly with their hands. Instead, surgeons sit at a console, several feet away from the operating table and use joy-sticks similar to those used in the video games. They perform surgical tasks by guiding the movement of the robotic arms in a process known as **telemanipulation.**

The **ZEUS** system is approved by USFDA in Oct 2001 to assist in control of blunt dissections during laparoscopic and thoracoscopic surgeries. It consists of a surgeon controlled console and three robotic arms. The right and left robotic arms replicate the arms of the surgeon and the third arm is an AESOP for visualization.

COMPARISON OF CONVENTIONAL LAPAROSCOPIC SURGERY vs ROBOTIC SURGERY (TABLE 24.1)

Laparoscopic surgery is technically more demanding than open surgery. The laparoscopic surgeon must view a distant monitor which provides 2D vision and changes the hand-eye coordination. But there is no stereoscopic depth perception. Moreover, the camera is being held by an assistant and hence the vision is not under surgeon's control and liable to fatigue and may cause an unsteady field of vision.

The instruments in laparoscopic surgery are rigid and provide only 4 degrees of motion as compared to the surgical robot, which provides 7 degrees, just like the human wrist does, in open surgery. Also, the tasks like ligation and suturing are much more complex. The other limitations of laparoscopy include limited instrument dexterity, tremor amplification and poor ergonomics.

However, the advantages of minimally invasive surgery are now confirmed beyond doubt with regard to oncologic safety, survival and recurrence rates for malignant diseases. The surgical robot can therefore be wisely used in gynecological malignancies with proper indications to provide the patient with the benefits of minimally invasive surgery, eliminating the pitfalls of conventional laparoscopy at the same time.

Table 24.1: Comparison among conventional, laparoscopic and robot-assisted surgeries

Attributes of Surgery	*Conventional Surgery*	*Laparoscopic Surgery*	*Robot-assisted Surgery*
Technology	Prone to tremor and fatigue	Good	Well-defined
Efficiency	Limited in difficult situations	Proven efficiency	Very efficient and approved by US-FDA
Hand-eye coordination	Strong, but limited dexterity outside natural scale	Compromised coordination and dexterity	Absence of haptic sensation but improved dexterity
Scalability	Human and operational limitation	Scalable	Better scalability
Integration of information	Can integrate extensive and diverse information. Good judgment	Unable to use qualitative information. No judgment	Unable to use qualitative information. No judgment
Costs	Reasonable	Affordable	Expensive

Table 24.2: Advantages and limitations of robotic surgery

Advantages of Robotic Surgery	*Limitations of Robotic Surgery*
New technology with 3D visualization	Absence of touch sensation
Improved dexterity and good precision	New technology, needs further studies
Seven degrees of freedom	Very expensive
Elimination of fulcrum effect	Requires trained staff
Elimination of psychological tremors	High start-up costs
Ability to scale motions	Benefits to be proved
Microanastomosis possible	
Telesurgery, ergonomics	

Table 24.2 casts light on the advantages and limitations of robotic surgery.

THE DA VINCI ROBOTIC SYSTEM (FIGS 24.1A TO C)

The da Vinci surgical system developed by Intuitive Surgical Systems (Inc Sunnyvale, CA) is the most significant advancement in the minimally invasive surgeries of this decade.

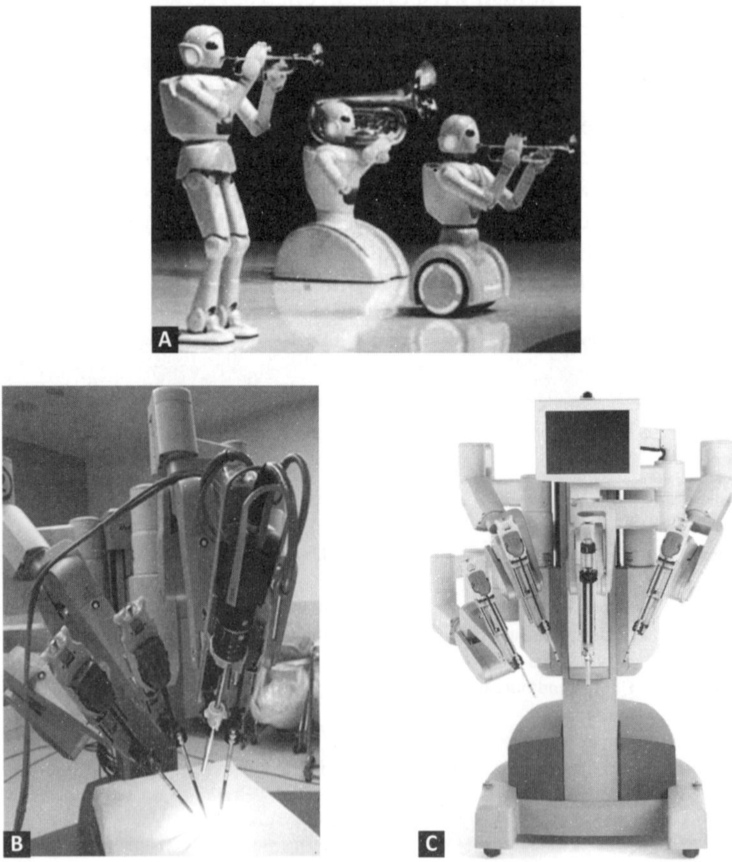

Figs 24.1A to C: Da Vinci robotic surgical system
(*Courtesy:* Intuitive Surgical Systems Inc, Sunnyvale, CA)

It is developed by Stanford Research Institute, the United States Defense Department and the National Aeronautics and Space Administration (NASA), with an attempt to allow telesurgery for wounded soldiers.

The main idea was to place the operating surgeon remote to the battlefield performing surgery through a robotic assistance in the battlefield operating room or a Mobile Advanced Surgical Hospital (MASH). It was hoped that this way of treating soldiers in the war, prevented them from being exsanguinated before they reached the hospital. But its practical use was limited by several factors including telecommunications, bandwidth requirements, etc.

Since its inception in 1997, the robot has been gradually upgraded from the first 3 arm system to the current 4 arms and light weight.

The system basically has 3 components (Fig. 24.2):

- The robotic cart
- The surgeon console
- The endoscopic stack.

The system delivers a high quality 3D vision to the surgeon manning the console and give improved depth perception. This technology allows Intuitive ***Telemanipulation with tremor abolition*** and ***endo-wristed movements.***

This is essentially, what gives a **cutting edge** over the conventional laparoscopy with limited capabilities of the surgeon in the field of minimally invasive surgery.

The Surgical Console (Fig. 24.3)

The computer system which controls the whole system resides in the surgeon's console. It consists of the binocular viewer of the Insite Vision System, the instrument controllers, the system setup and five foot control pedals.

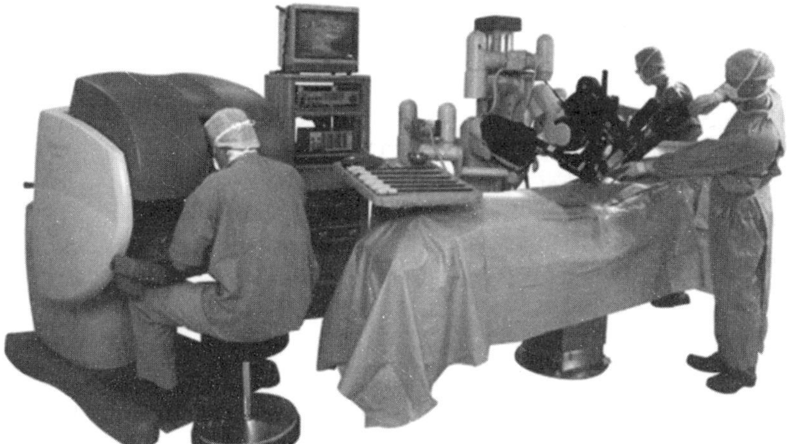

Fig. 24.2: Console and cart of the robotic system
(*Courtesy:* Intuitive Surgical Systems Inc, Sunnyvale, CA)

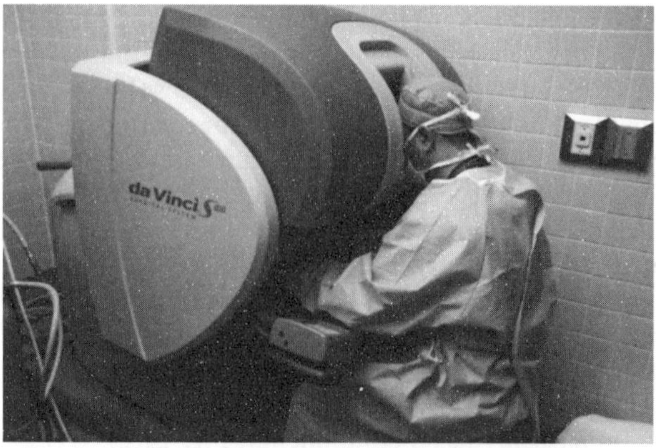

Fig. 24.3: Surgeons console (*Courtesy:* Intuitive Surgical Systems Inc, Sunnyvale, CA)

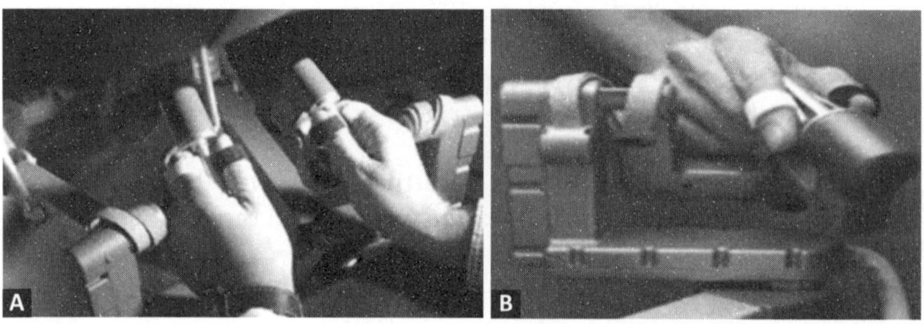

Figs 24.4A and B: Handcontrol (*Courtesy:* Intuitive Surgical System Inc, Sunnyvale, CA)

The camera system (Insite Vision System) has a dual lens system, representing left and right eyes. The instruments can be easily and rapidly changeable by assistant surgeon at the patient side. Except for the ultrasonic dissection, all the instruments are endowristed. The camera provides three dimensional views with upto 10-12 times magnification. The robotic arms and instruments together provide seven degrees of freedom, replicating that of the surgeon's hands. This master device consists of 2 finger controlled handles that control 4 robotic arms with different surgical instruments (Figs 24.4A and B).

Foot Pedals and Control Panels (Fig. 24.5)

Foot pedals are five in number and help in disengaging the instruments from the controllers to adjust focus, for bipolar coagulation and monopolar cautery. There are two panels on either sides of the surgeon, one on the left includes camera and endoscopic calibration and motion scaling; the other on the right hand side controls the system start, emergency stop and stand-by buttons.

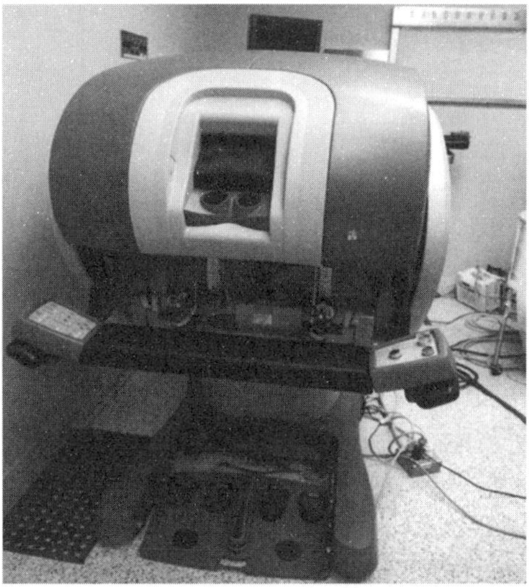

Fig. 24.5: Foot pedals and control panels
(*Courtesy:* Intuitive Surgical Systems Inc, Sunhyvale, CA)

The Endoscopic Stack

It has all the features of a standard laparoscopic stack, viz. the monitor, CO_2 insufflators, a dual high intensity light source and a dual CCD camera unit.

Set-up Procedures

System start-up sequence takes approximately one minute. Once the camera and endoscope are connected and calibrated, patient has to be placed in the position desired. Now the robotic ports can be placed and the arms attached to start the procedure. The surgeon takes his position at the console after the desired instruments are placed in the arms by assistant surgeon. Surgeon places his fingers in the adjustable loops and head in the binocular view and begins performing the surgery.

A large operating room is essential to house the robot and its components along with the routine equipment.

APPLICATIONS OF THE DA VINCI IN THE TREATMENT OF TUMORS AND CANCERS

Across the globe, there are almost a 1000 robotic systems and majority of them are in USA. Da Vinci system is designed to use in Minimally Invasive Surgeries and can also be used for open surgery. In addition to gynecologists, general surgeons, urologists, cardiothoracic and pediatric surgeons are using the system. It is best used for minimal invasive surgeries, which are seemingly impossible and difficult to perform with conventional laparoscopic techniques (Figs 24.6A and B).

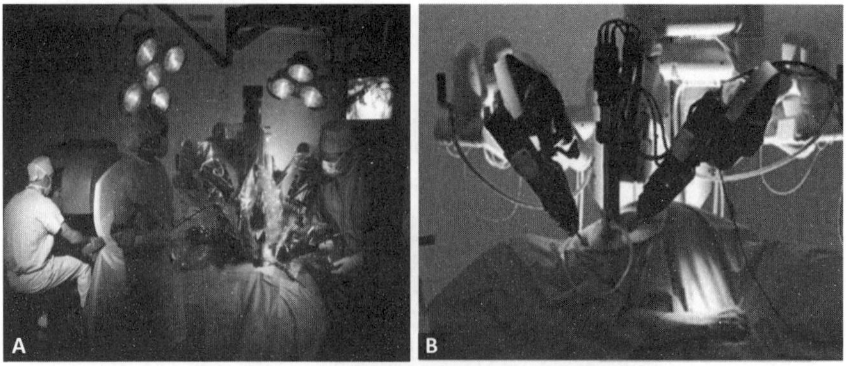

Figs 24.6A and B: Robotic surgery (*Contributed by*: Robospecs, Workmates, Peter Menzel, Sean Hayes, Jeff Chamberlein)

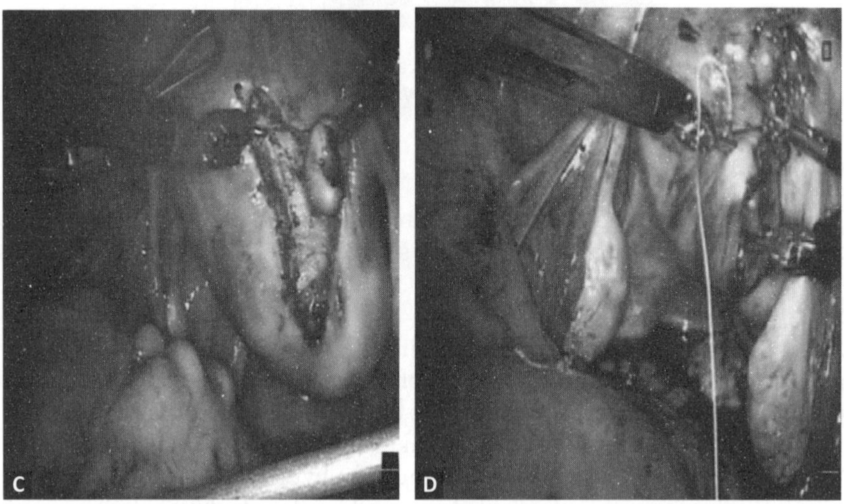

Figs 24.6C and D: Robotic surgery (*Courtesy*: Paul D Indman, OBGYN.NET) *(For color version, see Plate 8)*

Robotic surgery has been successful for esophageal tumors, retromediastinal tumors, and gastric cancer in addition to gynecological tumors. The application of Robotic systems is now efficiently applied in treating Breast lesions like invasive ductal carcinoma, adenocarcinoma and fibroadenoma (Figs 24.6C and D).

Robotics have superhuman capabilities that make surgery easier. For instance they do not tire. Robotics arms don't have a tremor, so they can remain steady at all times and robotic wrists make it easier for surgeons to manipulate tissue and work from all kinds of angles.

Each instrument has only 10 lives following which it needs to be discarded, as there may be a possibility of the instrument cable breaking off.

ROBOTIC SURGERY IN ADOLESCENT GYNECOLOGY (TABLE 24.3)

Robotic surgery is an already well established technology being used across the globe. Urologists and general surgeons are the front runners in using robotics but gynecologists are taking the cue. The application of these techniques in selected gynecological cancers is safe and effective alternative to laparotomy. The new robotic procedures tend to reduce blood loss, cut hospital stays and also offers advantages of faster post-op recovery, decreased pain and improved quality of life.

One of the areas where robotic surgery is creating stirring interest and excitement is the minimally invasive gynecological surgeries. With the report of management of uterine rhabdomyosarcoma, with robotic radical hysterectomy and pelvic lymphadenectomy, gynecological oncologists are keen on using robotic surgeries in all aspects of adolescent gynecological tumor management.

Emphasis on radical surgery has declined over the past decade with the efficacy of multi-agent chemotherapy, in these adolescents as most of the tumors have good prognosis. However, surgery remains an important treatment option if chemotherapy or radiotherapy fail to achieve local control. Radical surgery is very debilitating to these young patients and recovery is also prolonged with serious psychological impact. Laparoscopic surgery uses small incisions, causes less discomfort with quick recovery and gives a positive body image. However, it has its own limitations with regard to decreased wrist motion, adequate visualization and sometimes surgeon's discomfort.

Robotic surgery uses same small incisions but allows full hand and wrist movements without compromising the surgical technique. For technically challenging operations in these patients, robotic technology better facilitates the surgical approach as compared to laparoscopy. Technological advances in robotic surgery provide a minimally invasive surgical approach in settings of complex pathology in these young adolescents.

Endoscopic surgery in the pediatric and adolescent patients offers **several challenges** above and beyond what a surgeon finds in the adult correlate. The body cavities are smaller, the impact of tremor and loss of dexterity are enhanced, and visibility is further limited. In recent reviews it has been

Table 24.3: Robotic surgery in gynecology

Operation	*Indication*
Hysterectomy	Myoma uterus
Robotic radical hysterectomy	Cervical intra epithelial neoplasia, endometrial cancer, ovarian cancer
Robotic radical hysterectomy and pelvic lymphadenectomy	Uterine rhabdomyosarcoma
Ovarian transposition	In patients undergoing pelvic irradiation
Salpingo-oophorectomy	Complex ovarian tumors in adolescents and adults
Ovariectomy	Ovarian serous cyst
Robotic microsurgeries	Tubal anastomosis

noted that both the Zeus® (Computer Motion, Goleta, California) and Da Vinci® (Intuitive Surgical, Mountain View, California) systems address many of the basic inconveniences of endoscopic surgery. By maintaining steady camera position, filtering tremor, scaling motion, and restoring lost degrees of freedom, these master-slave systems enhance the dexterity and, in turn, the capabilities of a robotically trained endoscopic surgeon.

While sharing their **early experiences of robotic surgeries in children**, Gutt CN, Marcus B and others from the Department of General and Vascular Surgery, Johann Wolfgang Goethe University, Germany, quoted that,they had applied Da Vinci robotic technique in eleven children with a mean age of 12 years. They concluded that compared to conventional laparoscopy, the three-dimensional high quality vision, advanced instrument movement and improved ergonomic position of the surgeon appeared to enhance surgical precision. Robotic surgery in children using Da Vinci seems to be **feasible and safe**. However, the technique is limited due to the fact that instruments adapted to the size of small children have to be developed. In adolescent and adult gynecological field, Da Vinci is used in surgeries for Gonado-blastomas, Endometriosis, Cervical Intraepithelial Neoplasia. However the benefits to the young patients must be carefully evaluated and proven before this technology can be widely accepted.

The widespread acceptance of this technology largely depends on solving the issues: learning curve; suitable machine size; ensuring efficacy and safety in all operations; and, most importantly, making this procedure cost effective, so as to cater for the needs of most, if not all, children and adolescents.

ROBOTIC SURGERY IN GYNECOLOGY

Hysterectomy is the most common non-pregnancy associated laparoscopic surgical procedure in USA. The history of robotic laparoscopic hysterectomy is short and still developing. The first successful robotic laparoscopic hysterectomy was performed by Diaz-Arrastia in 2002.

Now the indications for robotic laparoscopic hysterectomy through Da Vinci surgical system are:

- Cervical intraepithelial neoplasia III
- Endometrial cancer
- Myoma of uterus
- Post-menopausal bleeding and
- Ovarian cancer.

Robotic and laparoscopic radical hysterectomy has shown to have advantages for patients over laparotomy approach in terms of blood loss, blood transfusion, complication and length of hospital stay, with the exception of prolonged operating time.

Robotic surgery for selected gynecological cancers is feasible and also associated with low morbidity. The difficult steps of gynecological surgeries such as unroofing and dissection of distal ureter are done with more precision.

Despite studies showing the feasibility of robotic surgery there is still much to be desired. More clinical trials are necessary and much more experience is needed to be obtained before the full potential of these systems can be realized.

The Future (Fig. 24.7)

As far as imagination, ideas, science and technology is concerned, surgical robotics is a deep fertile soil. Already development of robotics is creating stirring interest in **new tissue anastomosis techniques, improving laparoscopic instruments and digital integration of already existing technologies.** A new **robotic tele collaborative medical device** made by makers of Zeus robotic surgical system is already in the market, which allows surgeons at remote sites to connect to operating room and interact with another surgeon anywhere in the world. This helps in extending training and mentoring opportunities for surgeons worldwide.

The possibility of programing the surgery and the surgeon merely supervising as Robo performs the task is not far way.

CONCLUSION

Much attention is now being paid to the promise of Robotic surgery. The application of these techniques, in selected gynecological cancers is safe and effective alternative to laparotomy.

For technically challenging operations in adolescent gynecological malignancies, robotic technology facilitates the surgical approach better in comparison to laparoscopy. Because of its steady three dimensional view, instrumentation with articulating tips and with wrist like movements which provides finer and more dexterous movements with tremor elimination, it facilitates surgical procedures which were impossible with conventional laparoscopy.

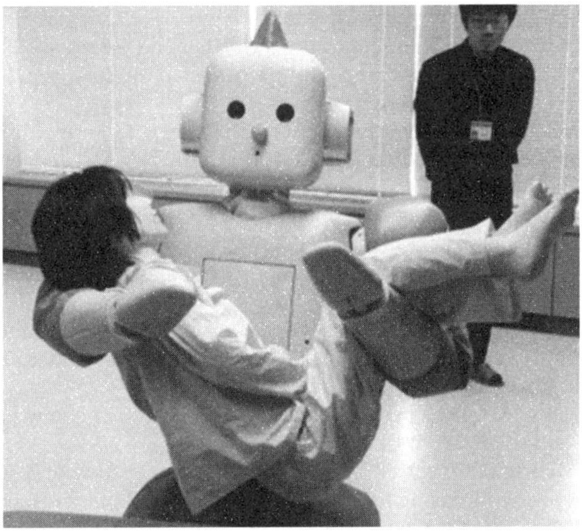

Fig. 24.7: The future (*Courtesy:* www.japancast.net/.../ robot_,robotsworldandhuman.com)

Robotic pediatric and adolescent gynecological surgery is feasible, but that smaller instrumentation and reduced costs are needed before routine robotic surgery can become a reality to them.

Although patient advantages are improved with Robotics, there are multiple advantages for surgeons as it is associated with faster performance times, increased accuracy and faster suturing. The skills to perform this procedure are acquired in short time.

Robotic technologies are being developed to guide surgical planning and execution in such a way that a surgeon may become more of a "General" guiding multiple robotic and virtual systems, rather than a "soldier" executing each individual cut.

No doubt that very soon, Robotics will become an important tool in the surgical armamentarium.

ACKNOWLEDGMENTS

My special thanks to Prof Javier F Magrina, Dept of Gynecology, Mayoclinic, Scottsdale, Arizona for guiding this article.

My special thanks to Intuitive Surgicals, Sunnyvale, CA; Zeus Surgicals; robotsworldandhuman.com; Paul D Indman, OBGYN.NET; Robospecs, workmates, Peter Menzel, Sean Hayes,Jeff Chamberlein, www.heart-valve-surgery.com/Images/davinci-robo; www.adventisthealthnw.com; www.urology.uci.edu/prostate/ Thomas Ahlering, MD, Professor and Vice Chairman, Department of Urology,

Special thanks to Prof Dr RA NAIK, Dept of Medicine, KGH, Visakhapatnam and Mr Srinivas Reddy, Wipro, APS, Phoenix, Arizona for editing the article.

SUGGESTED READING

1. A Najmaldin. Paediatric telerobotic surgery: Where do we stand? The International Journal of Medical Robotics and Computer Assisted Surgery. Sep 2007, Vol. 3, No. 3: 183-86.
   Early experience of tele-robotic surgery in children A Najmaldin, B Antao. The International Journal of Medical Robotics and Computer Assisted Surgery. Sep 2007, Vol. 3, No. 3: 199-202.
2. Advincula AP, Falcone T. Laparoscopic robotic gynecologic surgery. Obstet Gynecol Clin North Am 2004;31:599-609, ix-x.
3. Bann S, Khan M, Hernandez J, Munz Y, Moorthy K, Datta V, et al. Robotics in surgery. J Am Coll Surg 2003.
4. Bell MC, Torgenson J, Seshadri-Kreaden U, et al. Comparison of outcomes and cost for endometrial cancer staging via traditional laparotomy, standard laparoscopy and robotic techniques. Gynecol Oncol 2008;111:407-11.
5. Beste TM, Nelson KH, Daucher JA. Total laparoscopic hysterectomy utilizing a robotic surgical system. JSLS 2005;9:13-15.
6. Boggess JF, Gehrig PA, Cantrell L, et al. A comparative study of 3 surgical methods for hysterectomy with staging for endometrial cancer: Robotic assistance, laparoscopy, laparotomy. Am J Obstet Gynecol 2008;199:360.e1-9.
7. Childers JM, Brzechffa PR, Hatch KD, et al. Laparoscopically assisted surgical staging (LASS) of endometrial cancer. Gynecol Oncol 1993;51:33-8.

8. Childers JM, Surwit EA. Combined laparoscopic and vaginal surgery for the management of two cases of stage I endometrial cancer. Gynecol Oncol 1992;45: 45-51.
9. DeNardis SA, Holloway RW, Bigsby GE IV, et al. Robotically assisted laparoscopic hysterectomy versus total abdominal hysterectomy and lymphadenectomy for endometrial cancer. Gynecol Oncol 2008;111:412-17.
10. Falcone T, Goldberg JM. Robotics in gynecology. Surg Clin North Am 2003;83:1483-89, xii.
11. Fiorentino RP, Zepeda MA, Goldstein BH, et al. Pilot study assessing robotic laparoscopic hysterectomy and patient out-comes. J Minim Invasive Gynecol 2006;13:60-3.
12. Fiorentino RP, Zepeda MA, Goldstein BH, John CR, Rettenmaier MA. Pilot study assessing robotic laparoscopic hysterectomy and patient outcomes. J Minim Invasive Gynecol 2006;13:60-3.
13. Frumovitz M, dos Reis R, Sun C, et al. Comparison of total laparoscopic and abdominal radical hysterectomy for patients with early-stage cervical cancer. Obstet Gynecol 2007;110:96-102.
14. Gehrig PA, Cantrell LA, Shafer A, et al. What is the optimal minimally invasive surgical procedure for endometrial cancer staging in the obese and morbidly obese woman? Gynecol Oncol 2008;111:41-5.
15. Holloway RW, Finkler NJ, Pikaart DP, et al. Comparison of total laparoscopic and abdominal radical hysterectomy for patients with early-stage cervical cancer. Obstet Gynecol 2007;110:1174-75.
16. Jemal A, Siegel R, Ward E, et al. Cancer statistics, 2008. CA Cancer J Clin 2008;58: 71-96.
17. Johnson N, Barlow D, Lethaby A, et al. Methods of hysterectomy: Systematic review and meta-analysis of randomized controlled trials. BMJ 2005;330:1478.
18. Kho RM, Hilger WS, Hentz JG, et al. Robotic hysterectomy: Technique and initial outcomes. Am J Obstet Gynecol 2007;197:113.e1-e4.
19. Kim YT, Kim SW, Yoon BS, Nahm EJ, Hur HW, Kim SH, et al. Robot-assisted total laparoscopic hysterectomy; initial experience in Korea. Korean J Obstet Gynecol 2006;49:2620-25.
20. Koh CH. A new technique and system for simplifying total laparoscopic hysterectomy. J Am Assoc Gynecol Laparosc 1998;5:187-92.
21. Leiserowitz GS, Xing GB, Parikh-Patel A, et al. Survival of endometrial cancer patients after laparoscopically assisted vaginal hysterectomy or total abdominal hysterectomy: Analysis of risk factors. Gynecol Oncol 2007;104 (Suppl. 1):A7.
22. Lenihan JP Jr, Kovanda C, Seshardi-Kreaden U. What is the learning curve for robotic assisted gynecologic surgery? J Minim Invasive Gynecol 2008;15:589-94.
23. Magrina JF, Kho R, Magtibay PM. Robotic radical hysterectomy: Technical aspects. Gynecol Oncol 2009;113:28-31.
24. Naumann RW, Coleman RL. The use of adjuvant therapy in early endometrial cancer by members of the Society of Gynecologic Oncologists in 2005. Gynecol Oncol 2007;105:7-12.
25. Payne TN, Dauterive FR. A comparison of total laparoscopic hysterectomy to robotically assisted hysterectomy: Surgical outcomes in a community practice. J Minim Invasive Gynecol 2008;15:286-91.
26. Pikaart DP, Holloway RW, Ahmad S, et al. Clinical-pathologic and morbidity analyses of types 2 and 3 abdominal radical hysterectomy for cervical cancer. Gynecol Oncol 2007;107:205-210.
27. Reich H. New techniques in advanced laparoscopic surgery. Baillieres Clin Obstet Gynaecol 1989;3:655-81. Falcone T, Goldberg J, Garcia-Ruiz A, Margossian H, Stevens L. Full robotic assistance for laparoscopic tubal anastomosis: A case report. J Laparoendosc Adv Surg Tech A 1999;9:107-13.

28. Reynolds RK, Advincula AP. Robot-assisted laparoscopic hysterectomy: Technique and initial experience. Am J Surg 2006;191:555–560. Wu JM, Wechter ME, Geller EJ, et al: Hysterectomy rates in the United States, 2003. Obstet Gynecol 2007;110:1091-95.
29. Robotic Surgery in Gynecologic Field. Young Tae Kim, Sang Wun Kim, and Yong Wook Jung. Department of Obstetrics and Gynecology, Women's Cancer Clinic, Yonsei University College of Medicine, Seoul, Korea. Capek K, Capek J. The Insect Play. In: Oxford MB, editor. 1st ed. New York: Oxford University Press; 1963.
30. Satava RM. Robotic surgery: from past to future—a personal journey. Surg Clin North Am 2003;83:1491-500, xii.
31. Seamon LG, Cohn DE, Richardson DL, et al. Robotic hysterectomy and pelvicaortic lymphadenectomy for endometrial cancer. Obstet Gynecol 2008;112:1207-13.
32. Spirtos NM, Eisekop SM, Boike G, et al. Laparoscopic staging in patients with incompletely staged cancers of the uterus, ovary, fallopian tube, and primary peritoneum: A Gynecologic Oncology Group (GOG) study. Am J Obstet Gynecol 2005;193:1645-49.
33. Spirtos NM, Schlaerth JB, Kimball RE, et al. Laparoscopic radical hysterectomy (type III) with aortic and pelvic lymph-adenectomy. Am J Obstet Gynecol 1996;174: 1763-67.
Li G, Yan X, Shang H, et al. A comparison of laparoscopic radical hysterectomy and pelvic lymphadenectomy and laparotomy in the treatment of IB–IIA cervical cancer. Gynecol Oncol 2007;105:176-180.
34. Veljovich DS, Paley PJ, Drescher CW, et al. Robotic surgery in gynecologic oncology: Program initiation and outcomes after the first year with comparison with laparotomy for endometrial cancer staging. Am J Obstet Gynecol 2008;198:679.e1-10.
35. Walker J, Mannel R, Piedmonte M, et al. Phase III trial of laparoscopy versus laparotomy for surgical resection and comprehensive surgical staging of uterine cancer. A Gynecologic Oncology Group study funded by the National Cancer Institute. Gynecol Oncol 2006;101 (Suppl. 1):A22.
36. Wattiez A, Cohen SB, Selvaggi L. Laparoscopic hysterectomy. Curr Opin Obstet Gynecol 2002;14:417-22.

Section 6

SOCIAL ISSUES, LIFE SKILLS AND COUNSELING

25 Adolescence and Life Skill Education

Preeti M Galagali

Education for life, Education through life, Education throughout life.

—Mahatma Gandhi

Life skills are tools to handle and face life boldly, happily and successfully. They open the closed doors of our mind. World Health Organization has defined life skills as abilities for positive and adaptive behavior to deal effectively with demands and challenges of everyday life.[1] These skills enhance the ability to get on with life smoothly. Life skills are needed for developing psychosocial competence. Psychosocial competence is the ability to maintain a state of well-being while interacting with others or dealing with oneself in various day-to-day situations.

Adolescents form 22% of India's population (Census 2001) and their health will determine the health of the nation. In the current era of media boom, deteriorating moral and social values and innumerable choices, adolescents are facing a number of challenges. Also lifestyle diseases like obesity, diabetes mellitus, AIDS, drug abuse and depression in the youth are on the rise. Adolescents, who are on the threshold of adulthood, are immature to handle such overwhelming challenges to their physical health and psychosocial well-being. They need help from parents, teachers and other knowledgeable nonjudgmental trustworthy adults to make a smooth transition into adulthood. Due to the emergence of double income nuclear families, there remains an inadequate mechanism for passing on life skills from generation to generation in a traditional manner. Hence there is a need of a structured life skill education program in this vulnerable age.

Life Skill Education empowers the adolescents to make the right choices about their lifestyle. Thus life skills promote healthy behavior and prevent diseases. Life skills have also been applied in various other settings like promotion of peace, human rights, promotion of self confidence, environmental issues and gender equality. In 1997, World Health Organization (WHO) stated that 'Life Skill Program' should be implemented universally in schools.

THEORETICAL BASIS OF LIFE SKILLS AND LIFE SKILL EDUCATION

Life skills are based on Bandura's social learning theory. Social learning theory promotes opportunities for processing life experiences, structuring experiences and gaining experiences.[2] A change in behavior can occur only if the knowledge, attitudes and values of an individual are translated into abilities or skills. UNICEF has defined life skills as being a behavior change or behavior development approach designed to address a balance of three areas: knowledge, attitude and skills. Adolescents need both information and skills to adopt a healthy lifestyle. For example, adolescents can stay away from cigarette smoking only, if they are educated about risks of smoking, their values are against smoking and if they have the skills to handle stress and resist negative peer pressure. Adolescents need to develop skills of self awareness, critical and creative thinking, problem solving and decision making, coping with stress and assertion to remain 'drug free'. Hence life skills modify behavior by converting 'what we know' and 'what we think/ feel and believe' into 'what to do' and 'how to do'.[1]

CATEGORIES OF LIFE SKILLS

Life skills are classified into three categories as under:[2]

1. *Core life skills:* These include basic ten important life skills.
2. *Specific life skills:* A combination of generic life skills are used to develop skills in handling specific situations like peer, media and family pressures, violence, gender discrimination, bullying, substance abuse, suicide, eating disorders, sexuality and assertive behavior.
3. *Area specific skills:* A combination of life skills are used to develop specific skills in a particular area like career development, study skills, time management and technical skills.

Core Life Skills

Core life skills are outlined below:

The most important and basic ten generic life skills are outlined below:

1. *Self-esteem and self-awareness:* This helps the adolescent to understand his/her self worth and builds his/her confidence to face life boldly. It also enables one to identify ones weaknesses or negative personality traits and consequently improve oneself.
2. *Empathy:* It helps an adolescent to understand and accept others who are different from him/her, like people with disability and AIDS patients.
3. *Effective communication:* It enables an adolescent to express his opinions, desires and fears clearly by using both verbal communication and non-verbal expressions. It also trains the adolescent to ask for advice and help from others in times of need.
4. *Interpersonal relationships:* It teaches an adolescent to relate to other people in a positive manner. It also helps him/her to develop the ability to end relationships constructively.
5. *Creative thinking:* It helps an adolescent to respond in a flexible manner to various challenges of life. It enables him/her to explore available possible alternatives and to assess their consequences. This skill helps in both problem solving and decision-making.

6. *Critical thinking:* This skill enables an adolescent to analyze information and experiences objectively. It also helps to recognize factors like family values, peer and media pressures that influence attitudes and behavior.
7. *Decision-making:* It enables an adolescent to make constructive decisions about one's life like choice of a career or marriage partner, type and quantity of dietary intake, etc. It teaches that decision be made only after assessing different options and their effects.
8. *Problem solving:* It helps an adolescent to solve his/her problems by using creative and critical thinking. If problems are not resolved, they can lead to mental stress and physical strain.
9. *Coping with emotions:* It enables an adolescent to recognize emotions in oneself and others, to realize its effects on behavior and to respond to emotions appropriately. Uncontrolled emotions like excessive sorrow and anger can have negative effects on health.
10. *Coping with stress:* It helps an adolescent to recognize sources of stress and its effects. It also teaches methods to control stress and to overcome it by relaxation techniques.

Three broad areas of life skills are social, thinking/reflective and negotiation skills.[3]

These are explained below:

- Social skills include establishing good interpersonal relationships, communicating effectively and empathy.
- Thinking/reflective skills include self awareness, social awareness, goal setting and planning, problem solving and decision making, creative and critical thinking.
- Negotiation skills with self and with others to resist peer or family pressure. These include assertive and advocacy skills.

Life Skills and Neurobiology of Adolescent Brain

The adolescent brain tends to use the amygdala for analysis of novel stimuli compared to adults who use the frontal brain. This makes the adolescent prone to experimentation and high risk behavior as the amygdala responds in an emotive manner while the frontal lobes tend to impose judgment. The dorsolateral prefrontal cortex and superior temporal gyrus are responsible for the ability to inhibit impulses, for critical thinking, to prioritize and strategize mature later than other areas of brain.[4] In stressful situations, this ability is further compromised and impulsive behavior in adolescents is common.[5] Learning and implementing life skills may hasten myelination of the 'frequently used' neuronal pathways and pruning of the less used one resulting in improved cognitive abilities of adolescents. Hence the 'storm' and 'stress' of adolescence can be considerably reduced by learning life skills that improve judgment and decision making ability of the adolescent.

RELEVANCE OF LIFE SKILL EDUCATION IN ADOLESCENCE

Adolescence, the period of life from 10 to18 years is the most challenging phase of one's life between childhood and adulthood. It is marked by rapid rates of growth and development. G Stanley Hall in 1904 first conceptualized the adolescent period. Hollingshead has precisely defined adolescence as that period in the life of an individual when the society no longer recognizes him as a child but does not as yet concede him the roles or functions inherent in the status of an adult.[6]

Adolescence proceeds across three distinct periods—early (10 to 13 years), middle (14-16 years) and late (16-18 years). Each period is characterized by a set of salient biological, psychological and social features. Hormones in conjunction with social structures like gender, culture, physical and social stressors foster this transition and account for substantial individual variation.[7] Life skills are relevant to each period of adolescence.

Early adolescence is characterized by changes in physical appearance. Adolescents are preoccupied with bodily changes in this phase. They also seek increased independence from family. Life skills including self esteem and self awareness, coping with stress, decision making, effective communication and interpersonal relationship are especially important in this phase.

Middle adolescence is the period when sexual drive surges, experimentation peaks and there is increasing concern with body image. The adolescents are usually act selfish in this period and are greatly influenced by the peer group. A few adolescents may undergo an identity crisis leading to low self esteem. This phase is marked by emergence of abstract thinking and formal logical operation. It is essential for the adolescence to understand consequences of indulging in high risk behavior. Hence teaching all the ten generic life skills assumes special importance in this phase.

Late adolescence is heralded by consolidation of sexual identity and formation of a stable body image. Independence, feelings of intimacy with possible commitment and important career decisions are the features of this phase. Hence teaching life skills of critical thinking, creative thinking, problem solving and decision making with effective communication and interpersonal relationship are important.

RATIONALE OF LAUNCHING AN ADOLESCENT LIFE SKILL PROGRAM IN INDIA TARGETING HIGH-RISK BEHAVIOR

Contemporary health problems in the adolescents are linked to lifestyle issues and are potentially preventable. Adolescent risk taking behavior contributes greatly to the morbidity and mortality in this age group.[8] Due to immaturity of frontal lobes of the brain, adolescents have poor impulse control. In addition, relative independence and decreased parental control with increasing peer influence, poor life skill education result in adolescents indulging high-risk behavior. These high-risk behaviors include poor nutrition, decreased physical activity, poor safety measures, unsafe sexual behavior, substance abuse, violence and suicide.[9]

This 'at risk behavior' is known to track into adulthood. Hence enabling the adolescent to make an informed decision regarding a healthy lifestyle is not only important for his current well-being but has implications on the future adult health. WHO has mentioned that 'most adults die of diseases that were preventable in adolescence'. Tobacco abuse, poor stress management and obesity are said to be major 'killers' of today—seeds of these are implanted in adolescence itself.

The most common cause of death in adolescence is injuries—intentional and unintentional.[10] Road traffic accidents and suicides form a major part of this group. Suicides usually occur due to academic stress, high parental expectations and undiagnosed depression. The mortality rates are higher among adolescent girls aged 15 to 24 years compared to boys. Gender discrimination, low nutritional status, early child bearing and death during child birth contribute to this differential mortality. Thus an adolescent life skill education program should include safety issues, traffic rules, coping with stress and emotions, sexuality and gender issues.

Malnutrition is widespread in adolescence—20% of the adolescents are obese in India while 70% adolescent girls are anemic.[11] This has both immediate and long-term repercussions. Obese adolescents are prone to develop metabolic syndrome, hypertension, hyperlipidemia, diabetes, fatty liver, depression and slipped capital femoral epiphysis. Zimmet, an internationally renowned diabetologist has commented that 'this is the first generation where children may die before their parents'. 50-80% of obese adolescents will continue to remain obese in adulthood with its risk of coronary artery disease and diabetes. Sedentary lifestyle and poor physical activity are associated with obesity. Undernutrition makes the adolescent stunted, makes him/her prone to diseases and also decreases performance in school. According to Barker's hypothesis, an undernourished adolescent girl becomes an undernourished mother to give birth to a low birth weight baby who is prone for infectious diseases and genetically programmed to develop metabolic syndrome on excessive weight gain. Hence poor nutrition in adolescent girls has an intergenerational effect. Life skill education about nutrition and physical activity is essential.

As per the Global Youth Tobacco Survey (GYTS) conducted by WHO and CDC, Atlanta during 2002-2004, the current prevalence of tobacco use among Indian school going youth (13 to15 years) is 17.5%, around 30% in boys and 16% in girls. 14.6% used smokeless tobacco (paan masala, gutka, zarda etc) while 8.3% were smokers.[12] This habit too tracks into adulthood, 90% of tobacco addicts begin drug use before 14 years. Tobacco and alcohol are gateway drugs and eventually lead to hard drug abuse. According to a UNODC and Ministry of Social Justice and Empowerment report 2004, 24% drug addicts are between 12-18 years.[13] Prevention of drug abuse is also an important component of an adolescent life skill program.

Mean age of marriage for girls in India is 18 years. Nearly 20% of girls under the age of 15 years are mothers. Early marriage and child bearing leads to increased mortality and morbidity and poor education level amongst girls. Adolescents contribute to 19% of total fertility rate and 27% married adolescent girls have an unmet need for contraception.[13] 50-60% of new cases of AIDS every year occur in 15-24 years age group. Many adolescents indulge in premarital sex. Hence, imparting age appropriate and culturally acceptable sexuality education to adolescents is needed.

Poor personal hygiene and immunization coverage in this age group leads to infectious diseases like hepatitis A and B, typhoid, chickenpox, tetanus, measles, mumps, rubella that results in school absenteeism, mortality and morbidity. In clinical practice, poor awareness and unwillingness to take a prick on the part of the adolescent are cited as reasons for incomplete immunization. Life skill education regarding immunization and personal hygiene should be imparted to all adolescents.

India has the largest child labor force in the world.[13] There are a large number of street adolescents. The high risk behavior is maximum in working and street adolescents. Special outreach life skill programs need to be implemented for these out of school adolescents.

Research has proved that media has a huge impact on adolescent behavior and lifestyle including substance use, sexual acts, violence, eating habits. Critical thinking life skill is essential to understand and analyze media messages. This forms an integral part of media literacy program.

CONTENTS AND METHODOLOGY OF AN ADOLESCENT LIFE SKILL EDUCATION

Adolescent life skill education program should include generic life skills, specific life skills targeting high risk behavior and area specific life skills. To combat high risk behavior, topics of nutrition, physical activity, suicide and violence prevention, substance abuse, immunization, personal hygiene, media literacy, safety and sexuality issues should be included. Area specific skills should cover time management and study skills. All the topics should be relevant to the adolescents and the methodology used should be socio-culturally and developmentally appropriate.

Life skill education is different from traditional teaching in the following ways:[1]

- It is based on experiential learning. The skills are taught and then the students are asked to experience their application in real life. Only those things are taught here which can be applied practically.
- The participatory interactive approach is adopted here. The students are actively involved in learning process through group discussions, brainstorming sessions, debates and role-plays. One way didactic lectures are found boring by the adolescent and do not help in combating 'at risk behavior.'

A life skill education class on a particular topic usually has four sections:[14]

- A knowledge enhancing session in which the life skill trainer imparts scientific knowledge in the form of an interactive talk.
- Skill session in which skills are demonstrated and practiced in a non-threatening 'safe' environment.

- Homework assignment is given to test the practical use of the learnt skills.
- Feedback is taken to assess the effectiveness of the session and trainer. A long-term change in behavior can be evaluated to test the efficacy of a life skill program.

Further details of the life skill sessions are beyond the scope of this article; the interested reader can look into the suggested life skill education modules section given at the end.

Implementation of a Life Skill Program

Educational institutions are the best places to implement a life skill program because of the following reasons:[1]

- Schools and colleges enjoy high credibility especially with parents
- Infrastructure is easily available
- There is presence of teachers who can be easily trained to conduct such a program.

For out of school adolescents life skill education programs can be implemented in anganwadis, district hospitals, government hospitals, Nehru Yuvak Kendra Sangathan, National Social Service Scheme centers, and community health centers by trained personnel.[9] Life skills are also imparted through National Open Schooling System curricula to out of school adolescents.[15]

EFFECTIVENESS OF A LIFE SKILL PROGRAM: CURRENT AND FUTURE RESEARCH

Life skill training results in decreased high-risk behavior and improved life skills of the trainers as is evident from the research studies enumerated below.[13] WHO states that life skill education improves school attendance and relationships between students and teachers. It also decreases school drop out rates.

- Dr Bharat has reported a positive feedback by teachers in the NIMHANS program launched for teachers.[16]
- Evidence for reduction in high risk behavior is present in various studies. In 1991, Prothrow-Sith in The 'Boston Violence Prevention Project' involving a community approach showed a decrease in violent attitude.
- In 1993, Walter and Vaughan evaluated a sexuality education program. A three month follow-up indicated that compared to control group, program participants reported fewer sexual contacts with high-risk partners, fewer partners and increase in consistent condom use.
- In 1983, Botvin, Renich and Baker reported a reduction in smoking amongst youth after using a life skill based program.
- In 2005, the Institute of Health Management, Pachod, Maharashtra, India reported that life skill programs have postponed the age of marriage by two years for the girls in Aurangabad.[12] The intervention also had a positive impact on the attitudes of the parents.

- Reddy et al proved the efficacy of a school based tobacco control programs in 2002 in New Delhi. In their study, they showed that the intervention group of school going adolescents was less likely to initiate tobacco use compared to the nonintervention group.[17]
- In 2009, Rao et al in their study on juveniles in conflict with law proved that a life skill program in conjunction with individual and parental counseling was effective in decreasing the criminal propensity scale and increasing the morality score and brought about significant behavior change.[18]

All the above studies focus on single risk behavior. A comprehensive health program can have an impact on multiple risk behaviors simultaneously. It is indeed a challenge to plan, implement and evaluate such a longitudinal program due to the presence of many confounding factors like socioeconomic status, in or out of school program, quality of trainers, etc. that may influence the statistical analysis to determine program effectiveness. Rajiv Gandhi National Institute of Youth Development, Sriperumbudur, is currently in the process of designing a validated instrument to evaluate the effectiveness of a life skill education program.

LIFE SKILL PROGRAMS: INTERNATIONAL AND NATIONAL

United Nation agencies like WHO, UNFPA, UNICEF and UNESCO are actively involved in launching life skill programs through out the world.[2] Various WHO departments like the department of mental health, substance abuse, child and adolescent health and health promotion have designed their life skill programs. Most of the UN agencies' life skills programs focus on enhancing reproductive health, preventing substance abuse and AIDS, human rights, gender equity, peace and encouraging young people's leadership. They aim at making these programs socioculturally relevant to a particular nation.

In India, adolescent education program in CBSE schools was launched in 2006 using a life skill approach. Later in 2009, bowing to public pressure, the government of India withdrew the program as the academia raised serious objections to the topics dealing with sexuality. This was a big blow to the life skill education movement in India. It was later decided to include the life skill approach in some chapters of the regular syllabi. Under the Reproductive and Child Health II program, life skills are to be imparted to both boys and girls by Aganwadi workers, nurses and medical officers at aganwadis, primary health centers and district hospitals.[13] Indian Academy of Pediatrics in 2006 adopted life skills as an important component of its Adolescent Friendly School Initiative. FOGSI too is at the forefront of organizing life skill sessions for adolescent girls. Many NGOs all over the country, catering to the needs of the adolescents continue to teach life skills especially to the socially deprived and street adolescents.

At the grassroot level, life skill education program is still in its infancy in India. There are many political, social and economic hurdles to be overcome in implementing such a program. Lack of political will, apathy of the educational department, myths held by the public, lack of trained life skill trainers, absence of a concise national comprehensive module and difficulties in evaluation of the program are some of the barriers.[19] Rajiv Gandhi National Institute of Youth Development, Sriperumbudur, a deemed university, run by the Ministry of Youth and Sports Affairs has a department of life skills and social harmony and offers MA and diploma courses in Life skills. This landmark department is involved in conducting research on life skills as well as designing, implementing and evaluating programs.

CONCLUSION

Life skills enhance the emotional intelligence and physical health of the adolescent. High emotional quotient (EQ) and not just a high intelligence quotient (IQ) is needed for success in life. Life skills develop one's self-esteem, confidence and to make health promoting decisions and thereby ensures well-being. This in turn keeps several physical and psychosocial problems at bay among adolescents resulting in continued promotion of good health in all its dimensions—physical, mental, social and spiritual. Adolescent life skill education needs to be implemented on a war footing basis in India, with a strong political will and social commitment.

SUGGESTED LIFE SKILL EDUCATION MODULES

a. Activity Manual for the Teachers on Health Promotion using Life Skills Approach (manuals for 8th, 9th and 10th std)
   Dr Srikala Bharat, Additional Professor of Psychiatry
   Dept of Psychiatry, NIMHANS
   Bangaluru 560029

b. Life Skills Interactive Sessions Minus two to Plus two
   Dr Jeesson C Unni, Consultant Pediatrician
   Dr Kunhalu's Nursing Home, TD Road, Kochi
   Kerala 682011

c. Facilitator's Manual on Enhancing Life Skills
   Dr Radhakrishan Nair, HOD Dept of Life Skills
   Rajiv Gandhi National Institute of Youth Development
   Sriperumbudur, Tamilnadu 602105

d. YUVA Module (for 6th to 12th std)
   Mr Sudhir Kumar Kapoor, SCERT
   Defence Colony, New Delhi 110024

e. On Track: A Series on Life Skills and Personal Safety (for 3rd to 9th std)
   By Drs Shekhar Seshadri, Sangeeta Saksena, Shoibya Saldanha
   www.macmillanindia.com

REFERENCES

1. WHO Life skills education for children and adolescents in schools 1997 WHO/MNH/PSF/93.7A.Rev.2.
2. Nair RV. Life Skills Personality and Leadership. RGNYID Sriperumbdur 2010.
3. Ministry of Youth Affairs and Sports, Govt of India. Facilitators Module on Adolescent Health and Development 2006.
4. White AM. Understanding adolescent brain development and its implications for the clinicians. Adolesc Med 2009;20:73-90.
5. Blythe, Rosenthal. Adolescent Sexuality. AM Stars 2007;18:3.
6. Bhave S (Chief Ed) ITPAH Course Manual for Adolescent Health. Indian perspective 2002.
7. Kleigman, Behrman, Jenson, Stanton Nelson Textbook of Pediatrics 18th ed. Vol 1. Saunders pub USA 2007;60-5.
8. Strasburger, et al. Adolescent Medicine. PCNA 1997:44.
9. Nair MKC. PGD AP Course Manual Paper 1. University of Kerala 2004.
10. Bharat S, Kumar KV. Activity Manual for teachers on health promotion using life skill approach. NIMHANS 2005.
11. Bhave S, et al. Recommendations of IAP National Task force for childhood prevention of adult diseases: Childhood obesity. Indian Pediatr 2004,41:559-75.
12. Arora M, Reddy KS. GYTS, Delhi. Indian Pediatr 2005;42:850-51.
13. Adolescent Health Module for Basic Health Functionaries- IEC div. Dept of FW, Ministry of HFW, GOI 2006.
14. Bhave SY. Innovative Methods of Life Skill Training. Indian Journal of Life Skill Education 2009;1:1,1-12.
15. Singh A. Life Skills for enhancing excellence in education and life long learning. Indian Journal of Life Skills Education 2010;1:2,165-86.
16. Bharat S. Life skill education/initiatives for adolescents in India. In Psychological therapies with children and adolescents. Proceedings of the seminar. Kapur M (Ed). NIMHANS 2001.
17. Reddy KS, et al. Tobacco and alcohol use outcomes of a school based intervention in New Delhi. American Journal of Health Behavior 2002;26:173-81.
18. Rao UNB, Sunitha S, Gupta R. Life skills education and its importance for the Juveniles in conflict with law. Indian Journal of Life Skills Education 2009;1:1, 13-26.
19. Galagali PM. Adolescent life skill education program: The Bangalore experience. Indian Journal of life skills education. 2010;1:2,124-44.

26 Stress in Adolescents and Coping

JS Tuteja, CP Bansal

INTRODUCTION

The human body is exposed everyday to different person, species, situations and stimuli. Some of the exposures are rewarding and certain others are hazardous. If the exposure is hazardous then the body prepares itself to face the situation—the reason being its 'Internal Homeostasis' and hence its normal functioning should not be affected. This response is called the "Fight or Flight response". This response is to make persons cope with the situation successfully.

Stress is the body's adaptation response to any demand or pressure. These demands or pressures are called *stressors*. A stressor is an event; *coping* is what one does as a result of the stressor. No one lives without some degree of stress in their lives. The tricky part is that what stresses one person may, in fact, invigorate another.

Teen stress is similar to the adult stress in terms of the signs and symptoms. But the causes of teen stress are totally different and they need somewhat different stress management programs for dealing stress.

ADOLESCENCE

It is estimated that teens form 20% of the total population. Yet they are a neglected group of the population. The adolescent group is the intermediate group between the dependent childhood and the independent adulthood. This transition from childhood to adulthood is never so easy. This group is a vulnerable group to both physical and emotional stress. There are problems everywhere for them:

Problems at home with their parents and siblings, problems may be in the school or with their friends and in education.

Adolescent medicine is a new concept in the field of medicine. The adolescents cannot be treated as either adults or kids because their problems are totally different.

Teens are not immune to stress; however, they are sometimes ill-equipped to cope with the stressors that they face leading to various manifestations of that stress in their daily lives. Psychologically changes in behavior such as moodiness, irritability, inability to concentrate, crying, changes in eating patterns, changes in sleeping patterns, worrying, mood swings, frustration, nervousness, depression, exhibiting a negative attitude, low productivity, confusion, lack of creativity, lethargy, forgetfulness, and/or boredom may become more prevalent than usual for your adolescent.

Socially increased stress levels may be exhibited through isolating his or herself from others, loneliness, decreased general communication skills, lashing out at others, nagging, or simply a refusal to engage verbally.

Some sources of stress for today's teens clued: school demands; negative thoughts and feelings about themselves; changes in their bodies; exploring his or her own identity; problems with peer group; unsafe living environment; separation/divorce of parents; chronic illness within the family unit; death of a loved one; moving or changing schools; being involved in too many activities; and family financial problems are some examples.

When teens react to a stressor in an attempt to minimize its emotional impact, it is considered *emotion-focused coping*. Emotion-focused coping is a defensive action and usually takes the form of denial, lying/exaggerating, or wishful thinking. It is generally seen as passive rather than active. If instead, your teen reacts to a stressor with an attempt to change the situation, it is considered *problem-focused coping*.

When utilizing coping skills that are problem-focused, adolescents seek additional information or alternative approaches to confront the stressor at hand. As adolescents acquire their toolbox of coping mechanisms and gain experience and maturity, they typically begin to move from emotion-focused coping to problem-focused coping behaviors.

PHYSIOLOGY OF STRESS

When a person is exposed to a 'dangerous' situation his body gets ready to face it. It needs more energy for that. The extra energy is got by the "Fight or Flight" response. The initial step is taken by the Hypothalamus of the brain which secretes Adrenocorticotrophic releasing hormone (ARH). ARH stimulates the adjacent pituitary gland to secrete Adrenocorticotrophic hormone (ACTH). This in turn stimulates the adrenal glands which are situated on the kidneys to secrete Adrenaline and Cortisol. Now these two hormones work together to see that the body gets more energy by providing more oxygen and glucose. For these things to occur, the following adjustments are done:

- Diversion of the blood from less vital to more vital organs
- Increase in the heart rate to supply more blood quickly
- Increase in the blood pressure to supply blood efficiently
- Increase in the respiratory rate to get more oxygen from the atmosphere
- Breakdown of glycogen stores in liver and muscle to get more glucose
- Formation of more glucose from non carbohydrate substances.

Hence at the end of the response, the body is well geared up and it tackles the situation. To put it in a nut shell—"The mind feels the danger and the body tackles it. These actions are coordinated by hormones".

Once the trigger is gone the hormonal levels drops and the body returns to normal. But if this happens repeatedly, then all the hormonal levels are persistently high not allowing the body to come back to normal .The body keeps experiencing the above mentioned 'adjustments'. Soon the hormonal and energy stores get exhausted. The vital link between the mind and the body is lost and the person suffers. The mind gets disturbed by the fact that the threat is there. But the body is too tired to handle it. The coordination between the two is disturbed.

Causes of Stress

Stress is a normal physiological phenomenon. So 'Undue or Unrelieved Stress' is the right term when we discuss about the pathological aspects of stress. 'Undue or Unrelieved Stress' can occur in any person in whom the normal 'Fight or Flight' response is overdone. It can occur as: a short term response, delayed response or a prolonged response. A lot of physical and emotional changes occur during this period, which are very significant in shaping of the person.

Physical Changes

The physical changes include:
- Increase in the weight
- Increase in the height
- Change in voice
- Development of secondary sexual characters
- Menarche (beginning of menstruation) in girls.

Mental Changes

These are equally significant which include:
- Feeling of independence
- Attraction towards opposite sex
- Aggressive behavior
- Experimenting new things including substance abuse.

Study Conducted

Surveys conducted shows that one third of the teenagers suffer at least one episode of stress every week. Though stress has the same kind of response in all the age groups, the stress factors are different. Stress in teens could be due to:
- Pubertal changes
- Changing relationship with peers
- New demands in the school
- Safety issues in their neighborhood
- Responsibilities to their families
- Negative thoughts and feelings
- Separation or divorce of parents
- Death of a loved one
- Chronic illnesses
- Changing schools
- Financial problems
- Holiday stress.

In a study conducted on the stress and related problem of teens in the city of Baltimore showed that the following figures:

The Major Causes of Stress

- School work (78%)
- Parents (78%)
- Romantic relationships (64%)
- Problems with friends (64%)
- Siblings (64%).

The Conclusion of the Study

- Girls are affected more than boys.
- Girls respond to stress by seeking help from others or by taking certain actions to reduce or remove stress.
- Boys respond to stress by not dealing with the stress at all or by engaging the mind away from the sources of stress.
- Family members and friends are both sources of stress and support for teenagers.
- Teenagers use both healthy and unhealthy ways to cope up with stress.

Physical Signs and Symptoms of Stress

a. **Diversion of the blood from less vital to more vital organs**: Blood is diverted from less vital structures like skin, gastrointestinal tract, liver, kidney, spleen, bone and muscle to more vital organs like brain, heart and adrenals. This is called '**Diving reflex**' though the term is mostly used in the context of newborns. The effects of this reflex are:
   - The skin becomes cold and clammy with gooseflesh standing out
   - There is frequent passing of stools—the Irritable Bowel Syndrome
   - Existing Peptic Ulcer aggravates
   - There is loss of appetite
   - There is severe muscular pain, especially muscles of posture causing back pain and neck pain
   - Dryness of throat and hence difficulty in speaking and swallowing.

b. **Increase in the heart rate to supply more blood quickly**: The normal heart rate in adults is 100 beats per minute supplying about 5 liters of blood. To provide more nutrient to the body the heart rate increases. There is associated dilatation of the blood vessels also. These result in:
   - Palpitation
   - Chest pain
   - Flushing and feeling of warmth.

c. **Increase in the blood pressure to pupply blood efficiently**: To supply the increased cardiac output efficiently, the blood pressure increases which results in:
   - Headache
   - Precipitation of heart attack along with collection of fluids in the lungs in a heart patient.

d. **Increase in the respiratory rate to get more oxygen from the atmosphere**: As more oxygen is needed during stress, body tries to increase the respiratory rate to trap more oxygen from atmosphere. This causes:
   - Breathlessness
   - Respiratory alkalosis—an acid-base disturbance in blood.

e. **Mobilization of energy stores as body needs more energy during stress**: extra amount of glucose is mobilized to for that purpose. Glucose is stored as glycogen in liver and muscle. The hormone cortisol breaks down glycogen into glucose. This causes:
   - Depletion of energy stores
   - Hyperglycemia—increased blood glucose levels.
   - Increased viscosity of blood and so more chances of vessel block.

f. **Depletion of proteins and fats**: The hormone cortisol converts non carbohydrate substrates like protein and fat into glucose which results in:
   - Weight loss

g. **Other symptoms**:
   - Suppression of immunity resulting in infection
   - Overreaction of immune system resulting in flare ups of Asthma, Psoriasis, Arthritis, Lupus and Urticaria.
   - Increased appetite leading to weight gain.
   - Sleeplessness
   - Loss of sexual drive
   - Memory disturbances.

Psychological Symptoms

These effects are due to increased cortisol and its metabolites and other accumulated metabolic products. The symptoms include:
- Mood swings
- Anxiety
- Depression
- Outbursts of anger
- Headache
- Irritability
- Dependence on alcohol
- Lack of concentration.

Coping with Stress

There are several things that you can communicate to your teenager client for the help when they are in need, to guide them where they can go for the help when they are in acute stress, sometime it can be life saving too.
People who can help teenager in need are:
- Parents, a family member or family friend
- A close friend or caretaker
- A school nurse, teacher or school counselor

- A social worker or youth counselor
- A priest, someone from your temple

Guidelines for teens if:

- They feel that stress is affecting their health
- They feel so desperate that they think about stopping school or running away
- They feel low, sad, tearful, or that life is not worth living
- They lose appetite and find it difficult to sleep
- They have worries, feelings and thoughts that are hard to talk about because they feel people won't understand them or will think they are 'weird'

Guidelines for gatekeepers of society (school teachers, doctors, parents): If you notice teen becoming "stressed out", these are some of the things you can do to help him or her deal with the stresses of life.

1. Be vigilant about how the stresses in teen's life are affecting his or her health, behavior, thoughts or feelings. If you notice a drastic change in any of these areas, seek medical attention for them.
2. Lines of communication should remain open between adolescent and gatekeepers. Never turn down a request to chat, no matter how busy you may be. Listen carefully to their concerns and remember what may seem trivial to you, may feel like the proverbial end of the world to teen.
3. Model stress management skills . As gatekeepers, we are our adolescent's first helper. How we react to our everyday stressors provides the model for how our teens think they should act.
4. Support involvement in sports or other prosocial activities. Interacting with others is a good way to learn that they are not alone in what they are experiencing. That knowledge is comforting and can alleviate some if not all of certain types of stress. Physical activity is also a good reliever of some forms of stress.

Remember our Experience of Stress in Life

How we deal with that stress in our daily lives helps determine how successful we will ultimately be in coping throughout our lives. As adolescents grow and begin to develop their own identities, helping them fill their coping skills toolbox is something that we, as gatekeepers can contribute in their lives.

How to Tackle Teen Stress?

The teen stress should be dealt with both at home and in school—

- There is a wrong notion among adults that there is no earthly reason for stress in teens. This should be avoided.
- The first step in tackling teen stress is to identify the signs and symptoms of stress in the teens. The teens should be allowed to talk freely about their problems.
- Parents and teachers should teach them stress relief methods.

- They should set only reasonable goals in both curricular and extra-curricular activities.

There are several treatment models to help the teens cope up with stress. The steps of one such model:

- Ask the teenager to define stress taking an example of an incident
- Ask the teens about the their response to that stressful event
- Explain to the teens about normal stress response and ways of tackling stress
- Identify the source of stress in teens and help them understand that the same event incites different responses in different persons
- Teach the teen the best stress relieving techniques.
- Advise them to avoid unhealthy methods of tackling stress like aggression, avoidance, etc.

One to One Model of Dealing with Stress

- *Step one:* Identify the potential sources of stress. Help the teen recognize them.
- *Step two:* Find out whether the teens have any stress related signs and symptoms. If they have any, then discuss with them about the physical and emotional stress and the ways to relieve them.
- *Step three:* Find out whether the teenager has increase in the stress and related problems. If so, it needs long-term treatment with the help of a counselor.

Small Group Model of Dealing with Stress

Exercises involving a small group of teens are done. The exercises are related to:

- Mind body connection
- Ways of reacting to stress.

Large Group Model of Dealing with Stress

In this model, a larger group of teens is involved. The exercises done are:

- Methods to cope up with stress
- Self-expression of their feelings in forms of poems, essays, drawings
- Finding solutions to problems narrated in small stories.
  Healthy stress relieving methods as framed by the American Academy of Child and Adolescent Psychiatry
- Eat a well-balanced nutritious diet
- Exercise regularly
- Avoid caffeine, tobacco and substance of abuse like alcohol, drugs, etc.
- Follow simple stress relief methods like deep breathing, listening to music, recreational sports, etc.
- Develop assertiveness training skills
- Learn to be practical. Look for an alternative if the task is very stressful
- Have high self-esteem

- Learn to say no. By doing this a teenager can sort out important things in his life.
- Have good sense of humor
- Watching stress relief cartoons
- Have a good social relationship
- Discuss the problems with a trusted person and try to find his view of the problem
- Engage in hobbies like drawing, writing singing or playing with pets.

Teen stress is very significant as today's teens are tomorrow's adults. The transition will be smooth if they know the causes of teen stress and their stress relief methods, communicate well with others and learn problem solving skills.

APPROACH TO STRESS RELIEF IN TEENS

Natural Techniques

Natural stress reduction techniques can be categorized under the following headings:

- Exercise
- Yoga
- Meditation
- Reiki
- Herbs
- Dietary adjustments
- Lifestyle changes.

Exercise and Diet

Exercise and diet are simplest of the remedies for stress. Exercise helps in relieving the stress in the following ways:

- The adrenaline store gets exhausted and results in relaxation.
- Exercise produces Beta endorphin in our brain which relieves stress by providing a sense of well-being.
- Exercise increases blood flow to brain which supplies more oxygen and eliminates toxic materials including carbon dioxide and lactate.
- Exercise relaxes tensed muscles.
- Exercise distracts us from the causes of stress.

Deep breathing itself is a good exercise. It helps the body in getting more oxygen and eliminates the unwanted carbon dioxide.

Deep Breathing Exercises

Deep breathing exercises are perhaps the most commonly thought of stress relief techniques. Deep breathing works well as one of your relaxation techniques for stress, as the flow of oxygen to your brain releases the hormones that help you calm down and deal with the stressful event. This tricks your mind and body into relaxing when you need to.

Yoga

Stressed individuals have great amount of tension in their bodies. Yoga, an ancient Indian practice helps in releasing this tension and aiding in deep breathing which provides more oxygen and eliminates the toxic carbon dioxide. Three components of Yoga are used for stress relief. They are the asanas, pranayamas and meditation. Meditation can be done separately also for stress relief.

Yogic Postures (Asana)

The corpses pose (Savasana), the crocodile pose (Makarasana) and the child's pose (Bal asana) are relaxation postures which help in dealing with stress.

Yogic Breathing (Pranayama)

One form of pranayama is Nadi shodhanam in which alternate nostril breathing is done. Pranayama should always be done in a suitable posture or asana in which the lung capacity is the highest and the muscle tension is lowest. It should always be done with the help of a teacher. It should be always done with empty stomach and one should never do it till exhaustion.

Meditation

Two methods need mention:

a. Meditation that needs focusing and
b. Meditation that does not need focusing.

Meditation that needs focusing: The affected person focuses on any object or image or sound or any thoughts. It takes the mind away from the source of stress and provides stress relief.

Meditation that does not need focusing: Transcendental meditation is one form of meditation that does not need focusing. It is done by sitting comfortably with the eyes closed. During the process the fluctuating mind gradually becomes still and attains a state of "Restful alertness". It is done for about 20 minutes everyday in the morning and evening.

Reiki

Reiki is a Japanese art of healing. Rei means "free passage" and ki means "universal energy". It involves transfer of energy from a practitioner to the patient to increase the body's natural ability to heal itself through the balance of energy. Reiki incorporates of most of the other alternate therapies like spiritual therapy, meditation, aroma therapy, etc. The hands are the tools of healing in Reiki.The position in which the hands are placed is important. Reiki can be done through clothing. But most prefer no barrier to the therapy. Reiki practitioners impart energy through a particular pattern. This induces deep relaxation, detoxifies the body and provides new vitality.

Hypnosis

Hypnosis as a relief method for stress has gained considerable credibility in recent years. Hypnosis for anxiety and stress is clinically proven and is an effective long-term solution for stress related conditions.

Stress Vitamins

Since the late 1970s, significant importance is being given for the so called stress vitamins. The vitamins which are considered to relieve stress are Vitamin B complex and Vitamin C along with Vitamin E and Vitamin A.

A Natural Method That Works (Dhayana)

Recent scientific experiments validate a new, natural, and very simple method of eliminating stress called Natural stress relief.

Natural stress relief (NSR) is an easily-learned, effortless mental technique, practiced for 15 minutes twice a day. It can be learned at home through lessons taken over a period of only three days.

NSR uses a natural procedure called transcending (which means "diving within") to bring about a unique state of deep rest in which alertness is maintained. This state of restful alertness allows the body to experience a state of rest deeper than that of sleep, allowing even deep-rooted stresses to be dissolved.

NSR involves no mysticism, religion, or changes to lifestyle. It is just a technique, so it is independent of and compatible with any religion or beliefs.

Stress Relief Games

Stress relief games are categorized as:
- Outdoor games like tennis, golf, soccer
- Indoor games like chess, checkers, rubik cube, darts, crossword puzzles, computer games, mobile phone games.

CONCLUSION

In adolescence stress is very common, teenagers who are in distress they show poor performance in their studies, in all aspect of life, while teens who are in stress show excellent performance, so it is the duty of the gatekeepers of the society to keep an eye on teenagers and guide them as role model by helping them and teaching them all required life skills for the healthy lives.

SUGGESTED READING

1. Adolescent Stress, Stressors, and Coping
   Guest Author: Stephanie K. Ferguson, http://www.bellaonline.com/articles/art13970.asp.
2. Coping with stress: information for young people
   http://www.rcpsych.ac.uk/mentalhealthinfo/mentalhealthandgrowingup/copingwithstress.aspx.

3. Coping Skills for Trauma http://www.ibiblio.org/rcip/copingskills.html.
4. http://www.m-a-h.net/support/article-grounding.htm.
5. http://www.m-a-h.net/support/article-grounding.htm.
6. http://www.psyke.org/coping/coping_skills.
7. http://www.pe2000.com/anx-breathe.htm.
8. http://www.ncptsd.va.gov/facts/treatment/fs_coping.html.
9. http://www.m-a-h.net/library/coping/article-containment.htm.
10. http://www.liferhymecoaching.com/tuneup4.html.
11. http://rainbow-hope.tripod.com/tricks1.html#to.
12. http://www.ibiblio.org/rcip/cognitivews.html.
13. http://www.dailyom.com/articles/2005/500.html.
14. http://www.ibiblio.org/rcip//safeplace.html.
15. http://ptsd.factsforhealth.org/anxiety.html.
16. Stress management http://www.associatedcontent.com/article/5229/stress_management_for_teens_101.html?cat=25.
17. Teens stress http://www.stressfocus.com/stress_focus_article/teen-stress-causes.htm.

27 Adolescent Counseling—Are We Well-Versed?

Pratima Mittal, Kirti Sharma

Adolescence is the threshold between childhood and adulthood. It is a period of rapid change in both the external and internal environment of the individual. The external include social, cultural and familial while the inner environment consists of the awareness of ones sexuality, the associated physical changes, the change in psychology and cognition. Adolescents try to keep pace with all of these factors. Needless to say it is a time that brings curiosity and excitement on the one hand but anxiety and confusion on the other. Adolescents have many questions and concerns about what is happening to their bodies but they are unable to share their questions and concerns, and do not seek answers from competent and caring adults.

In a country like India where adolescent girls are one-tenth of the population, the situation is further complicated by a rapidly changing social and economic situation. In spite of rapid changes we remain a patriarchal society where the girls are discriminated against and required to play multiple roles. This leads to a serious compromise on their physical, mental and emotional health which can lead to long-term effects.

While adolescence is generally considered as a healthy time of life, it is also a period when adult behavior patterns develop, some of which may negatively affect health both during adolescence and later in life. Furthermore, many adolescents die every year—mostly from unintentional injuries (e.g. car crashes), intentional injuries (suicide and interpersonal violence) and pregnancy-related causes.

Many of the adolescent problems are due to incorrect information, lack of communication and due to inaccessible health services. These problems can be effectively handled by proper counseling.

Counseling in its most literal sense means one person trying to help another as they talk person-to-person. *It is helping people to identify a problem, making informed decisions and giving them the confidence to put their decisions in practice.* It requires good communication skills especially with adolescents who are likely to be intimidated, defensive and even resistant during the session.

They are acutely self-conscious with a limited perspective of the future and limited understanding of abstract concepts hence leading to the need for patience and understanding on the part of the counselor.

Healthcare providers especially gynecologists are in the position to counsel this age group effectively and with far-reaching effects. Gynecologists may have direct interaction with adolescents due to some menstrual problem or problems related to pregnancy, indirect interaction can be through the mother/guardian of adolescents. Healthcare providers can help healthy adolescents to stay that way and help those with health problems get back to good health. They can:

- Provide them with information, counseling and clinical services aimed at helping them maintain safe behaviors and modify unsafe ones (i.e. those that put them at risk of negative health outcomes).
- Diagnose/detect and manage health problems and behaviors that put them at risk of negative health outcomes; and can refer them to other health and social service providers, when necessary.
- Help community leaders and members understand the needs of adolescents, and the importance of working together to respond to these needs.

After understanding the special situation of the adolescents, the health care provider should analyze whether he or she is competent for providing effective and appropriate counseling, which is one of the most important aspects of managing the adolescents? Does he/she has the knowledge and the requisite skill? If answer is "No", one has to make an effort to imbibe adolescent friendly attributes in his/her practice. Some of the important points in counseling the adolescents are highlighted here.

PROVIDERS ATTRIBUTES

The provider should be trained, dedicated personnel with adolescent friendly characteristics as he/she should:

- Be welcoming and friendly
- Be knowledgeable and presentable
- Have good communication skills
- Maintain confidentiality and privacy
- Be punctual
- Be understanding
- Be a good listener
- Be nonjudgmental.

COUNSELING APPROACH

A systematic approach helps. One can use the GATHER approach. (G: Greet, A: Ask about the issue bothering him/her, T: Tell all the options, H: Help her choose one, E: Explain her regarding the chosen option, R: Return for follow-up.)

1. **Establish rapport (Greet)**—It is essential to start the session in a polite, friendly and helpful way. The clients should be given full attention; one may explain the course of the visit in brief in the beginning. The need for *interaction* as against a monologue should be stressed upon from the beginning.
2. **Create an appropriate atmosphere (Greet)**—One should always start with *nonthreatening* questions on the background of the client, for

example, questions about school, friends and how she spends her time during the day. Adolescents are often shy about discussing their problems and starting with questions on sexuality, or addiction habits early in the session might make them resistant to the session. One has to first *build up trust*.

3. **Maintain confidentiality (Ask)**—The client should be reassured of *confidentiality* and the session must be carried out as a *one-to-one*. The parent or guardian accompanying the adolescent also needs to be addressed and this can be done either at the beginning of the session or at the end of the session in the presence of the adolescent. One should try to engage the guardian, but the adolescent has to be reassured that they are the ones who are being addressed primarily and any information divulged during the session would stay confidential.
4. **Obtain complete information (Ask)**—One should ask the relevant questions in a leading manner, without being intrusive or forcing any information. One should listen patiently and attentively to the client and avoid being judgmental. One may begin with asking them their reasons for coming, help them define their problems and express their feelings and needs. Ask them about any previous experience with reproductive health care. The questions should be kept simple and brief.
5. **HEADS assessment (Ask)**—Adolescents may not volunteer information about a health problem or concern because they may be embarrassed or scared to do so, or because they may not be comfortable either with the health worker or the situation they are in. One could consider using the HEADS assessment which could detect health and development problems that the adolescent has not presented with; detect whether the adolescent engages in behaviors that could put one at risk of negative health outcome (such as injecting drugs or having unprotected sex); detect important factors in their environment that increase the likelihood of their engaging in these behaviors. This provides a full picture of the adolescent as an individual and not just a case of this or that condition. The HEADS assessment is structured—it starts by examining the home and the educational/employment setting. It then goes on to eating, and then to activities. Only then does it deal with more sensitive issues such as drugs, sexuality, safety and suicide/depression.

   If time does not permit to do a full HEADS assessment, one will need to prioritize which sections of the HEADS assessment to do. One may choose to prioritize the sections which are most related to presenting complaint:

   HEADS is an acronym for:
   - Home
   - Education/Employment/Eating
   - Activity
   - Drugs
   - Sexuality/Safety/Suicide.

6. **Recognize and adjust to barriers in doctor-patient communication (Tell)**—Nonverbal communication also plays a role and one must try to avoid negative nonverbal signs, like interrupting the session to attend to other matters or phone calls, appearing distracted, referring to notes, etc. One must look the client in the eye and express understanding and empathy.
7. **Decision making (Tell/Help)**—The clients should be given clear, accurate, specific information regarding their choices in the course of the session. The information should be tailored and personalized and the client should be helped to understand the nature of the choice. It should be made amply clear that the choice is theirs, and they are the ones responsible, and that the counselor is there to help them make it in an informed way and help them in the execution. The counselor should take special care, especially in matters of sexual behavior, to not to project ones' own opinions and inhibitions in the process of decision making. At the same time, the results of all possible choices must be explained.
8. **Implementation/explain**—At the end of the session one must summarize the key points and explain the client regarding the instructions and how they must be followed. If possible, printed material should be given with the instructions written clearly and the date and time for follow-up specified. All medical advice should be given while explaining the basis for it so that the client understands the need to follow it effectively.
9. **Physical examination**—The physical examination should be carried out after a level of comfort has been established. The examination should be carried out in a different room. The client should be explained need and the procedure. The client should be appropriately draped. One should try and maintain conversation while the examination is being conducted. This will make the client comfortable and more receptive to talk about issues like sexuality and reproductive health. Examination of breasts and genitalia must be carried out gently and normal stages of development may be explained so the client is reassured if everything is normal.
10. **Age appropriate counseling**—The health care provider should further acknowledge that adolescence is not a homogeneous phase and while early adolescents (10-14 yrs) might have different needs as compared to mid (15-17 yrs) and late adolescence (above 17 yrs). The counselor should be sensitive to the young person's development level and it should be remembered that physical appearance and chronological age may be misleading measures of cognitive development. Those in early adolescence may have issues regarding body image and growth and development, while those in late adolescence may have issues regarding intimacy.
11. **Parental/Guardian counseling**—The parent or the guardian accompanying the adolescent should also be counseled either in the beginning or preferably at the end of the session taking the adolescent in confidence.

CASE STUDY 1

A 19 years old girl comes to you because she had unprotected sex last night and she is worried about getting pregnant.

How will you counsel her?

- Be nonjudgmental—Do not say it is wrong to do so even if you feel so
- Tell her about consequences of unsafe sex
- Provide her with emergency contraception
- Screen for STI
- Must talk about next visit, after periods or after missed periods
- Discuss about diet, exercises, hygiene, etc. at an appropriate time.

COMPONENTS OF ADOLESCENT COUNSELING

Can be divided into the Preventive measures and the Promotive measures. They include:

1. **Prevention of anemia and other nutritional deficiencies**: Advice regarding appropriate diet and dietary habits, with relevant history regarding chronic infections or worm infestation and treatment for the same. Dietary supplementation, if required.
2. **Adolescent growth, development and nutrition monitoring and counseling**: Maintain growth charts or adolescent cards so the client has a personal record and feels more capable. Give visual aids with advice regarding appropriate diet and diet charts.
3. **Personal hygiene and menstrual hygiene**: Information regarding importance of daily bath, keeping the genitals clean, use of clean dry, cotton undergarments, etc. can be provided. Young girls should be prepared for menstruation and young boys' anxiety related to ejaculation must be addressed.
4. **Sexual issues**: Importance of abstinence before marriage and avoidance of risk taking behavior (due to peer pressure and media influences) should be encouraged. Practice of safe sex with appropriate contraceptive advice, risk of reproductive tract infections and sexually transmitted infections like HIV, chances of pregnancy, dangers of unsafe abortion and the increased risk in this age group, should be explained and emphasized. One should be particularly careful to keep out personal biases while counseling or appearing judgmental and opinionated.
5. **Unwanted adolescent pregnancy and unsafe abortion**: Preventive measures should be advocated, in the form of contraceptive advice, avoidance of unsafe abortion by explaining consequences and making MTP services available. One must explain increased risk of fetal and maternal morbidity associated with adolescent pregnancy and responsibility associated with parenting.
6. **HIV/AIDS**: The association of HIV/AIDS with increased risk taking behavior, the chances of acquiring the disease and the morbidity associated along with contraceptive advice should be explained.
7. **Body image issues:** (I am too fat or I am too thin, I am short). These issues should be addressed using graphic and visual aids besides explaining normal growth and development and where the adolescent

exactly stands. The need for a healthy body and mind should be explained along with the other detrimental effects on the body. Need for adequate, balanced diet and exercise should be explained.

8. **Immunization**: Vaccination against diseases like Rubella is a service that should be provided to all girls of adolescent age group to prevent further morbidity. HPV vaccination to protect against diseases like Carcinoma cervix should also be provided to this age group and appropriate information regarding the same must be provided and clients counseled regarding the benefits of these measures.
9. Issues like literacy, pre-marital counseling and gender bias may also be addressed depending on the social and cultural background of the client.

CASE STUDY 2

An 18 years old unmarried girl comes to you. She explains that she is engaged to be married and her fiancée is pressing her to have sex with him. How will you counsel her?

- Promote concept of marriage and abstinence before marriage
- Explain risk of premarital sex
- Explain to her the uncertainty of future
- Explain feelings are involuntary, behavior is a voluntary action
- Explain mutual respect for each other is important
- Let them decide (if decision is yes, promote safe sex).

CHALLENGES IN ADOLESCENT COUNSELING

Adolescent counseling is a minefield. There can be challenges as:

1. **The client is silent**: Silence can be sign of shyness or may signify anger or anxiety.
   - If it occurs at the beginning of a session, the provider can say, "I realize it's hard for you to talk. This often happens to people who come for the first time."
   - If she/he seems angry, the counselor can say, "Sometimes when someone comes to see me against her/his will and doesn't want to be here, it is difficult to speak."
   - If the client is shy, the provider can legitimize the feeling by saying, "I'd feel the same way in your place. I understand that it's not easy to talk to a person you've just met."
   - If the adolescent has difficulty expressing her/his feelings or ideas, the counselor can use some brochures or posters to encourage discussions or refer to a story or anecdote so the adolescent can talk about other than her/himself.
   - If the adolescent cannot or will not talk, the counselors should propose another meeting.
2. **The client cries**: The counselor should try to evaluate what provoked the tears and assess if it makes sense in the given situation.
   - If the crying is consistent with the situation, the counselor should allow her/him to freely express emotions and not try to stop the feeling or belittle its importance.

- If the Client is crying to relieve tension, the counselor gives the adolescent permission to express her/ his feeling by saying, "It's okay to cry since it's the normal thing to do when you're sad."
- If the Client is using crying as manipulation, the counselors can say "Although I'm sorry you feel sad. It's good to express your feelings."

3. **The counselor cannot see a solution to the client's problem—**
   - Counselors may feel anxious if they are not sure what to advice. The counselor is a reproductive health expert but does not have to solve every problem for the client. Express understanding. Sometimes this is what the client really wants. Also, suggest others who could help.
4. **The counselor does not know the answer to a client's question—**
   - Say honestly and openly that you do not know the answer but together you can find out. Check with a supervisor, a knowledgeable co-worker, or reference materials, and give the client the accurate answer.
5. **The counselor makes a mistake—**
   - Correct the mistake and say you are sorry. It is important to be accurate. It is not important to look perfect. Admitting a mistake shows respect for the client.
   - Be honest. The more honestly you express your own feelings when appropriate (without revealing your personal life), the easier for the client to do the same.
6. **Counselor and client already know each other—**
   - Emphasize confidentiality and ensure privacy
   - If the client wishes, arrange for another counselor.
7. **The client asks a personal question—**
   - In general, try not to talk about yourself. It takes attention away from the client.
   - You do not have to answer personal questions. The relationship between client and counselor is a professional one, not a social one.
   - It can help to talk about your own experience if you wish or you can describe what happened to someone else, without using names or identifying them as other clients.
   - Sometimes the client asks if the counselor has the same problem. It is best not to say yes or no. Instead, you can say something such as, "I'm familiar with that kind of situation. Please tell me more."
8. **The client threatens to commit suicide—**
   - *All suicide threats or attempts must be taken seriously*. It is essential to determine if attempts were made in the past, she/he is really considering suicide and the reasons for doing so—or if it's something that was said without thinking.
   - It is the best to refer the adolescent to a psychiatrist or psychologist and accompany her/him to the appointment.

9. **The client wants the counselor to make the decision—**
   - This client may actually be asking for help. You can ask questions such as these: "You seem to be having trouble reaching a decision. Perhaps you are not quite ready? Would you like to discuss this further? Do you need more information? More time to think? Would you like to talk this over with someone else, perhaps your friend or your parents?"
   - You can say, "I can answer your questions and help you think about your choices, but you know your own life best. The best decisions will be the decisions you make yourself."

SOME COMMON MISTAKES

1. **We patronize**: The adolescent has enough of that in her daily life and will only raise barriers between the counselor and the client.
2. **We preach**: The adolescent has a developing set of moral values that are uniquely her own. Being in a position of relative power does not authorize the counselor to impose a sense of morality.
3. **We do not listen**: A common complaint among adolescents is that no one listens to them. To understand their problems we must listen, listen and listen.
4. **We treat them as children**: Adolescents are not big children—Accord the adolescent the same respect and confidentiality due to an adult. Their sense of dignity must not feel threatened.

TIME REQUIREMENT FOR COUNSELING

Usually 30 minutes are sufficient for the initial interview, first 5 minutes can be spent with parent and the adolescent, then 10 minutes with teenager for exploring, 10 minutes for examination and 5 minutes for treatment. In follow-up visits, 15 minutes are sufficient. For complex psychosocial problems, two or three 30 minutes sessions, one week apart are more productive than one long session. This way, both the adolescent and the health care provider can look back and think about their assessment and responses given in the previous session.

ADOLESCENT FRIENDLY HEALTH SERVICES

Crowding and absence of dedicated space for adolescent counseling can be a significant hurdle in establishing rapport between the counselor and the client. Hence, it is essential to make the center an Adolescent friendly health center. This can be done by guiding and training the staff involved, dedicating adequate space which is quiet and ensures privacy with a positive atmosphere. Various charts highlighting the services provided for adolescents and educational charts may be used. An adolescent health card which monitors growth, provides guidelines regarding diet can be provided. Cards and various

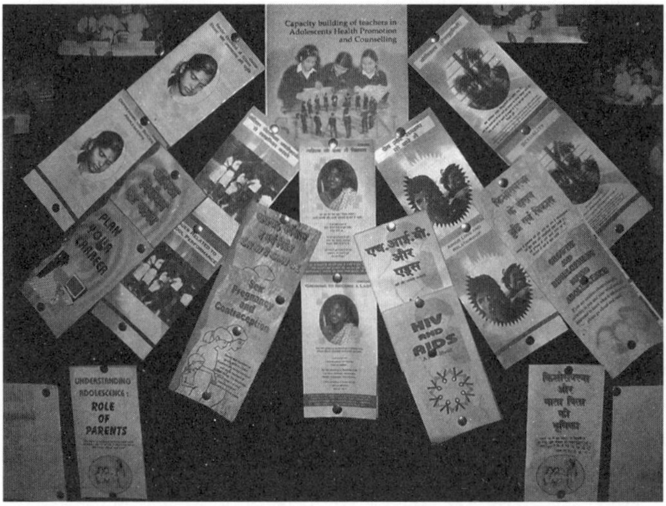

Fig. 27.1: Safdarjung Hospital, New Delhi, Adolescent Healthcare Network (Shahn) Pamphlets on Display for Adolescents (*Courtesy:* Shahn)

tools may also be provided giving guidance regarding when a healthcare personnel should be approached, especially in matters of reproductive and sexual health to avoid delay in the clients seeking care. These services should provide comprehensive healthcare to adolescents that includes preventive, promotive care besides treating the biomedical illnesses and counseling. An example of displayed pamphlets for further reference for adolescents is given in Figure 27.1 (*Courtesy*: Shahn).

SUMMARY AND CONCLUSION

As a society and as individuals, we now identify adolescence as an important time in a person's life. It is full of doubts and anxiety, hopes and ambition, the period when one looks at the world around to identify ones place in it. One's actions, habits and impulses which develop during this time have a long-term bearing on ones future life. This is especially true of the issues concerning health. A healthcare provider as a counselor for adolescents must have a sincere fondness for youth, the willingness to lend an ear, be nonjudgmental and the courage to be honest and fair. The healthcare provider should also be well-informed and a good communicator with the ability to engage the adolescents interest. Adolescent counseling, if conducted with enthusiasm, in a dedicated manner and on a large scale could go a long way in improving the health of our adolescents, ensuring a healthy future for the people and the society.

KEY POINTS

- Adolescent counseling is an important measure for preventing and promoting good health in the adolescents.

- It requires commitment on the part of the health counselor in terms of time, space and patience.
- Confidentiality and a nonjudgmental attitude has to be maintained.
- Communication barriers whether on the part of client, provider or policy should be recognized and dealt with in a subtle manner.
- It should focus on personality development, growth and development, nutrition, literacy and sex education.
- Counseling should be preventive and promotive in order to prevent high-risk behavior and should promote healthy sexual behavior. It should impart knowledge regarding contraceptive measures and avoidance of pregnancy. Adolescents should know risk of STIs and RTIs including HIV and AIDS.
- Youth and adolescent friendly centers can provide ideal set-up for counseling.

SUGGESTED READING

1. A handy desk reference tool for primary level health workers: Adolescent Job Aid published by World Health Organisation 2008.
2. Agarwal N, Suneja A. Counselling for adolescent girls: Pediatric and Adolescent Gynecology, Jaypee Publications, New Delhi, 2003.
3. Counselling skills training in adolescent sexuality and reproductive health—A Facilitator's Guide: Adolescent Health Programme, Division of Family Health, World Health Organisation 1998.
4. Gandhi AB. Gynecological Manual on Adolescent Girls and Young Women. A FOGSI Publication, 2009.
5. Hertweck S, Rayburn Williams. The Adolescent Sexual Health Visit, Obst and Gyne Clinics of North America; Pediatric and Adolescent Gynecology. 2009;36(1):99-118.
6. Orientation programme for medical officers to provide adolescent friendly reproductive and sexual health services. Published by IEC division, Ministry of Health and Family Welfare, Govt of India 2006.

28 Handling Peer Pressure: Learn to Say No!

Rajiv Mohta

Peers—they are people your age or close to it, who have experiences and interests similar to yours and you identify with them. Peer pressure occurs when the individual experiences implicit or explicit persuasion, sometimes amounting to coercion, to adopt similar values, beliefs, and goals, or to participate in the same activities as those in the peer group.

Peer pressure is one thing that all teens have in common. Peer pressure can turn the best person into a coward and can lead us to do things we would never choose to do on our own. No matter how old you are, peer pressure can affect your daily life. As a teenager, there is peer pressure to fit in, peer pressure to do silly dares, peer pressure to smoke, and peer pressure to be the cool kid in school. As an adult, there's peer pressure to pick the right job, form cliques with people in the work place, pressure to confirm with social norms and the same peer pressures as a kid—to fit in, to try something new or dangerous.

While it is hard to overcome these pressures as an adult, it can be twice as hard as an adolescent. While not all peer pressure is bad, the type of peer pressure that leaves you feeling confused or hurt is never good. When peer pressure is good it is very, very good, but when it is bad, peer pressure can be devastating. The difference between negative and positive peer pressure is 'the outcome'.

WHEN PEER PRESSURE IS GOOD

Peers can enforce a profoundly positive influence on each other and play important roles in each other's lives:

- **Friendship:** Among peers you can find friendship and acceptance, and share experiences that can build lasting bonds.
- **Positive examples:** Peers set plenty of good examples for each other. Having peers, who are committed to doing well in school, can influence you to be more goal-oriented, too. Even peers you've never met can be role models! For example, watching someone your age compete in the Olympics, give a piano concert, etc.
- **Feedback and advice:** Your friends listen and give you feedback as you try out new ideas, explore belief, and discuss problems. Peers can help you make decisions, too. Peers often give each other good advice. Your friends will be quick to tell you when they think you're making a mistake or doing something risky.

- **Socializing:** Your peer group gives you opportunities to try out new social skills. Getting to know lots of different people, such as classmates or teammates; gives you a chance to learn how to expand your circle of friends, build relationships, and work out differences. You may have peers you agree or disagree with, compete with, or team with, peers you admire, and peers you don't want to be like.
- **Encouragement:** Peers encourage you to work hard to get the solo in the concert, help you study, listen and support you when you're upset or troubled, and empathize with you when they've experienced similar difficulties.
- **New experiences:** Your peers might get you involved in clubs, sports, or religious groups. Your world would be far less rich without peers to encourage you listen to a CD you've never heard before, or to offer moral support when you audition for the school play.

When the Pressure is not Good

Sometimes, though, the stresses in your life can actually come from your peers. They may pressure you into doing something you're uncomfortable with, such as shoplifting, doing drugs or drinking, taking dangerous risks when driving a car, or having sex before you feel ready. This pressure may be expressed openly ("Oh, come on friend, it's just one beer, and everyone else is having one") or more indirectly by simply making beer available at a party, for instance. Most peer pressure is less easy to define. Sometimes a group can make subtle signals without saying anything at all—letting you know that you must dress or talk a certain way or adopt particular attitudes toward school, other students, parents, and teachers in order to win acceptance and approval.

Peer Pressure: Risk Factors

There are certain risk factors for peer pressure, personality traits that make you more prone to give in to pressure. The traits that put you at higher risk for falling in to the peer pressure trap include:

- Low selfesteem
- Lack of confidence
- Uncertainty about ones place within a given peer group
- No personal interests exclusive of one's peer group
- Feeling isolated from peers and/or family
- Poor academic abilities or performance
- Fear of one's peers
- Lack of strong ties to friends
- Feeling that friends could turn on you
- Close bond with a bully.

FACTS ABOUT THE TEEN-PARENT RELATIONSHIP

- Parent relationships are not necessarily undermined by peer relationships. During adolescence, relationships between parents and teens are more often re-negotiated rather than rejected .What this means is that they are beginning to shift the relationship to incorporate their increasing independence and maturity.

- While it seems that teens are influenced by their peers, parents continue to be the most influential factor in their lives. Positive relationships between parents and teens also equip youth to have healthy relationships with friends. Teens who have high-quality relationships with parents also report having a positive relationship with their peers.
- Parent-adolescent conflict increases between childhood and early adolescence; although in most families, its frequency and intensity remain low. Parents need to include adolescents in decision-making and rule-setting that affects their lives.
- Parents who continue to communicate with their teens, even when there are conflicts, actually maintain closer relationships. So parents need to continue talking to their teens and maintaining an open line of communication, rather than simply trying to avoid disagreements.

FACTS ABOUT PEER FRIENDSHIPS

- Teens often have multiple layers and groups of friendships. Unlike in childhood, when friendships usually meant two or more close friends, teens often have multiple friends and belong to multiple groups.
- Peer friendships are dynamic. This simply means that peer friendships may change. For instance, while teens can have friendships that are long term, they often move from one clique to another, and they might develop new friendships and lose others.
- Peers tend to choose those who are similar to themselves. Whether it is gender, age, socioeconomic status, ethnicity, or interests, teens tend to gravitate towards those who are more similar to them.
- Peer friendships can be a healthy venue for positive youth development. Peer friendships can be a safe place for youth to explore their identity, learn about social norms, and practice their autonomy. Healthy friendships provide youth with social support for dealing with some of the challenges of adolescence, and can also provide youth with some of the most positive experiences during those years. Many teens report having some of the happiest and most fun moments with their peers, likely due to shared interests as well close relationships.

When Peer Pressure Becomes a Problem

Handling Peer Pressure

The influence of peer pressure is usually addressed in relation to the relative influence of the family on an individual. Some characteristics that peer groups offer and which families may be lacking are: (1) a strong belief structure; (2) a clear system of rules; and (3) communication and discussion about taboo subjects such as drugs, sex, and religion. In the following paragraphs some tips are given for the doctors to use while counseling the Adolescents and their parents which will in turn help in their decision making.

Ways to Handle Peer Pressure

For the Adolescents

- Script out the reaction you want to have in a given situation and play that script out in your head over and over again.
- Know where you stand on key issues like sex, drugs and alcohol and do not allow anybody to make you deviate from your position. Never be afraid to speak up and let others know your boundaries. You may get a bit of teasing at first but most people respect the boundaries of others when they know what they are.
- Think of yourself as a leader and act accordingly. The more you see yourself in a leadership role the more comfortable you will feel. Always stand up for what you think is right. Peer pressure sometimes gets the better of you but chances are when it does it is because you don't really know where you stand on whatever the issue at hand. This comes from a lack of self awareness and a willingness to be led rather than think for self.
- Always be comfortable with your choices. It is very easy to get caught up in the moment and forget that you will have to live with the choices you make. If you give in and do something that is contrary to your character or core value system it will cause you distress later and you will feel regret.
- Some people may not like it when you go against the group but doing the right thing is rewarding. Peer pressure only works if you let it, if you refuse to let it intimidate you, it loses its power. The secret is to be assertive without becoming preachy or self-righteous. Remember, peer pressure can only win if you let it.

Learn to Say NO

- As a parent, it's important to talk to your children about being direct, and that it's Okay to say—"No, thanks!" or "No, I'm not interested". No explanation is needed, no matter how much others may pry.
- If they are being pressured to smoke, it's advised to use humor to try and combat the pressure. For example, if a child is pressured to try smoking, they can respond with "No thanks, I'm not a chimney". While humorous, the others around may laugh or at least take it in stride that you're not interested.
- If the child may think it may become a situation, make sure they know of a place they can go to if they start to feel uncomfortable. If they are with a friend, they may want to talk beforehand about what they would do if they encountered a situation where peer pressure may occur.
- Consider offering a valid excuse. For example, if it is stemming from pressure to do drugs or smoke, it's Okay for them to say that they have a dentist appointment While lying is normally not a good thing to encourage your child to do, in this case, it may be better for them to lie than to start smoking at a young age or doing drugs.

- Arrange a "bail-out" code phrase you can use with your parents without losing face with your peers. You might call home from a party at which you're feeling pressured to drink alcohol and say, for instance, "Can you come and drive me home? I have a terrible earache."
- Hang with people who feel the same way you do. Choose friends who will speak up with you when you're in need of moral support, and be quick to speak up for a friend in the same way. Just having one other person stand with you against peer pressure makes it much easier for both people to resist.
- Blame your parents: Are you kidding? If my mom found out, she'd kill me.
- If a situation seems dangerous, don't hesitate to get an adult's help.

For Parents

- Talk to your teen. State clearly that you do not have a problem with their friends as people. You understand that that your teen's friends can make mistakes – just like your teen made a mistake. But you do have a problem with the risk-taking behavior and there needs to be a change on your teen's part and on their friend's part in order for you to be comfortable with them hanging out again.
- Open up the lines of communication with the other parents. Let them in on what is going on so that there is no miscommunication happening. Keep in mind that everyone has their own perspective, so there is no need to argue any points on who may have done what. Simply let them know that you are an involved parent and you wish to be informed if your teen is mixed up in any more harmful behaviors.
- Build an action plan with your teen. Address changing the behaviors that are concerning you in the plan and allow your teen to come up with different options to these behaviors. Learn more about the problem behavior and use your discipline skills as necessary. Limit your teens unsupervised time with the friends that were involved until you feel comfortable to slowly give back more of these privileges. You will need to be more involved with your teen at this time and offer more supervised activities with their friends.
- Take caution. Don't allow your teen to place all of the blame at their friend's feet. This is an easy out and may be the way to even bigger problems for your teenager down the road. Even if your teen's friend was 90% accountable for the misbehavior, you still need to hold your teen accountable so that he can actively deal with the problem and move on.
- Encourage your teenager not to belong to 'the popular' crowd. Many-a-times teens that belong to this crowd become overly stressed. They become so involved with what others want from them that they never explore what genuine friendship is all about.
- Don't get caught up in the discipline battles. If your teen and their friends do something wrong, even if it is a serious issue, you will need to apply

the auto rewind-repeat discipline. Teenagers learn by making choices, so they need to have the situations to be able to make their choices. If your teen gets into trouble with a friend, they will learn if you take the privilege away of seeing that friend for one week and then being allowed to make the same choices again. If you take the privilege of seeing that friend away forever, there will be nothing for them to learn from.

- Don't nit-pick their social life. Now this one is a thin line! Yes, going out with friends is a privilege, and one that should be taken away at times when your teenager does not live up to his responsibilities at home and at school. But, you need to remember that learning social skills can only happen in a social setting. It is very important that they learn these skills before they head off on their own. Therefore, try different forms of discipline instead of always taking social events away.
- Try not to make your teen feel bad about who they are. If they are left out of a certain group that you would like to see them be involved in, remember that it may be their choice not to be involved with that group and it is their choice to make. Allow them to be true to who they are. Give them constructive choices, show them what they can become involved in and then let them make the choice.
- Encourage diverse relationships by encouraging youth from diverse backgrounds to work and play together.
- Support parent education programs for families with teenagers. Parents need to be better informed about the dynamics of adolescent peer groups and the demands and expectations teenagers face in peer relationships. Seeking information is not a sign of weakness, and showing interest in these issues might actually show your teens that you are concerned about them.
- Encourage positive relationships between significant adults and teens. Youth should know that they can go to these caring adults for help or advice about their peer relationships.

CONCLUSION

During adolescence, peers play a large part in a young person's life even while the family continues to be significant. In general, peer friendships offer youth with many positive opportunities despite the negative connotations that peer relationships have to many of us. Peer relationships are actually important for healthy development and essential for youth to develop into healthy adults.

Nonetheless, peer relationships also have the potential to encourage problem behaviors. Although the negative influence of peers is often over-emphasized, more can be done to help teenagers experience the family and the peer group as mutually constructive environments. To accomplish this, families, communities, schools, can all contribute to helping youth develop positive peer relationships, and deflect negative peer pressures and influences.

SUGGESTED READING

1. Brown, BB. Adolescents relationships with peers. In RM Lerner and L Steinberg (Eds.), Handbook of Adolescent Psychology, 2nd edition. New York: Wiley, 2004; 363-94.
2. Brown BB, Klute C. Friendships, cliques, and crowds. In GR Adams and MD Berzonsky (Eds). Blackwell Handbook of Adolescence. Malden, MA: Blackwell Publishing, 2006;330-48.
3. Brown, BB. Peer groups and peer cultures. In SS Feldman and GR Elliott (Eds). At the threshold: The developing adolescent. Cambridge, MA: Harvard University Press, 1990;171-98.
4. Denise Witmer. Pressure The Difference Between Negative and Positive Peer.
5. Hallie Bourne. Encyclopedia of Psychology, Apr 06, 2001.
6. Mike Hardcastle. How to Combat Peer Pressure.
7. Preparing Youth for Peer Pressure From US Dept of Health and Human Services.
8. Steinberg L. Adolescence. New York, NY: McGraw-Hill, 2005.

29 Risk Taking Behaviors by Adolescents

Atul Kanikar

The most crucial yet vulnerable period of human life is between 10-19 years is a phase of life which has recently gained recognition as a phase with its own special needs,[1] a period aptly named as the period of storm and stress. Teenage is when the core personality and development of basic philosophies of life take shape. If an individual can sail through this vital span rather smoothly, the life is made. Most of the youngsters do overcome the challenges with some teething troubles; however few succumb to the ill effects and fall prey to the so called high risk behaviors with probably lifelong consequences.[6] The present article aims at listing, causation, clinical features, early identification, treatment, consequences and prevention of most of the common risk taking behaviors in teens. The role of gatekeepers, i.e. parents, teachers and policy makers also will be emphasized as and when deemed necessary. The risk taking behaviors of violence, poor conduct, and surviving on streets being less common in adolescent girls; will not be discussed here in detail. Poor stress management and anemia in teenagers have been discussed elsewhere. Table 29.1 summarizes the various risk taking behaviors commonly exhibited by teenagers.

Table 29.1: Various risk taking behaviors commonly exhibited by teenagers

Behaviors	*Boys*	*Girls*
1. Sexual experimentations	Usual initiators	Usual sufferers
2. Sexual abuse and rape	Perpetrators	Usual victims
3. Substance abuse	Very common	Usually imposed upon
4. Careless driving	Almost universal	Increasing these days
5. Media addictions and crimes	Common	Rare
6. Loss of interest in schools and colleges	Secondary to other factors	Not so common
7. Inappropriate financial management	Common in hostels	Rarely obvious
8. Violence	Very common	Exceptional
9. Poor conduct	Usual to some extent	Uncommon
10. Surviving on streets	Antisocial behavior	Early prostitution
11. Poor eating habits	Obesity is common	Undernutririon mainly
12. Incorrect stress management	Variety of manifestations	Depression and suicide

SEXUAL EXPERIMENTATION AND UNSAFE SEXUAL ACTIVITY (TABLE 29.2)

Sexual health may be defined as the absence of illness and injury associated with sexual behavior, and a sense of sexual well-being.[1] The 3 'E's of adolescence are: Expanding, Experiencing and Experimenting.[3] In addition to the physical growth and certain areas in brain, the teenager experiences lot of hormonal impacts on the newly appreciated body organs. The genitalia which were till now merely the excretory outlets suddenly are considered as pleasure points. The world of the teenager is studded with sexually explicit messages given by peers and media. Lethargy and ignorance of parents and teachers in imparting age-appropriate information, further worsens the problem. The amalgamation of nature and nurture takes form.

The timing and speed of puberty determines the outcome of sexual behavior in early teens. Boys who attain puberty earlier than the peer group (early bloomers) turn out to be leaders in the group. They are looked upon as the best source of sexual information by the peer group. In girls however, early puberty is not an advantage. The height gain after menarche is minimal and the girl takes an adult form although mentally she may be still a child. Thus, early blooming in girl poses her the risk of social isolation, parental restrictions and even sexual abuse which she may not be able to handle at least initially.

Table 29.2: Factors in adolescent sexual activity

Risk factor	*Various implications*
1. Early puberty and delayed age of marriage	Prolonged abstinence due to cultural factors.
2. Increased desire and libido	More pleasure and frequency
3. Curiosity	Tendency to experiment, peer influence
4. Ignorance and misconception	Unhealthy sexual activity
5. Low contraception usage	Pregnancy, Sexually transmitted infections.
6. Partner is likely to be high risk	STI and HIV
7. Multiple partners	STI and HIV, emotional stress
8. Peer pressure and coercive sex	Physical and emotional trauma
9. Unprotected and unplanned sexual activity	Pregnancy, STI, mental trauma
10. Lack of life skills	Inability to say "No", inability to negotiate
11. Physical, emotional and social consequences	Pregnancy, unsafe abortions, STI, depression, prostitution, early and forced marriages, school and college drop-outs, economic burden, etc

Role of Gatekeepers in Sexual Behaviors of Teenagers (Table 29.3)

Parents, school and college teachers along with policy makers have a lot of scope in preventing the increasing problems of teenage sexual activity and its consequences. The only flaw is lethargy, ignorance and inability to join hands for a comprehensive program. Everybody finds it easier to put the responsibility and blame on others. Teachers are overburdened with school curriculum and have practically no knowledge of imparting the least essential family life education to students. Even the lessons on reproduction are at times skipped wishfully to avoid embarrassing situations. The adolescents are actually now looking at human sexuality as something dirty and not to be talked about. The parents on other hand have given too much significance to scholastics alone and even discussions over issues like sexuality and life skills are labeled as hindrances to studies. Policy makers have no single program at national level for this 23.5% Indian population,[1] the largest in the world. All that is desired is a productive population at minimum or no cost. In view of these wishful lethargies by the gatekeepers, today's adolescent has to rely only on media and peers for the vital scientific information on sexuality issues. Both actually give a misleading and fictitious picture of the same. Hence it is not incorrect to mention that the gatekeepers are more responsible than the teenagers themselves for the worsening scenario of human sexual behavior in the delicate years of life.

Table 29.3: Teaching sexuality to children

	Hurdles	*Method to solve the problem*
1.	You don't know the exact answer.	Be honest and comfortable with yourself. Buy time if necessary. Teenager is likely to accept.
2.	Teenager wants to know about sex.	Ask what he/she already knows. Give age appropriate information.
3.	Teenager wants to share information.	Talk less—listen more. Use non-verbal tools.
4.	Timid and shy teenager.	Encourage queries.
5.	You are scared that teenager will ask difficult questions.	Anticipate and be prepared.
6.	Teenager wants to know about condoms or emergency pill.	Stay calm. Be non-judgmental. Let the teenager express his/her knowledge and opinion.
7.	You are worried about the teenager's knowledge and attitude towards sex.	Ask open ended questions. Use why, how, can you describe type of questions.
8.	You feel that a particular issue is important but the teenager doesn't want to talk to you about sexual matters.	Use teachable moments. Discussions can be opened with newspaper cuttings, advertisements, stories, films, etc.
9.	Teenager is concerned about puberty changes, interest in opposite sex, body image, pornography, etc.	Identify question behind the question. The usual question is "Am I normal or not".
10.	Teenager tends to assign sex specific roles and expects the same.	Gender sensitization and changing roles of boys and girls needs to be emphasized.
11.	Adolescent is inclined to break family and social norms.	Imbibe values whenever possible but at the end of the discussion.

Most of the adolescents are receptive to the appropriate information imparted by parents and teachers.[2] The key is to give a listening ear, being non-judgmental and non-formal in our approach.

SEXUAL ABUSE AND RAPE

Sexual abuse is when an adult makes sexual contact with a child or teenager in a harmful and unwanted way. Sexual abuse includes forced sex or rape; incest or sexual molesting. Sexual molesting means unwanted sexual activities such as kissing or fondling the breasts or genitals. Sexual abuse is a global problem mainly because children are scared to talk about it.[4] The main fear is that nobody will believe them and the abuser will make some harm. Children further find it difficult to talk because in 80% cases, the abuser is commonly a family member or someone whom they know well.[2] Both boys and girls are vulnerable to the brutal invasion of their privacy, although girls are at a very high risk. Boys tend to hide the problem whereas girls at least disclose it to the mother.[3] The problem is more in early maturing girls who still have the innocence of a child. Unfortunately the perpetrator is usually a trusted person (uncle, cousin, grandfather, father, brother, autorickshaw driver or neighbor) known to the child and probably the mother also. The so called 'sugar daddy' takes advantage of the economic dependence of the family on him and the victim can hardly oppose. In more common situations, episodic abuse occurs in many adolescents who do not report to the parents or teachers for the fear of getting ill fame. In another situation, in an existing love affair, a girl may be victimized through forced sex or drugged unknowingly, leading to the so called date rape. Many girls also succumb to the false promises about marriage by their boyfriends leading to misery.

Causal Factors in Sexual Abuse

- Evolving sexual urges and early physical maturation
- Ignorance of the teenager and parents
- Tendency to disregard and hide
- Economic dependence on the abuser
- Too many opportunities these days
- Parental conflicts and neglect
- Changing social norms and family structure
- Media influence especially on boys
- Provoking and revealing tendencies of girls
- Peer acceptance and pressure
- Victim may be labeled as being easily 'available'
- Influence of date rape drugs like flunitrazepam, ketamine, barbiturates, etc
- Increasing incidence of substance abuse, mainly alcohol, even in girls
- Poor attachment of the adolescent with the parents and family
- Street children

Consequences of Sexual Abuse in Adolescents

The effects of sexual abuse on teenagers could be varied and in combination. They may be short lasting or have a lifelong pathetic journey of self blame, guilt and revengefulness making the life of not only the teenager but many significant people in his/her life. The principal four categories of the impact on the victim of sexual abuse could be roughly summarized as follows:

a. ***Traumatic sexualization:*** It is an aversive feeling about sex including sexual identity problems. The teenager may exhibit extremes of sexual behaviors from total avoidance to hypersexual encounters.
b. ***Betrayal:*** The teenager feels betrayed and severely hurt by the perpetrator who is or was so close and dependable. The teenager may then start confusing sex with love or an exchange means of care and attention. The teenager learns to sexualize all future relationships leading to sexual promiscuity, prostitution and even inappropriate and unethical relationships with own children. There is an obvious impaired ability to judge people with a lot of mistrust. On the other hand, the victim may develop total aversion about sex leading to sexual dysfunction and

complete avoidance of future sexual activity making even the life of future partner miserable.

c. ***Stigmatization:*** The so called "damaged good syndrome" described by Sgroi include the combination of guilt and self blame. There is a tendency to even repent the act of disclosure of sexual abuse. The teenager carries around this stigma like a heavy weight attached to self leading to a feeling of worthlessness and poor self esteem. Eventually this may lead to self destructive behaviors in the form of drug abuse, self mutilation, suicidal ideation/acts and provoking behaviors which will lead to punishment.
d. ***Powerlessness:*** The weak teenager having realized that abuse cannot be stopped, feels powerless and fails to control his/her life. As this teenager grows, there is poor coping with stress, despair, depression, tendency for repeated abuse, inclination to run away from real life situations and potentiality for aggression and becoming an abuser in later life.

The prognosis of a victim of sexual abuse depends mainly on the ability to boldly refuse the responsibility for the act. If the teenager has a self blaming thought process, the prognosis is guarded with a constant feeling of being trapped in own thoughts and negative sense of self. On the other hand, if the victim takes to reclaim the self, he or she is likely to praise self for being a survivor of the abuse, feel proud not to be responsible for the unfortunate act and hence feel positive towards his/her future actions in life.

Role of Gatekeepers in Prevention of Sexual Abuse in Adolescents

1. Identify the precipitating factors and manage these whenever possible.
2. Encourage self-protection skills by giving age appropriate information and means to identify inappropriate touch. It is mandatory to mention that boys too need to be educated.
3. Teach the teenagers that he/she is the custodian of body, mind and spirit and nobody except the mother and doctor (in the presence of mother) has the right to touch them against their will.[3]
4. In case someone tries to abuse a teenager, all that he/she needs to do is shout "No, don't do this to me." and get help. Most perpetrators are scared by a big "No" from a teenager and further problems can be easily avoided. Let the teenager actually practice saying big "No" once in a while. It may look funny but can actually be very useful when needed.
5. Teenager should be taught that it is the abuser and not the victim who is responsible for the act of abuse.[2]
6. Create an environment where the teenager will not be scared and uncomfortable to share his/her feelings. Take steps to enhance teenager's attachment to home or school.[5]
7. Teenager should be helped to demarcate clear boundaries between friendships and sex. Girls should be convinced that defending yourself is not offending the boyfriend (Fig. 29.1). Alcohol and substance abuse is to be strictly avoided and caution should be observed while in parties or on a date.

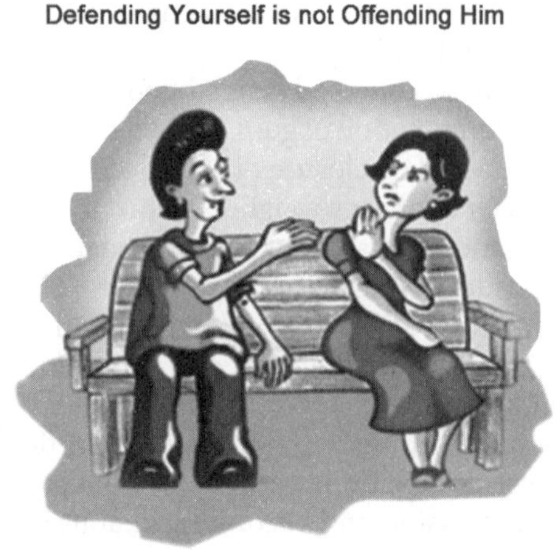

Fig. 29.1: WHO poster on prevention of sexual abuse in girls

In spite of all the preventive measures mentioned above, an occasional bitter incidence should not demoralize the teenager and parents and teachers should provide a listening ear, lot of support and prevent the self blaming by teenager or parents themselves. A warm family milieu, positive parental behavior towards one another, proper rehabilitation of street children and life skills education made mandatory to all the teenagers will go a long way in preventing sexual abuse in the society.

SUBSTANCE ABUSE

Substance abuse is a 'medico-socioeconomic disease' with a high mortality and morbidity.[5] Substance abuse in most of the cases has its onset in adolescence (70% adults start substance abuse during teenage) and has both short-term and long-term implications on physical and mental and social well-being. Drug abuse is associated with high-risk sexual behavior, HIV, hepatitis, endocarditis and other high-risk behaviors like road traffic accidents, homicide and suicide. With a growing economy, loss of traditional 'societal buffers', changing lifestyles and family structure and norms, the problem of adolescent drug abuse will attain unimaginable dimensions in the next few years.

The nonmedical use of chemical substances in order to achieve alteration in psychological functioning has been termed substance use.[5] The adolescents use these substances to stimulate, depress or otherwise affect mental faculties usually to conform to peer standards and to relieve emotional pain such as despair, hopelessness and loneliness. Various Indian and Western studies highlight that male, illiterate and semiliterate, unemployed, street children and school dropouts are at the highest risk of drug abuse. The age of initiation is early in this group. They mostly indulge in hard drugs and are likely to engage in other high-risk behavior. Recent trends have shown a drop in age of initiation of alcohol from 28 years in 1920 to 19 years in 2005.[5] There has been an increase in use of opium products, narcotics and synthetic drugs especially in rave parties.

Characteristics of Substance Abuse in Adolescence (Fig. 29.2)

- Use of tobacco and alcohol at an early age is a predictive factor for the use of other drugs, a variety of drugs and more potent drugs.
- Tobacco and alcohol are considered 'gateway drugs'.
- Most of the adolescent drug users are experimental or recreational users and can be treated as outpatients.
- The interval between first use of tobacco and development of nicotine addiction appears to be two years. This time period offers a good 'window of opportunity' to initiate a tobacco cessation program.
- 74% youth with substance use disorder have comorbid disorders that usually occurs first either in childhood or early adolescence followed by substance use 5-10 years later, thereby offering another 'window of opportunity'. These disorders include conduct disorders, ADHD, depression, anxiety, adjustment disorder, specific learning disability, social phobia, and eating disorder.
- Drug abusing adolescents suffer from poor health, liver, lung disease and neuropsychological deficits. Even infrequent casual use of alcohol, marijuana and other hard drugs can cause abuse, date rape, injuries and even death due to risk taking behavior.

Determinants of Adolescent Substance Abuse

Factors that predispose to substance abuse are called 'risk factors' and those that reduce the potential for drug abuse are called 'protective' factors. Adolescents function in five principle domains that include individual, family, school, peer and community. These domains interact with each other to either promote or protect against drug abuse. The various determinants of drug abuse are as follows:

1. *Community:* In India, this is the most important factor influencing adolescent drug use. Easy availability, accessibility of drugs and poor law enforcement, glamorized media portrayal, disorganized and violent neighborhood as in slums and streets, extreme poverty, high rates of illiteracy and unemployment facilitate drug abuse. Changing social norms and worsening relationships with neighbors also contributes to the free substance abuse by the teenager.
2. *Individual:* Adolescents who are impulsive, sensation seeking, with low self-esteem, aggressive and with drug abusing role models are particularly vulnerable. Another class includes victims of dating violence and sexual abuse. Those who are early initiators and gamblers and street children form a major group. As mentioned earlier, existing co-morbid conditions predispose the teenager for drug abuse. The protective factors include having high aspirations in life, resilience, involvement in religious activities.

3. ***Family:*** Parental conflict and divorce, permissive/authoritarian parenting, parental approval of drug use, parental and sibling drug use, family history of drug abuse, poor parental connectedness, availability and monitoring, faulty discipline techniques and parents with 'a pill for every ill' attitude increase the risk of substance abuse in the teenager.
4. ***School:*** Poor school connectedness, early school failure, truancy, school adjustment problems, school dropout and drug use by teachers make the adolescent more vulnerable for drug abuse. Adolescents with high academic achievement and a drug free environment at school are protected against drug use.
5. ***Peers:*** Peer use and/or approval of drug use and delinquent and violent peer group make the teenager easily susceptible.
   There are some drug specific indicators as follows:
   Amnesia: Date rape drugs, e.g. flunitrazepam, ketamine, barbiturates, gamma hydroxybutrate, etc.
   Black outs, gastritis, body odor: Alcohol
   'Flu like symptoms': Marijuana, cocaine, inhalants
   Red conjunctiva, abnormal pupils: Marijuana
   Paint stains on face and clothes: Inhalants
   Chest pain, tachycardia: Cocaine, amphetamine
   Bronchospasm, constipation: Opiates, marijuana
   Increased appetite for sweets: Marijuana

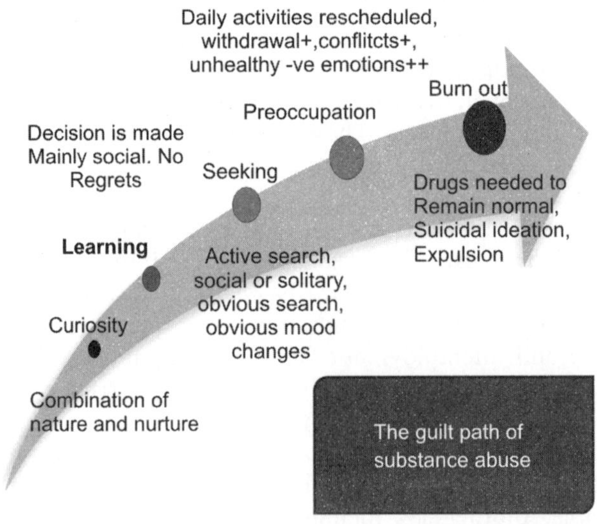

Fig. 29.2: Staging of substance abuse: (Based on AFSI module)

It is important to remember that earlier the teenager is brought to the clinician, the better. Most parents tend to hide the problem initially. This makes the treatment more difficult.

Early Indicators of Drug Abuse

- Efforts to mask the smell as evidenced by frequent rinsing and washing hands, use of perfume or deodorant, chewing mint, etc.
- Avoiding eye contact and hug by parents.
- New set of (senior) friends.
- Social isolation with loss of interest in activities which the teenager was enjoying earlier.
- Scholastic deterioration.
- Poor hygiene, altered appetite and sleep pattern.
- Changed preference for movies and music which depict high action and drug abuse.
- Unexplained irritability and increasing conflicts with parents and teachers.
- Spending extra time in toilet.
- Stealing money/valuables from the house.

Parents, especially the mother can and should sense the initiation of substance abuse in the teen. Subtle changes in the behavior if picked up early can prevent the natural curiosity of teenager taking a bad turn.

Role of Gatekeepers in Prevention of Substance Abuse in Teenagers

1. Keep a vigilance over teenager's routine. Know his/her peer group and their family background.
2. Guide and limit the adolescent's behavior which you do not approve.
3. Be a good role model yourself.
4. Discuss the incidences like rave parties openly with the teenagers or the class and obtain their opinions. Mention the preventive measures for mishaps during such incidences.
5. Teach assertive skills with lot of practice sessions and role plays.
6. Define a clear and usable drug abuse prevention module in the school and implement it. Involve the students and parents in the formulation, implementation and follow-up process. The authorities should do, all that is possible before considering expulsion from school.
7. In case the teenager is already using drug, give lot of support and encouragement to help him win over the guilt factor associated with it. Let him/her experience regret for the same. Help the teenager to help himself. In advanced stages go for professional assistance. Urgent intervention and possibly referral are needed in the situations of Stage 3 and Stage 4 of drug use, multiple high risk behavior, comorbid disorders with drug use, preadolescent drug abuse and relapse of drug abuse.
8. Medical practitioners should not miss clinical features like weight loss, hypertension, jaundice, HIV, red eyes, nasal irritation, hoarseness, chronic cough, hymoptysis, chest pain, wheezing, unexplained injuries, needle tracks, blank stares, tattoos, scratch marks, excessive acne, testicular atrophy, etc. as markers of substance abuse in an adolescent client.

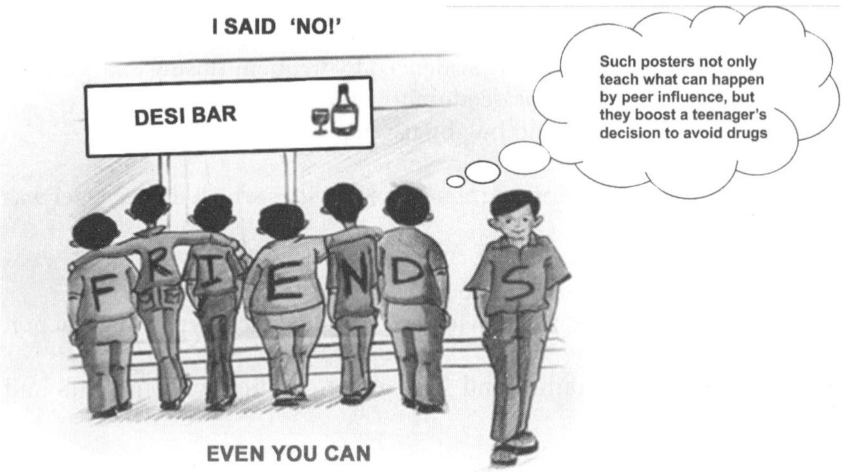

Fig. 29.3: Adolescent health posters on substance abuse published by WHO

Figure 29.3 shows an adolescent health poster on substance abuse published by WHO. Such posters not only teach what can happen by peer influence, but they boost a teenager's decision to avoid drugs.

CARELESS DRIVING

Road traffic accidents are the leading cause of mortality and morbidity in teenagers. There is no parent in the community who is not concerned about this vital issue. Nearly all adults have had at least one road accident in their teenage. The problem is exponentially increasing in amount and severity due to increase in the number of vehicles, time constraints, too many appointments, poor traffic conditions and pathetic control by the authorities. Boys tend to attempt careless driving in order to seek attention and impress friends and opposite sex. Slow and careful driving is taken as a negative trait. Girls want to be no less than boys and due to inherent poor skills tend to meet accidents easily. Youth under 19 years are at the greatest risk of motor vehicle fatalities, more so under the influence of alcohol and other drugs. The mechanism, of increasing number of accidents is depicted in Figure 29.4.

Role of Gatekeepers in Prevention of Risky Driving by Teenagers

1. Parents should have strict vigilance on teenager's driving skills. It is advisable to practically teach the adolescent the safety rules emphasizing the fact that in spite of teenager being careful, the rest of the people on the street may not obey the traffic rules. In either case, the looser will be the teenager only.
2. The alarming incidence of mortality and morbidity should be told to the teenager mentioning the importance of priceless life and its quality. Parents may actually take this opportunity to convey their own feelings for the adolescent.

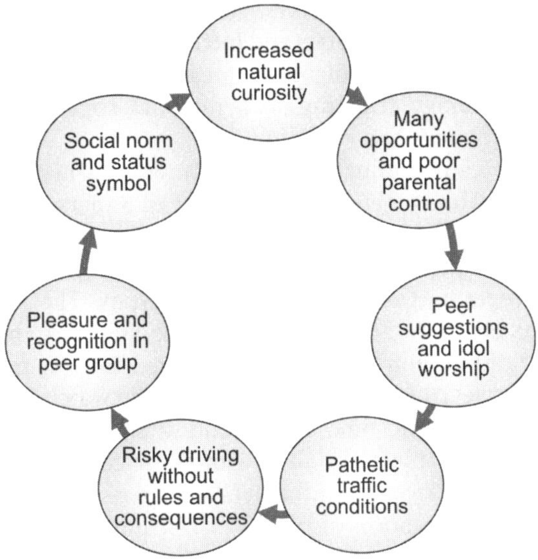

Fig. 29.4: Mechanism of increasing number of accidents

3. Giving away high speed vehicles even as a reward should be withheld till the teenager has understood the safety norms and agrees to follow them.
4. Negative reinforcement in the form of withdrawing the privilege of driving should follow irresponsible driving immediately.
5. Law enforcement is mandatory with a periodic update. Routine as well as surprise scrutiny of driving license, vehicle documents and insurance is essential and any defaulter be punished without bias. Parents and politicians should not try to needlessly protect the defaulter since it may actually give a wrong message, adding further to the irresponsible driving.
6. School curriculum should include teaching safety measures and traffic rules as a part of value education.
7. The family life education program should also emphasize road traffic accidents as a leading cause of teenage loss.
8. Finally parents should themselves set a very good role model by observing traffic rules especially when a teenager accompanies them.

MEDIA ADDICTIONS AND CRIME

No other thing has a greater impact than media on today's adolescents. Media is the thread which binds the routine and has a decisive role on the future of our generation. This very powerful and useful tool for education, information and entertainment has influenced the lives of nearly all the human beings on this planet probably more than God Almighty himself. The visual medium has more impact on adolescents than any other medium.[5] Life without a television is unimaginable these days. With the explosive developments in information technology, Computers and Internet have brought in a sea change in the information media available to present day teenagers. With these advances in technology, teaching academic and social skills to children became very convenient and efficient.

While its educative influences are enormous, its negative impacts are also innumerable. Young viewers up to the age of 8 years cannot distinguish hype from normalcy. Research has shown a correlation between watching television and maladaptive behavior. TV's influence on kids is subtle and reinforced by repetition of images and stereotypes. The media pressures adolescents to be more adult-like. Evidence suggests that television's influence on children and adolescents is related to how much time they spend watching television. Children on an average watch 28 hours of TV a week, spending twice the time they spend at school.[5] Often violence is depicted as an acceptable solution to simple or complex problem in TV programs. Marketing strongly influences children's food preferences that may lead on to consumption of plenty of fast foods/processed foods that cause obesity.

The primary effects of media exposure are increased violent and aggressive behavior, increased high-risk behaviors, including alcohol and tobacco use, and accelerated onset of sexual activity. Among adolescents, the prevalence of obesity increases by 2% for each additional hour per day spent on viewing TV. Another cause is in the advertising that goes on in the programs. The main targets of advertising for younger kids are fast foods, snacks and sugar coated cereals. TV is effective in provoking kids to request for the advertised foods. Girls and boys who frequently thought about wanting toned or well-defined muscles were at increased risk for using potentially unhealthy products to enhance their physique. Exposure to sexual content in music, movies, television, and magazines accelerates adolescents' sexual activity and increases their risk of engaging in early sexual intercourse. Less than one third of parents discuss sexuality with their children. Many schools do not offer comprehensive sex education. By default, TV may be the leading sex educator for most of the children these days. Unfortunately such an influential medium often presents sex in most inappropriate way. Reporting and portrayal of suicidal behavior in the media may have potentially negative influences and facilitate suicidal acts by people exposed to such stimuli. Excessive amounts of time at a computer can contribute undeveloped social skills and a form of addictive behavior. Although rare, some children with seizure disorders are more prone to attacks brought on by a flickering television or computer screen.

The adverse effects of all electronic media are described below:

1. Prolonged sitting in front of TV or computer can affect child's postural development.
2. Eating junk food while with media can increase obesity, lead to underdeveloped socialization and internet addiction syndrome.

3. Pedophiles may use the internet to hook young and innocent teenagers into a perverted relationship.
4. Intentional or accidental exposure to pornographic sites even through internet games can pollute the adolescent's image of a woman as a mother, sister, friend or companion. Soon the teenager may start treating the opposite sex as a sex toy which he/she can use and throw away at will.
5. Instant messaging and e-mail can interfere with more meaningful work like school assignments.
6. Media takes away the valuable time which the family has for its members.
7. Information given by the media need not be always true and accurate. A teenager thus can get false beliefs on very important issues like sexuality, growth, nutrition, body image, etc.
8. The advertising gimmicks on the media can actually persuade the teenager to use or even steal a credit card to pay off for the product without parental consent. Online gambling also may be attempted.
9. The violence shown in media including cartoon channels and video games has deleterious effects on a teenager's mind.
10. Girls also develop a negative image of self due to constant depiction of women as pleasure tools. Paradoxically, some adolescent girls may use electronic media for financial gains.

Role of Gatekeepers

1. Admit that media is a very powerful tool. Discuss the beneficial effects of media with teenagers.
2. Allow teenager to enlist the adverse effects with the strategies which teenager already knows to combat these side effects. Know his/her opinions before parents start the preaching.
3. Keep TV and computer in a central place in the house. Use various net nannies and other tools to restrict access to pornographic sites.
4. Eating with media should be strictly avoided.
5. Make a family rule for watching TV and internet. See that every member of the family including grandparents has understood the rule correctly and then implement it religiously. Strong consequences should follow if anyone doesn't follow what has been agreed upon.
6. Get a consensus on what should be watched in a given week. Stick to the time-table and praise the teenager if he/she abides by the parent's suggestions.
7. Monitor teenager's routine and time with peers to avoid being fooled by him/her.
8. Adverse effects of media especially on advertising and pornography should be highlighted in the family life education programs in school. Media education should be made compulsory as a part of value education.
9. Strengthening existing legislations and strictest punishments for inadvertent use of electronic and print media by the authorities is the need of the time.

LOSS OF INTEREST IN SCHOOL AND STUDIES (FIG. 29.5)

Abrupt worsening in scholastic performance is an uncommon but alarming condition. Parents and teachers prefer to put the blame on one another initially and later on the peer group. Coaching classes are looked upon as an immediate rescue and there is a panic situation. Poor scholastic performance could be a symptom of many underlying problems in the child, family or school. Sudden deterioration in scholastics should arouse suspicion for the following reasons:

- Health related issues
- Maladjustments with peers/teacher
- Study related stresses
- Bad company
- Money—easy come, easy go
- Broken heart
- Drugs or sexual experimentation
- Cyber addictions
- Domestic problems
- The blues.

Before blaming each other, parents and teachers should look for any of the above mentioned possibilities. Some reasons need immediate attention and if addressed effectively can save the teenager's career and mental health. At times, many factors come into picture together and gatekeepers cannot solve the issue. Professional help may be taken in these cases in the form of

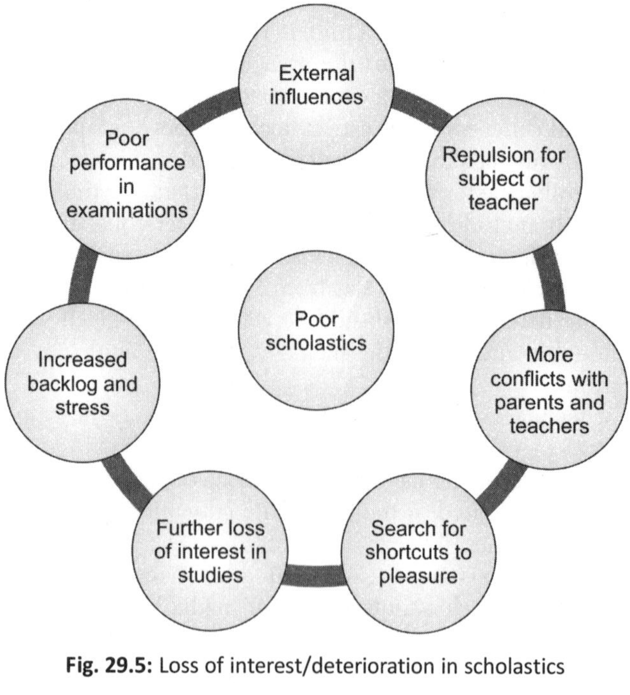

Fig. 29.5: Loss of interest/deterioration in scholastics

a counselor or educationist. Certain emotional and behavioral problems can emerge in adolescence.[3]

Delayed puberty in boys and early menarche in girls can put the teenagers at a particular risk of bullying by the peer group. Most of the adult psychiatric disorders have their roots in adolescence.[3] A detailed perosnality testing (MMPI) assessed by a clinical psychologist may be needed in rare instances.

By far the common pathway to scholastic deterioration in most of the adolescents has a typical emergence as depicted in Figure 29.5.

Role of Gatekeepers in Improving Scholastic Performance of Teenagers[5]

Motivation

Even if an adolescent has normal or above average intelligence, it is unlikely that he/she will do well, without a desire or motivation to succeed at school. To help a teenager develop a positive attitude and motivation toward working hard at school, the gatekeepers should:

- Praise and reward the adolescent for doing something well or working hard towards a difficult or challenging problem.
- Help build self-confidence by avoiding frequent criticism and praising hard work.
- Communicate to the teenager about school and ask him/her about the day at school, to show that you are interested.
- Help the teenager to find something that he/she has a skill or special interest in, such as music, sports, reading, etc.
- Help to understand that success has a lot to do with how much time and effort you put into a task, and is not just about how smart or strong he/she is. Children who believe this are more likely to take on new challenges and work harder on difficult tasks.
- Set realistic goals and expectations for the adolescent and set up consequences for not meeting these expectations and rewards or privileges, when he/she does.
- If the teenager is not doing well in spite of working hard and doing homework, then it may be unreasonable to expect beyond his/her capacity. Gatekeepers should instead reward and praise the hard work and not punish the teenager for not living up to their expectations. Search and treatment for specific learning difficulties be made at this point.

Some Steps that Parents can Take to Help the Teenager are:

- Become actively involved in your adolescent's schoolwork, by talking with teachers, reviewing homework, and helping with study strategies.
- Develop a daily study routine for after-school, during which the teenager can study and do the homework. Adolescents up to the age of 13 may need the presence of mother while doing school work.
- Help the teenager become better organized; use clear directions, use colors, heading size or highlighting to help important concepts stand out, vary the type of activities to keep the interest.

- Consider getting a tutor at school or a private tutor to help boost performance.
- Prepare a quite environment for the teenager to do the homework, without the distraction of a TV, stereo or siblings.
- Make sure that the adolescent has enough time to complete the homework and that he/she isn't too involved in extracurricular activities or an after-school job.
- For teenagers with below average intelligence, learning disabilities or ADHD is a possibility. Be an advocate for your teenager by making sure that the school is providing the proper education modifications to help him/her succeed.
- Avoid creating a power struggle over homework and school performance.

School Strategies

There are many classroom modifications that can be put in place to help improve school performance, memory and attention, impulse control, organization, and self esteem. Parents should discuss implementing these techniques with school authorities.

Improving Memory and Attention Span

- Provide teenager with an area with the least amount of distractions, near the teacher if possible. Consider using a study carrel, especially for independent work and keep the work area uncluttered.
- Make instructions clear and unambiguous.
- Keep oral instructions brief and repeat them at least once.
- Consider providing written instructions and directions to supplement oral instructions.
- Use visual aids.
- Break up instructions, assignments and homework into small steps.
- Improve reading comprehension by teaching the adolescent to underline key words or topics with a highlighter.
- Improve listening comprehension by teaching to take notes of key concepts.
- Provide special signals or cues to remind the adolescent to get back on task.

Improving Organizational Skills

- Establish a daily checklist of assignments.
- Keep a special notebook in which he/she can record homework assignments, project or report due dates, and test schedules.

Improving Productivity

- Divide work sheets and assignments into sections.
- Reduce the amount of homework and written class work, especially repetitive assignments such as math problems and spelling words that the teenager can do accurately.

- Vary the type of activities that he/she is doing.
- Vary the way that material is presented.
- Provide one on one instruction or small groups to introduce major concepts.

Improving Performance

- Provide extra time to complete assignments and tests.
- Consider providing oral testing instead of or in addition to written tests.
- Remind the student to slow down.
- Give extra weight to the content of an assignment when grading, and do not take off points for poor handwriting or minor spelling errors.

Protecting Self-esteem

- Avoid humiliating the adolescent who performs poorly in front of the other students.
- Give positive feedback when he/she stays on task, pays attention or works hard at an assignment.
- Find things that the adolescent has special interest or strength in and encourage him/her to do these activities.

Improving Behavior and Impulse Control

- Provide special signals or cues when the teenager is beginning to misbehave.
- Give clear expectations of what behaviors are expected in the classroom and school premises.
- Be consistent and unanimous in the expectations and in the consequences for misbehavior.

It is sometimes difficult to figure out if a child's problems at school are caused by their other medical problems, such as depression, or if these problems began because of their poor school performance. Children who do poorly at school may be under a lot of stress, and will develop different ways to cope with this stress. Some may externalize their feelings, which can lead to acting out and behavior problems or becoming the class clown. Other children will internalize their feelings, and will develop almost daily complaints of headaches or stomachaches. A thorough evaluation by an experienced professional is usually needed to correctly diagnose children with complex problems. Thus in any sudden deterioration in adolescent's scholastics, parents and teachers should join hands instead of blaming one another. Specific management for certain causative factors should be considered and the teenager's confidence to come back to normalcy be boosted.

INAPPROPRIATE FINANCIAL MANAGEMENT

Owing to the struggle for independence, a teenager is at times inclined to spend money out of proportion. When asked for explanations, he/she may feel offended and throw a temper tantrum. Parents on one hand want the teenager to be responsible and a mature decision maker and hence may offer some freedom to the growing teenager who may actually fall prey to the external influences and variety of temptations and experimentations, thus demoralizing the parents. Many parents thus feel confused whether pocket-money should be given to the teenager or not.

Occasional stealing of small amounts is quite common and usually is for instant gratification. The adolescent however needs aggressive intervention when it turns into a habit and a compulsive behavior. Coexisting conditions such as conduct disorder, substance abuse, attention deficit hyperactive disorder, or thought disorders, severe peer dependence should be ruled out.

Typical parental reaction is initial disregard followed by lectures on importance of earning and spending money. These hardly change the teenager's behavior. Instead, parents should have a close vigilance on the teenager's expenses and pocket money without being too inquisitive. This is a tricky step and both parents should stick to what has been agreed upon. Another strategy that works is giving the adolescent the responsibility of managing daily expenses of all the family members. This makes the adolescent feel important and responsible and the value of money is indirectly understood.[2]

POOR EATING HABITS

The two most important manifestations of teenager's poor eating habits include under nutrition (Protein, calories, fats, vitamins and minerals) leading to various deficiencies and low body mass index and when these underweight girls conceive, the net result is intrauterine growth retardation and the vicious cycle continues through generations. On the other hand, due to sedentary lifestyles, media influence and plenty of junk food available in addition to poor parental control over teenager's dietary habits, a new epidemic of adolescent obesity is obvious. especially in the cities and towns. Obesity has its own serious consequences in adult life in the form of coronary artery disease, hypertension, type-2 diabetes, postural problems and body image concerns including depression. Anemia in adolescents is discussed elsewhere.

A significant number of adolescent girls opt for weight losing maneuvers. Out of proportion dieting and fasting, with or without strenuous exercise, in order to remain slim and thin has become a latest craze in teenager girls. The 'zero figure' look becomes the ultimate goal in spite of multiple advices given by parents and medical professionals.

Eating patterns of Teenagers[1]

- Adolescence is independent phase of life and parental control diminishes.
- Breakaway from family eating patterns and family meals.
- Limited future perspectives of current eating patterns.

- Influence of peers, media and body image concerns.
- Tendency for missing meals and snacking and junk foods.
- Junk foods are dangerously high on calories and low on nutritive value.
- Food selection is based mainly on availability, convenience and time rather than food value.

Recommendations for Gatekeepers

- Take out time to eat with your teenager. This ensures at least one healthy meal under parent's supervision.
- Parents should curtail down ready to eat food products. Bakery products and foods from restaurants should be only occasional. The difference between good food and bad food should be taught from a very early age.
- Breakfast is a food for brain.[3] Breakfast prepared by the parents must be made compulsory. Choice of item selection may be kept with the teenagers themselves.
- Eating and television watching must never be combined. Television watching also increases obesity through incorrect advertisements about junk food products.
- Eating habits of the peer group modifies teenager's food choices. Health talk on healthy nutrition may be attempted in small groups including the wrong media messages which influence the eating habits of young generation.
- Other aspects of beauty and personality should be highlighted to an anorectic adolescent girl, mentioning the importance of correlation between mother's health and the health of the unborn baby.
- Parents should be a good role model to the teenagers as regards dietary habits and physical fitness.

Adolescent risk taking behaviors are thus directly or indirectly related to the behaviors of gatekeepers. Teenage being an era of experiencing and experimenting, adolescents are bound to opt for many risk taking behaviors. Many will sail through these fantastic years of life rather smoothly provided parents and teachers stick to their responsibilities. Only a few will need extra guidance and professional assistance. Family-life education in schools along with life skills education and a lot of parental support and guidance is the need of the hour.

REFERENCES

1. Facilitator's guide, orientation program for medical officers to provide adolescent friendly reproductive and sexual health services.
2. Bhave's textbook of adolescent medicine, Jaypee Brothers.
3. Nair MKC. Manual of adolescent health, CDCTrivandrum.
4. "Choices"– a guide for young people, Gill Gorden 1999, Macmillan Education Ltd.
5. Adolescent Friendly School Initiative (AFSI) manual under IAP vision 2007.
6. Atul Kanikar, Swati Bhave. Parenting of adolescents, Bhave's textbook of adolescent medicine, Jaypee Brothers.

Section 7

ADOLESCENT FRIENDLY HEALTH SERVICES: BUILDING CAPACITY

30 Ready to Decide? Evolving Capacities, Young Women and Sexual and Reproductive Health

Kat Watson, Arushi Singh

INTRODUCTION

Imagine a girl of 17 who walks into a clinic wanting to get an abortion. She consults with the doctor who tells her that she needs to bring a parent or guardian along to avail the service as she is under 18. The girl walks out of the clinic and doesn't come back.

What might have happened to her after she left the clinic? She may have decided not to have an abortion. She may have gone to another clinic or service delivery point. She may not have been able to tell a parent or guardian or even a friend. She may have gone to a backstreet abortion provider. She may have had an unsafe abortion. She may have lifelong complications. She may even have died.

What it is it that makes an 18 year old girl more capable of taking the decision to have an abortion than a 17 year old? Does her 18th birthday equip her with the capacity, information, problem solving and decision making skills that are required to deal with an unwanted pregnancy and an abortion? Age is not the only determinant of capacity. And this is a crucial aspect of providing youth-friendly sexual and reproductive health services that all service providers need to recognize.

Adolescents and young people have varied lives and live in diverse circumstances, with age being but one commonality that cuts across. Other factors that affect them include:

- Family—The kind of family, the relationships within this family, the status of the young person in the family, etc.
- Community—The kind of leaders there are, the hierarchies that exist or not, the external influences on the community, etc.
- Education—Received or not, to what level, in what setting, with what biases, etc.
- Gender—Prevalent roles and expectations, discrimination, effects of this discrimination on access to nutrition, health, education, sanitation, etc.
- Religion—Dominant beliefs, interpretations, denominations, its dictates on practices, attitudes and ability to gain knowledge, etc.
- Culture—Extent of conservatism, external influences, openness, values held, etc.

In order to assess capacity, we need to look at the composite effect of these factors on a young person's life and decision-making capacities. For example, in India, a young woman who is married may have more or less agency with regard to certain sexual or reproductive decisions as compared with a young woman who is unmarried. While the young, married woman may be able to access STI management services without hesitation, the young, unmarried woman of the same age may not be able to do so or even have adequate information. On the other hand, while the unmarried young woman may be able to insist on condom use, the married young woman may not have the agency to do so. Therefore, it is important to consider that 17-year old girl's life circumstances, not only for the purpose of assessing her decision-making capacity, but also for tailoring the information and services provided, to ensure that they meet her specific needs.

If we are able to examine all angles of her life circumstances, we may actually prevent all the other (possibly negative) eventualities that come about from her walking out of the clinic without receiving treatment, information or care. She may not have known about contraception. She may have been coerced into sex. Her contraceptive method may have failed. She may not be able to talk about her unwanted pregnancy to anyone. She may be in fear of her life and liberty if she reveals her situation to anyone. After all, as a service provider, it would be a missed opportunity for ensuring that one young person leads a healthy and satisfying sexual and reproductive life and shares the same with her partner(s) and offspring. Certainly, there are no laws against providing information about all of the above-mentioned issues.

The other important question is—how much courage, information and awareness, analysis and introspection does it take for a 17-year old girl, in such circumstances, to walk into a clinic and ask for an abortion? A reasonable answer would be—quite a lot. It should be remembered that seeking health services and contraceptive advice is a very good indicator of competency to make such decisions.

EVOLVING CAPACITIES

In their book *Rethinking Youth*, Drs Johanna Wyn and Rob White identify one of the greatest challenges as maintaining *a balance between recognizing the importance of physical and psychological changes that occur in young people's lives and recognizing the extent to which these are constructed by social institutions and negotiated by individuals*. Simply put, it's striking a balance between providing young people with the support/guidance that they need and want as a result of their relative inexperience and empowering young people to exercise their autonomous decision-making power.

The concept being deliberated upon here is that of the **evolving capacity of the child**—a concept that is embedded in the United Nations Convention on the Rights of the Child (CRC), *in particular articles 5 and 12*. As a legal principle, evolving capacity occupies the middle ground between protection and autonomy when it comes to young women's choices about sex and pregnancy. The benefit of such an approach is that it allows for contextual factors, such as those mentioned earlier, to be taken into account when determining the capacity of each individual young person.

The 2009 UNICEF's State of the World's Children special edition report (for the 20th anniversary of the CRC) helpfully outlined the evolution of children's rights starting from the protective approach, embodied in such documents as the 1924 Geneva Convention and (to an extent) the 1959 Universal Declaration of Human Rights, that focuses more on what children should be 'free from' rather than what they have a 'right to.' Things began to change in 1959 with the UN Declaration on the Rights of the Child, which recognized children's rights to such things as education and healthcare. However, as we all know, it was not until the ratification of the Convention on the Rights of the Child in 1989 that (in theory) children's and young people's capacities to exercise, fulfil and realise their own human rights were recognized.

The so-called 'mature minor' doctrine has its legal roots in the 1986 English House of Lords decision, *Gillick vs West Norfolk and Wisbech Area Health Authority*. Mrs Gillick, mother of five daughters, challenged her local authority's policy to provide contraception to under-16s without parental consent. The judges deemed that '*to allow the law to impose fixed borders, particularly in an area as sensitive as a reproductive case, would be to let formalism trump realism.*[1] Further, the judges recognized *adolescence as a developmental and evolutionary period of life*.

Lord Fraser's judgment in the *Gillick* case led to the formation of the so-called Fraser Guidelines, a specific set of criteria used by health practitioners to assess the capacity of young clients to make autonomous decisions and provide informed consent to treatment. The Guidelines place young people's **best interests** at the centre of the decision-making process, thus providing a good model of how to strike the balance between protection and autonomy.

The Fraser Guidelines

1. The young person understands the advice being given.
2. The young person cannot be convinced to involve parents/carers or allow the medical practitioner to do so on their behalf.
3. It is likely that the young person will begin or continue having intercourse with or without treatment/contraception.
4. Unless he or she receives treatment/contraception, their physical or mental health (or both) is likely to suffer.
5. The young person's best interests require contraceptive advice, treatment or supplies to be given without parental consent.

From: http://www.nspcc.org.uk/Inform/research/questions/gillick_wda61289.html.

Many jurisdictions continue to draw definitive boundaries by instituting age limitations on young people's ability to make autonomous decisions about their sexual and reproductive lives. For example, in India, the age of sexual consent is not defined for boys and is 16 for girls, whilst girls under the age of 18 need their parents' or guardian's consent to access safe abortion services. These age demarcations are arbitrary at best and, at worst, prevent adolescents and young people from participating meaningfully in decisions related to their sexual and reproductive lives.

An example of a 'middle ground' approach can be found in the UK. Although age limitations still exist in the UK, the application of the Fraser Guidelines means that if a young woman under the age of consent to medical treatment (16 years old) presents herself at a clinic, the health professional can provide her with services so long as she is deemed to be 'Gillick competent.' This approach seems to be a good compromise between the age limitation approach, which provides certainty and predictability for young people who are 16 or older, and the evolving capacities approach, which provides competent under-16s with the opportunity to participate in and/or make decisions related to their sexual and reproductive health.

However, it should be pointed out that in applying the 'middle ground' approach, the burden of proof of competency should not be placed solely on the young person. The lone fact that a young woman seeks out clinical services and the assistance of health professionals signals a maturity that should suffice in establishing her competency to give informed consent to treatment. In this situation, the young client should be presumed competent until proven otherwise.

At the same time, the 'middle ground' approach requires health professionals to be avid advocates for young people's sexual rights. This is crucial in the creation of a supportive environment that eliminates the fear and shame young people can feel in accessing sexual and reproductive health services.[2] Young people who are not confident in making autonomous decisions should be encouraged and supported in becoming active agents in the exercise of their own sexual rights. Without the commitment of health professionals to young people's sexual rights, young people will continue to face major barriers in accessing sexual and reproductive health services.

CONCLUSION

When young women make choices about sex (when, where, with whom, how, why, for how long, for what purpose) and when they make choices about pregnancy (I don't want to get pregnant; I don't want to remain pregnant; I want to get pregnant), these decisions are not taken in the abstract. In other words, it is not helpful to think about young women's decisions around sex and pregnancy as being taken in a vacuum, devoid of consequences (social and personal, positive and negative) or even coercion.

Nor is it the case that all young people want to take decisions by themselves or navigate the consequences of those decisions without support from friends, family and organizations. Therefore, it is good practice for service providers to give young clients the option of involving a parent or another trusted adult in their life in the decision-making process. However, this option needs to be backed up with the support to enable this involvement. In addition to this support, service providers need to be prepared to identify and respond to situations in which young people are being abused, exploited or harmed.

Gerison Lansdown[3] argues that we, as adults, need to recognize the extent to which over-protection by adults increases young people's vulnerabilities, by failing to equip them with the information needed to make informed decisions, the agency/status to act upon those decisions and the services available to respond to them. If we recognize that young people's vulnerability derives in part from their lack of status and power, how do we respond to that? How do we equip young people and women with the status and power they need within the clinic to realize their sexual rights?

If service providers are able to internalize the concept of evolving capacity, more young people will be enabled to access life-saving services, exercise their choices and have a better quality of life. The 17-year-old girl we started with may actually be able to come back to the clinic and receive the service she wanted, get comprehensive information on contraceptives and choose the one best for her. She may also be protected from harm and empowered to enjoy a healthy, satisfying and pleasurable sexual life.

REFERENCES

1. Kelly, Lisa and IPPF. '*Developing Young People's Capacities for Autonomous Decision-making*', 2010 (to be published).
2. Bankole A, Malarchers. (2010). Removing Barriers to Adolescents' Access to Contraceptive Information and Services. *Studies in Family Planning*, 41(2). Based on a study in four African countries.
3. Lansdown, Gerison and IPPF. Are autonomy and protection opposing concepts? 2010 (to be bublished).

31 Adolescent Health and Role of the Corporate Social Responsibility

AK Khanna

CHALLENGES FOR THE YOUTH TODAY AND TOMORROW

Societies evolve, nations progress, but each tomorrow is a reflection of what we are today. A healthier society and a progressive nation need to take care of its adolescents, for they are the future of the nation.

Today about 30% of the Indian population is below the age of 14 years, where as the adult population is about 64% and geriatric population percentage being 5.2%.

The age structure of a population affects a nation's key socioeconomic issues. Since 1/3rd of our population is adolescent, our need to invest in the welfare of this age group is most vital, be it child care heath, primary education, counseling centers, employment, all these are concerns that today need to be addressed on all levels of planning and execution by the government and private sector alike.

India will age in 2040 and thus it becomes imperative for us to take care of the youth. The dynamics of life-expectancy too have a deep impact on the health care sector of the country.

Urbanization is a key factor that brings about major structural and social-economic changes in any society. In recession hit times when the rest of the world is hardly growing, India is expected to grow by 8.4%, i.e to 1.16 trillions in 2010.

Where urbanization is considered synonymous to development and opportunities, it has its fair share of challenges to deal with. Youths are a significant component of the urbanization process.

The Retail, BPO age that has brought in much financial independence in the younger lot and at an early age has also added to the increased stress levels, peer pressure, competitive edge, irregular and unhealthy life styles in them. With their changing lifestyle, cultural values and ethics one must also be sensitive to the fact that there is an ever increasing risk of sexually transmitted diseases in this group and hence the importance of counseling and awareness.

Several positive and negative lifelong behaviors are established during adolescence. The complex issues that adolescents deal with on a daily basis can turn into health problems that persist throughout adulthood. Unfortunately the adolescents who are frequently the most disconnected from routine health care services are often the ones with greatest risk for multiple and chronic health problems.

With an invasion of multimedia in our day to day lives, the exposure that adolescents have to information has made it imperative to make them release the implications of their actions. Today's youth are inquisitive and seek answers for all their queries and through an expert. Isn't it our responsibility to give them this information in the right way, through a reliable source? This is all the more relevant today since the value system is lot more different. The parent – child relationship has undergone a metamorphosis and today a parent is more of a friend.

Literacy is one way of empowering the young. Literacy in India grew to 68% in 2007 from 12% before Independence. According to the survey by the National Sample Survey Office (NSSO) in June 2008, the literacy rate among the population with age 7 and above was 72% whereas the adult population (age, 15 and above) had a literacy rate of 66%.

The education system has undergone a sea change in the last 20 years. The ethos, the values that were built in, probably 20 years back, are not seen in today's youth, as now the outlook is more objective.

With a wide gender disparity in the literacy rate of India, 76.9% of adult men and 54.5% of women are literate. Studies have indicated that female literacy is a strong predictor of the use of contraception among married Indian couples, even when women do not otherwise have economic independence, thus emphasizing on the fact that adolescent girls need to looked after in terms of providing education and empowering them to take decisions on their own for their benefit.

Hence, Emcure in an effort to do some thing for the society that it operates in, has taken up a few Corporate Social Responsibility (CSR) efforts. However, some could reason as to why should corporate support social responsibility, well, for a few simple reasons:

1. Corporate as an organization of responsible citizen must conduct the affairs in ways to solve or at least ameliorate some of the serious social problems.
2. It can and should improve the corporate and local image of the company.
3. It is in the stockholders best interest. By making communities a better place to live, it can entice superior and happier workers to the company who in turn will put out better products and increase profits.

But the biggest reason being that CSR is in the long-run interest of the business, to become intimately involved in and to promote and improve the communities in which it does its business.

There is another point to ponder upon, as it may be alluring to connect social responsibility with profitability with many of the corporates shying away from CSR thinking, whether there is a link between corporate social performance and corporate financial performance.

Profitability should not be the primary rationale for Corporate Social Responsibility.

None of this is to suggest that companies should not engage in activities that generate social good. However, we should not expect to be handsomely rewarded against these activities. Social responsible behavior may not bring in the mullah, but if the goal is return on investment, there are many other ways to spend money that can deliver a greater payoff.

Keeping this philosophy in mind, Emcure has initiated a total of 11 CSR activities with FOGSI on the subject of maternal and adolescent health care in India.

Emcure, in association with the Adolescent health committee of Federation of Obstetrics and Gynecology societies of India has formulated a program *'Challenges for Youth Today and Tomorrow'* which addresses some of the burning health issues like the importance of correct diet, regular exercise, ill effects of smoking and drinking, safe sexual practices, personal hygiene, mental, spiritual and social health.

Under this association, Emcure, has conducted educative programs in schools and colleges across the country. In these programs, the correct information is disseminated through gynecologists who are WHO-trained on ASRH issues and the youth is sensitized on the lurking health concerns. More than 7000 school and college girls, in the last 2 years have been covered under this program.

Through these programs, each girl is counseled by doctors and given a booklet as a ready reference for her. This has far reaching benefit, as it serves as an information tool for the girl's family and are thus aware of her health care needs.

The school/college programs also provide a platform to the girls to discuss their 'growing up' problems with the gynecologist rather than peers who are as clueless as them.

Under this program, another distinctive effort from Emcure was to get a young celebrity as an ambassador to spread the right messages to the youth, an Icon that is looked upon and is acceptable to them. Emcure had brought in the iconic youth musical band, Agnee. Through this model as well the message of positive social behavior was imparted to the school and college youth. More of such activities would bring much more interest in youth to understand the challenges.

The success of any Corporate Social Responsibility depends on the team and the right partnership. Adolescence CSR—Challenges for Youth Today and Tomorrow – became a grand success due to the excellent partnership between Emcure and FOGSI. As the Chairperson of Adolescent Health Committee FOGSI, Dr Roza Olyai and her team played a very vital role to take this initiative to the next level. Dr Roza Olyai and team completely owned up the initiative and gave valuable inputs.

Anemia is one of the very common problems seen in our girls and women. Anemia eradication is one of Emcure's core CSR. Currently there are ongoing 5 different programs in association with FOGSI 12 by 12 initiative, Village Adoption Program, Ankur, Adolescent Health Program, Eradicate Anemia Everyday 24 × 7 × 365.

The above CSR initiatives in the field of adolescence and women healthcare are Emcure's efforts in giving back to the society to build up a healthier nation.

Emcure in its endeavor to bring upon some change for the better and improving women healthcare is committed to its partnership with FOGSI and is willing to take up any additional projects identified by them on the same.

32 Adolescent Friendly Health Centers

Roza Olyai

INTRODUCTION

WHO defines "**adolescents**" as individuals in the 10-19 years age group and "**youth**" as the 15-24 years age group. These two overlapping age groups are combined in the group "**young people**" covering the age range 10-24 years.

These age definitions are useful for a common understanding but do not convey strict age compartments. It should be realized that adolescence is a phase of life that has biological and socio-cultural hallmarks that vary from case to case and society to society.

WHY FOCUS ON ADOLESCENTS?

The number of adolescents (age 10-19) is increasing and comprises over one-fifth of the population in our country. They are not only in large numbers but are the future citizens and drivers of economic growth as the productive workers of tomorrow. Adolescents are not homogeneous population but exist in a variety of circumstances. A large number of them are out of school, get married early, work in vulnerable situations, are likely to be sexually active, and are exposed to several health risks. These have serious social, economic and public health implications for the nation.

Their needs vary by their age, sex, stage of development, life circumstances, socio-economic status, marital status, class, region and cultural context. This calls for interventions that are flexible and responsive to their desperate needs. Some of the public health challenges for adolescents are related to early pregnancy, with associated higher risk of maternal and infant mortality, sexually transmitted infections (including HIV) and reproductive tract infections, under-nutrition and anemia, substance abuse, injuries, etc. It is important to health of adolescents as their situation will be central in determining India's health, mortality and morbidity; and the population growth scenario.

Ministry of Health and Family Welfare

Responding to these considerations, the Ministry of Health and Family Welfare, Government of India has included Adolescent Reproductive and Sexual Health (ARSH) as a key technical strategy under the National RCH II program. This strategy focuses on reorganizing and strengthening the existing public health system in order to meet the reproductive and sexual health needs of adolescents. The primary focus is on meeting the national targets of reduction of Total Fertility Rate (TFR), Maternal and Infant Mortality Rates (MMR and IMR), and the incidence of STI and HIV.

FOGSI and FIGO collaboration

Seeing to the present health scenario of the adolescent's health in today's fast moving world, the International Federation of Obstetric and Gynecology (FIGO) is now focusing on adolescent sexual and reproductive health (ASRH) issues. Following the various Regional ASRH workshops by FIGO, the Adolescent Health Committee FOGSI has developed standard guidelines to enable the members to initiate adolescent health services within their existing practices. Some salient features of the guidelines are explained in this chapter.

ADOLESCENT FRIENDLY HEALTH SERVICES

What are Adolescent Friendly Health Services?

Healthcare providers and health services have an important role to play in promoting healthy development and preventing health problems amongst adolescents; specialized services dedicated to adolescents can definitely help in detecting them early and in responding to them promptly and effectively—if and when they do arise. However, adolescents often face constraints in seeking help from the existing health services. The well known barriers to access of services are related to their personal issues related to shyness; need to deal with shame and embarrassment in disclosing their problems. Some barriers are related to the health facility like crowding, absence of dedicated space or services for adolescents, policies that make privacy and confidentiality difficult to ensure. Healthcare provider's unsupportive and judgmental attitude is an important barrier that prevents adolescents from accessing services.

Health services that are able to minimize these barriers are likely to attract adolescent and young clients. Several attributes of adolescent /young people friendly health services are well known. These are summarized in the following Table 32.1:

Table 32.1: Attributes of adolescent/young people friendly health services

Criteria for Adolescent Friendly Health Worker	*Criteria for a Adolescent Friendly Health Center*	*Program Design Characteristics*
Be welcoming and friendly Be knowledgeable Be presentable Have good communication skills Maintain confidentiality Be punctual Be understanding Be a good listener Be non-judgmental	Be welcoming to all Have enough facilities to use Be accessible Provide quality care and trained people Be presentable and clean Provide privacy Have a conducive environment Educational material is available	No overcrowding Short waiting times Drop in clients welcomed and appointments arranged rapidly Affordable fees Boys and young men welcomed and served Wide range of services available Necessary referrals available Involve adolescents in design and continuing feedback

Standards for Adolescent Friendly Health Centers

Based on these attributes, the Ministry of Health and Family Welfare, Government of India has developed National Standards for the proposed Adolescent Friendly Health Services (AFHS) under the RCH-II ARSH strategy. The National Standards for AFHS define criteria that help define and ensure quality of services. These standards are presently being implemented in the public health facilities across the states.

In line with these national standards, Adolescent Health Committee of FOGSI recommends the following specifications and guidelines for organizing adolescent friendly health centers in the clinics/nursing homes and hospitals of our members:

Reorganize existing clinic space

- Allocate convenient time slot for the provision of services to adolescents and youth. Depending upon the availability of time, the clinic specifically for adolescents may be fixed once/twice or thrice a week and ensure that the clinic timings suit the needs of adolescents. In case this is not possible, be prepared to offer appointments to adolescent young people at a time when you can offer longer interaction time and dedicated attention to them. You could choose time for them at the beginning or end of the usual OPD session.
- Consider consultations with adolescent clients both by prior appointment as well as a walk-in arrangement.
- If possible, allocate separate working area for adolescent clients. This could be achieved by reserving fixed dedicated time for them (first point above) when adolescents will have exclusive access to the services.
- Ensure that privacy (audio and visual) and confidentiality are maintained all the time during the consultation and subsequently as well.
- Ensure that the premises are clean; lighting and ventilation adequate; drinking water available; and the toilets are functional and clean.
- Decorate (color scheme, posters, etc.) the adolescent clinic area in confirmation with trends currently prevalent among adolescents.
- Prepare and maintain in good condition a signboard displaying the timings of the clinic, services provided, and fee structure.
- Ensure that the necessary equipments (Weight and Height equipment, BP apparatus, orchidometer, etc.) required to provide services are always available.
- Ensure that informational and educational pamphlets are displayed and made available to adolescents and youth to take away. The Adolescent Health Committee FOGSI has developed some prototypes that can be accessed from the committee website.

Decide service package

Depending on your capacity and interest, decide a package of services that would be provided in your clinic and through referral services. Such a package could include several or all adolescent problems that are prevalent in your area. A list of common adolescent concerns has been given in Table 32.2.

Develop standard clinic procedures

- Develop clear procedure on how the client will be received and by whom.
- Registration procedure for the client should be simple, quick and follow privacy.
- Ensure that anonymous interview and treatment is possible.
- Develop and maintain standard history taking, physical examination protocols case records. Samples are provided with these guidelines. Make sure that these client records are maintained in confidentiality.
- Develop/adapt standard treatment protocols to manage common clinical conditions with which adolescents come to your clinic.
- Develop referral procedures for laboratory, radiology work-up and for clinical specialities.
- A resource directory of organizations/clinics/specialists providing health services not provided by you should be available at the center to ensure referral linkages.
- Develop an adolescent health card (personal health record and important health messages) that would remain with the client.

Strengthen skills of the team of health care providers

- Ensure adequate support staff with appropriate profile is in place and are present during the working hours of the Adolescent Clinic.
- Ensure that Doctors (including yourself) and support staff at your clinic have received orientation/training on the importance of non-judgmental, caring with strong inter-personal skills and supportive attitude towards adolescents and young clients.
- Ensure that colleagues/staff involved in peer educator training and school linked programmes, if any, are also appropriately trained (if applicable).
- Supervise your staff to ensure that they practice appropriate technical and interpersonal competencies and positive attitudes to provide adolescent health services effectively with sensitivity.
- Develop a network of adolescent friendly experts in other clinical specialities and counseling for ensuring referral services.

Outreach activities for demand generation and provide services beyond the clinic

- Identify community organizations in the catchment area to promote adolescent health and organize community camps for creating, enabling social environment for promoting adolescent health.
- Identify schools in your neighborhood to interact with teachers and students periodically to promote adolescent health and inform about services available. Develop such an initiative with prior consultation and concurrence of the principal, teachers and parents. You could choose to offer annual check-up for students.
- Disseminate messages and communication materials on priority adolescent health issues in schools, youth clubs, youth centers, youth

associations and different community organizations to support awareness generation. Also inform about where and when they can access adolescent friendly health services.

Monitoring performance of the clinic

- Monitor the performance of your clinic regularly in terms of number of clients, their age and sex, types of problems they come to you with and treatment/referral offered. All the records must be kept confidential.
- Self-assessment of the quality of services at your clinic should be carried out periodically with the purpose of continuous improvement in quality.
- Periodically assess yourself to ensure that the standard guidelines provided here are being followed in your clinic. Such periodic self-assessment would help you constantly improve the quality of services provided by you in your clinic.

Table 32.2 : List of common adolescent concerns to help decide service package

• Pubertal issues: – Adolescent growth and development – Pubertal delay or precocity – Weight and height issues • Sexual and reproductive health: – Gynecological and menstrual problems – Contraception – Pregnancy testing and option – MTP – STD/HIV screening, counseling and treatment – Sexual and reproductive health education	• Psycho-social issues: – Relationship development – Adjustment problems – Growing-up issues • Nutrition issues: – Healthy eating during adolescence – Anemia prevention and management – Undernutrition and obesity – Eating disorders (anorexia nervosa, Bulimia nervosa, Binge disorder) • Immunization • Safety and injury prevention
• Chronic conditions like asthma, diabetes, hypertension, renal disorders • Eye care, ENT care, Dental care • Preventive health checkups, like annual checkup, pre-college health checkup, pre-marital counseling, etc.	• Adolescent mental health – Psychiatric disorders: depression, anxiety, bipolar, personality disorders – Substance abuse including tobacco and alcohol

Peer Group Approach

Experience shows that most of the times, adolescents/young people prefer talking with their peers about sensitive issues. Keeping this in mind, PGEs (both females and males) are selected and oriented to promote AFHS. This approach is easier in the school settings but is also effective in the out-of-school settings in the community and neighborhoods. In addition to their orientation, they need to be followed up regularly to assess the work done, identify the problems, provide training and motivate them for further work. A peer group educator should be a good communicator, acceptable to the group, interested in the work, able to understand the problems of adolescents, having a good personality, and be confident. Peer led approach is usually based on volunteerism.

ADOLESCENT FRIENDLY HEALTH CLINICS

Clinic within Existing Solo Practice

Most common option for practicing gynecologists and obstetricians who have their own OPD clinics would be to consider an adolescent friendly clinic at a designated time on particular days (if not daily) exclusively to provide quality services to adolescent girls and, if possible, boys. Boys and young men should be welcome in the gynecologist's clinic since it has been observed that at times they want to help their female partners by seeking advice on their behalf or accompany their partners. In case you are comfortable and confident, you could also provide services to these boys and young men.

Understandably, an individual gynecologist would be able to limit number/type of services at her clinic that she/he must decide before hand depending on her capacity. For additional services and clinical requirements, there should be an arrangement to refer such clients to appropriate experts/ specialists who are equally respectful and friendly to adolescents.

Multi-specialty Adolescent Friendly Clinic at Big Nursing Homes and Hospitals

At bigger setups, where several specialists are attached or available, it may be possible to develop a multi-specialty adolescent friendly clinic that provides single window services.

Multi-specialty Team

In such a clinic, a team of some or all of the specialists may be considered: Gynecologist, Pediatrician specializing in adolescent medicine, Professional Counselor, Endocrinologist, Trained Nurse, Health Educator, Psychologist, and Social Worker.

Location of the Adolescent Health Clinic

Such a multi-specialty center in a big hospital should be located in an accessible location that does not hinder the movements by adolescent clients. If it is planned to initiate a new independent unit in a private or NGO setting it should be centrally located in the city, easily approachable to teenagers from every corner. In a big city several centers/clinics are required to serve a large portion of adolescent population.

EXPECTED CHALLENGES IN SETTING UP ADOLESCENT CENTERS

The foremost factor for ensuring success of adolescent clinic is a motivated provider. Several established gynecologists/pediatricians may not feel motivated to practice adolescent medicine. This may be because of lack of knowledge and experience in attending to the special needs of adolescent clients, lack of financial reward or due to discomfort in handling sexuality related issues that some of the clients may come with.

Unavailability or irregular availability of doctors and staff at the appointed hour are important roadblocks in the proper functioning of adolescent clinics. It is observed that booked appointments drop when the provider of adolescent services was unavailable or had insufficient time to offer.

Another problem is missed appointments on part of the clients. Typical adolescent behavioral characteristics result in cancellation of booked appointments, because either the problem has resolved or something arose that the adolescent considered more pressing. Owing to the confidential nature of appointments, reminder notices or phone calls are rarely used, and this contributes to the likelihood of missed appointments.

SUMMARY

Guidelines have been developed and designed to ensure uniform standards of good quality of health services for adolescents and youth. The Adolescent Health Committee, FOGSI, plans to disseminate these guidelines for establishing adolescent friendly health centers/clinics. In addition, a brief package for an Orientation Programme would be offered to orient interested members.

Many members are already conducting school and community based activities towards promotion of adolescent health. Those who are interested in starting adolescent friendly health centers are encouraged to develop a defined plan for such activities. The overall goal of this plan is to *"help young people form a strong moral identity in their early adolescent years and empower them to contribute to the well-being of their communities...."*

SUGGESTED READING

1. Adolescent Friendly Concept, Chapter 27, in Bhave's textbook of adolescent medicine 1st Edition 2006, Chief Editor Swati Y Bhave, Jaypee Publishers, New Delhi. 988-1048.
2. Guidelines for Establishing Adolescent Friendly Health Center_FOGSI, visit **Website:** http://adolescenthealthindia.org/

Index